Degenerative Disc Disease

Degenerative Disc Disease

Editors

Robert Gunzburg, M.D., Ph.D.
*Senior Consultant
Department of Orthopedics
Centenary Clinic
Antwerp, Belgium*

Marek Szpalski, M.D.
*Associate Professor
Free University of Brussels
Chairman, Department of Orthopedics
Iris South Teaching Hospitals
Brussels, Belgium*

Gunnar B.J. Andersson, M.D., Ph.D.
*Professor and Chairman
Department of Orthopedic Surgery
Rush Medical College
Senior Vice President, Medical Affairs
Chairman, Department of Orthopedic Surgery
Rush–Presbyterian–St. Luke's Medical Center
Chicago, Illinois*

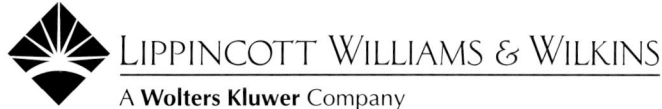

A **Wolters Kluwer** Company
Philadelphia • Baltimore • New York • London
Buenos Aires • Hong Kong • Sydney • Tokyo

Acquisitions Editor: Robert Hurley
Developmental Editor: Julia Seto
Production Editor: Jonathan Geffner
Manufacturing Manager: Benjamin Rivera
Cover Designer: Christine Jenny
Compositor: Lippincott Williams & Wilkins Desktop Division
Printer: Maple Press

© 2004 by LIPPINCOTT WILLIAMS & WILKINS
530 Walnut Street
Philadelphia, PA 19106 USA
LWW.com

Chapter 7 © Henry V. Crock

All rights reserved. This book is protected by copyright. No part of this book may be reproduced in any form or by any means, including photocopying, or utilized by any information storage and retrieval system without written permission from the copyright owner, except for brief quotations embodied in critical articles and reviews. Materials appearing in this book prepared by individuals as part of their official duties as U.S. government employees are not covered by the above-mentioned copyright.

Printed in the USA

Library of Congress Cataloging-in-Publication Data
Degenerative disc disease / editors, Robert Gunzburg, Marek Szpalski, Gunnar B.J. Andersson.
　　p. ; cm.
　　Includes bibliographical references and index.
　　ISBN 0-7817-5073-3
　　1. Intervertebral disk—Diseases.　I. Gunzburg, Robert.　II. Szpalski, Marek.　III. Andersson, Gunnar, 1942–
　　[DNLM: 1. Intervertebral Disk—pathology.　2. Spinal Diseases.　3. Intervertebral Disk Displacement. WE 740 D317 2004]
　　RD771.I6D446 2004
　　616.7′3—dc22

2003058809

Care has been taken to confirm the accuracy of the information presented and to describe generally accepted practices. However, the authors, editors, and publisher are not responsible for errors or omissions or for any consequences from application of the information in this book and make no warranty, expressed or implied, with respect to the currency, completeness, or accuracy of the contents of the publication. Application of this information in a particular situation remains the professional responsibility of the practitioner.

The authors, editors, and publisher have exerted every effort to ensure that drug selection and dosage set forth in this text are in accordance with current recommendations and practice at the time of publication. However, in view of ongoing research, changes in government regulations, and the constant flow of information relating to drug therapy and drug reactions, the reader is urged to check the package insert for each drug for any change in indications and dosage and for added warnings and precautions. This is particularly important when the recommended agent is a new or infrequently employed drug.

Some drugs and medical devices presented in this publication have Food and Drug Administration (FDA) clearance for limited use in restricted research settings. It is the responsibility of the health care provider to ascertain the FDA status of each drug or device planned for use in their clinical practice.

10　9　8　7　6　5　4　3　2　1

Contents

Contributing Authors ix
Preface xv

Basics

1. Is There Such a Thing as Degenerative Disc Disease? 1
   Alf Nachemson

2. Morphologic Changes of Endplates in Degenerative Disc Disease 7
   Robert J. Moore

3. Biochemical Changes in Degenerative Disc Disease 15
   Sally Roberts and Bruce Caterson

4. The Physiology of Intervertebral Disc Degeneration 23
   Susan R. S. Bibby, Jing Yu, and Jill P. G. Urban

5. Degenerative Disc Disease and Occupational Exposure 35
   Malcolm H. Pope

6. Disc Degeneration and Segmental Instability 53
   Tommy Hansson

7. Internal Disc Disruption 63
   Henry V. Crock

Diagnosis

8. Imaging of Degenerative Disc Disease 75
   Jean-Louis Dietemann

9. Behavior of the Disc in Upright Magnetic Resonance Imaging 91
   Francis W. Smith, J. Randy Jinkins, and Malcolm H. Pope

10. Lumbar Discography 99
    Asif Saifuddin

Clinical Presentation

11. Disc Degeneration and Low Back Pain 111
    Michel Benoist and Philippe Boulu

12. Disc Degeneration in Children and Adolescents 121
    Federico Balagué and Jean Dudler

Conservative Treatment Modalities

13. Gene Therapy Approach for the Treatment of Disc Degeneration 133
S. Tim Yoon

Biologic Aspects of Surgical Fusion

14. Bone Graft Alternatives in Spinal Surgery 139
Angelo M. Ciminiello, David H. Kim, and Alexander R. Vaccaro

15. Inducing Spine Fusion with Osteoinductive Molecules 155
S. Tim Yoon

Surgical Treatment Modalities

16. Intradiscal Electrothermal Therapy 163
Gunnar B. J. Andersson

17. Anterior Lumbar Interbody Fusion Versus Posterior Lumbar Interbody Fusion for Degenerative Disc Disease 169
Jean-Charles Le Huec, Stéphane Aunoble, and Thomas A. Zdeblick

18. Posterolateral Fusion 181
Norbert Passuti, Joël Delécrin, Mostafa Romih, and Dominique Brossard

19. A New Concept in Spinal Stabilization: OptiMesh 189
Stephen D. Kuslich

20. The Graf Ligament System 197
Norbert Passuti, Joël Delécrin, Mostafa Romih, and Dominique Brossard

21. Characterization of a Synthetic Bioactive Spinal Interbody Device 207
Gina M. Nagvajara, James P. Murphy, Theodore D. Clineff, and Erik M. Erbe

22. K-Centrum, a "Zero-Profile" Anterior Spinal Intramedullary Rod Fixation System: Preclinical Testing and Clinical Experience 215
Matthew D. Garner and Stephen D. Kuslich

23. Dynamic Neutralization System for the Spine in Degenerative Disc Disease 227
Thomas M. Stoll, Gilles G. Dubois, and Othmar Schwarzenbach

24. Cervical Interbody Fusion with a New Composite in Degenerative Disc Disease: A Preliminary Experience 239
Richard Assaker, Véronique Tonelle, Stéphane Aunoble, and Jean-Charles Le Huec

Disc Replacements: Total Disc Replacements

25. Ten Years On 245
E. Raymond S. Ross, Zahid Asker, and David G. Hughes

26. Total Disc Replacement for Low Back Pain of Discogenic Origin 249
H. Michael Mayer, Karsten Wiechert, and Andreas Korge

27. The PDN Prosthetic Disc Nucleus Device: Product Design
and Clinical Results 257
Sinéad A. Kavanagh and Charles D. Ray

Economic and Ethical Considerations

28. The Evidence Base for Treatment of—not Degenerative
Disc Disease—but Back Pain 263
Alf Nachemson

29. The Need for Central Registration: Spine Tango. A European
Spine Registry 273
*Christoph P. Roeder, Amer I. EL-Kerdi, Dieter Grob, and
Max Aebi*

30. Assessment of Health-Related Quality of Life 279
Christian Mélot

31. Rationale for the Surgical Treatment of Degenerative Disc Disease
from the Cochrane Review 291
J.N. Alastair Gibson and Gordon Waddell

32. Animal Models in the Study of Degenerative Disc Disease 303
Robert J. Moore

33. Epidemiology, Outcome, and Costs of Surgery for Lumbar
Disc Herniation 313
Marc G. Du Bois and Peter Donceel

34. Clinical Outcome, Measurements, and Languages: Some
Cultural Aspects 321
Margareta Nordin

Subject Index 327

Contributing Authors

Max Aebi, M.D.
Professor and Chair
Center of Orthopaedic Research
University of Bern
Chief of Staff
Orthopedic Department
Salem Hospital
Bern, Switzerland

Gunnar B. J. Andersson, M.D., Ph.D.
Professor and Chairman
Department of Orthopedic Surgery
Rush Medical College
Senior Vice President, Medical Affairs
Chairman, Department of Orthopedic Surgery
Rush–Presbyterian–St. Luke's Medical Center
Chicago, Illinois

Zahid Asker, M.B.B.S.
Spinal Fellow
Department of Surgery
Hope Hospital
Salford, United Kingdom

Richard Assaker, M.D.
Department of Neurosurgery
Salengro University Hospital
Lille, France

Stéphane Aunoble, M.D.
Associate Professor
Department of Orthopedic Surgery
Orthopedic Surgeon
Spine Unit
Centre Hospitalier Universitaire Pellegrin
Bordeaux, France

Federico Balagué, M.D.
Medicine Chief Adjoint
Department of Rheumatology, Physical Medicine, and Rehabilitation
Cantonal Hospital
Fribourg, Switzerland
Adjunct Associate Professor
Department of Orthopedic Surgery
New York University School of Medicine
New York, New York

Michel Benoist, M.D.
Consultant of Paris Hospitals
University of Paris VII
Paris, France
Consultant in Rheumatology
Department of Rheumatology
Hôpital Beaujon
Clichy, France

Susan R. S. Bibby, D.Phil.
University Laboratory of Physiology
Oxford University
Oxford, United Kingdom

Philippe Boulu, M.D.
Consultant in Neurology
Department of Neurology
Hopital Beaujou
Clichy, France

Dominique Brossard, M.D.
Senior Resident
Department of Orthopedic Surgery
Nantes University
Senior Resident
Department of Orthopedic Surgery
Nantes Hospital
Nantes, France

Bruce Caterson, Ph.D
Professor
Cardiff School of Biosciences
Cardiff University
Associate Director of Musculoskeletal Disease
Department of Orthopedics and Trauma
University of Wales College of Medicine
Cardiff, United Kingdom

Angelo M. Ciminiello, M.D.
Resident
Department of Orthopedic Surgery
University of Connecticut Health Center
Farmington, Connecticut

CONTRIBUTING AUTHORS

Theodore D. Clineff, M.S.
Senior Analytical Engineer
Department of Product Development
Orthovita, Inc.
Malvern, Pennsylvania

Henry V. Crock, A.O., M.D., M.S.
Honorary Consultant Surgeon
Senior Lecturer
Department of Orthopedic Surgery
Imperial College of Science and Medicine
Hammersmith Hospital
Director (Retired)
Spinal Disorders Unit
Cromwell Hospital
London, United Kingdom

Joël Delécrin, M.D., Ph.D.
Associate Professor
Clinic of Orthopedic Surgery
Centre Hospitalier Universitaire Hôtel Dieu
Nantes, France

Jean-Louis Dietemann, M.D.
Professor
Department of Radiology
University Louis Pasteur
Chief
Department of Radiology
University Hospital of Strasbourg
Strasbourg, France

Peter Donceel, M.D., Ph. D.
Professor
Department of Occupational and Insurance
  Medicine
School of Public Health
Catholic University of Leuven
Leuven, Belgium

Gilles G. Dubois, M.D.
Head
Department of Neurosurgery
Clinique de l'Union
St. Jean, France

Marc G. Du Bois, M.D.
Research Fellow
Department of Occupational and Insurance
  Medicine
School of Public Health
Catholic University of Leuven
Leuven, Belgium

Jean Dudler, M.D.
Associate Professor
Department of Rheumatology, Physical
  Medicine, and Rehabilitation
University of Lausanne
Attending Physician
Department of Rheumatology, Physical
  Medicine, and Rehabilitation
Central Hospitalier Universitaire Vaudois
Lausanne, Switzerland

**Amer I. EL-Kerdi, M.Sc., Ph.D.
  candidate**
Group Head, Medical Informatics
Institute for Evaluative Research in
  Orthopaedic Surgery
University of Bern
Bern, Switzerland

Erik M. Erbe, Ph.D.
Chief Scientific Officer
Orthovita, Inc.
Malvern, Pennsylvania

Matthew D. Garner, PA-C
Research Assistant
Spineology Research Group
Stillwater, Minnesota

J. N. Alastair Gibson, M.D.
Senior Lecturer
Department of Orthopedic Surgery
The University of Edinburgh
Consultant Spinal Surgeon
Spinal Unit
The Royal Infirmary of Edinburgh
Edinburgh, United Kingdom

Dieter Grob, P.D. D.Med.
Professor
Department of Orthopedic Surgery
Zurich University
Chief
Department of Spine Surgery
Division of Orthopedics
Schulthess Clinic
Zurich, Switzerland

Tommy Hansson, M.D., Ph.D.
Vice Dean
Faculty of Medicine
Sahlgrenska Academy
Professor
Department of Orthopedics
Sahlgren University Hospital
Göteborg, Sweden

CONTRIBUTING AUTHORS

David G. Hughes, M.B.B.S.
Honorary Lecturer
Department of Radiology
University of Manchester
Manchester, United Kingdom
Consultant Neuroradiologist
Department of Neuroradiology
Hope Hospital
Salford, United Kingdom

J. Randy Jinkins, M.D.
Senior Research Fellow
Fonar Corporation
Melville, New York

Sinéad A. Kavanagh, B.Eng.
Ph.D. Candidate
Department of Mechanical Engineering
National University of Ireland, Galway
Galway, Ireland

David H. Kim, M.D.
Attending Spinal Surgeon
The Boston Spine Group
New England Baptist Hospital
Boston, Massachusetts

Andreas Korge, M.D.
Chief Staff Surgeon
Spine Center
Orthozentrum Munich
Munich, Germany

Stephen D. Kuslich, M.D.
Associate Clinical Professor
Department of Orthopedics
University of Minnesota
Minneapolis, Minnesota
Medical Director
Spineology Research Group
Spineology Inc.
Stillwater, Minnesota

Jean-Charles Le Huec, M.D., Ph.D.
Professor
Department of Orthopedic Surgery
Chief, Spine Unit
Centre Hospitalier Universitaire Pellegrin
  Bordeaux
Bordeaux, France

H. Michael Mayer, M.D., Ph.D.
Associate Professor and Chief
Spine Center
Orthozentrum Munich
Munich, Germany

Christian Mélot, M.D., Ph.D., M.Sci.
  Biostat, M.Sci. Health Manag.
Professor of Biostatistics
Faculty of Medicine
Free University of Brussels
Associate Professor of Medicine
Department of Intensive Care
Erasme University Hospital
Brussels, Belgium

Robert J. Moore, Ph.D.
Affiliate Senior Lecturer
Department of Pathology
The University of Adelaide
Head
The Adelaide Centre for Spinal Research
Institute of Medical and Veterinary Science
Adelaide, Australia

James P. Murphy, M.S.Eng.
Senior Product Development Engineer
Department of Research and Development
Orthovita, Inc.
Malvern, Pennsylvania

Alf Nachemson, M.D., Ph.D.
Professor Emeritus
Department of Orthopedics
Göteborg University
Göteborg, Sweden
Research Professor
Department of Orthopedics
Georgetown University
Washington, DC
Sahlgrenska University Hospital
Göteborg, Sweden

Gina M. Nagvajara, Ph.D.
Director of Research and Intellectual Property
Department of Research and Development
Orthovita, Inc.
Malvern, Pennyslvania

Margareta Nordin, Dr. Sci.
Professor
Departments of Occupational and
  Environmental Medicine
School of Medicine
New York University
Director
Occupational and Industrial Orthopedic Center
Hospital for Joint Diseases
New York, New York

Norbert Passuti, M.D., Ph.D.
Professor
Department of Orthopedic Surgery
Nantes University
Chief
Department of Orthopedic Surgery
Nantes Hospital
Nantes, France

Malcolm H. Pope, M.S., Dr.Med.Sc., Ph.D., D.Sc.
Professor
Department of Environmental and
 Occupational Medicine
University of Aberdeen
Honorary Consultant
Department of Biomedical Physics
Aberdeen Royal Infirmary
Aberdeen, United Kingdom

Charles D. Ray, M.D.
President
American College of Spine Surgery
Jacksonville, Florida
President
International Spine Arthroplasty Society
West Palm Beach, Florida
Past President
North American Spine Society
La Grange, Illinois

Sally Roberts, Ph.D.
Reader
Centre for Science and Technology in
 Medicine
Keele University
Staffordshire, United Kingdom
Director of Spinal Research
Centre for Spinal Studies
Robert Jones & Agnes Hunt Orthopaedic
 Hospital
Shropshire, United Kingdom

Christoph P. Roeder, M.D.
Clinical Research Associate
Institute for Evaluative Research in
 Orthopaedic Surgery
University of Bern
Bern, Switzerland

Mostafa Romih, M.D.
Senior Resident
Department of Orthopedic Surgery
Nantes University
Senior Resident
Department of Orthopedic Surgery
Nantes Hospital
Nantes, France

E. Raymond S. Ross, M.B.Ch.B.
Honorary Assistant Lecturer
Department of Orthopedics
University of Manchester
Manchester, United Kingdom
Consultant Spinal Surgeon
Department of Spinal Surgery
Hope Hospital
Salford, United Kingdom

Asif Saifuddin, B.Sc., M.B.Ch.B.
Consultant Radiologist
Department of Radiology
Royal National Orthopedic Hospital Trust
NHS Trust
Middlesex, United Kingdom

Othmar Schwarzenbach, M.D.
Das Ruckenzentrum
Thun, Switzerland

Francis W. Smith, M.D.
Senior Lecturer
Department of Radiology
University of Aberdeen
Consultant Radiologist
MRI Centre
Woodend Hospital
Aberdeen, United Kingdom

Thomas M. Stoll, M.D.
Department of Orthopedic Spine Surgery
Bethesda Spital
Basel, Switzerland

Véronique Tonelle, M.D.
Department of Neurosurgery
Salengro University Hospital
Lille, France

Jill P. G. Urban, Ph.D.
Senior Arthritis and Rheumatism Campaign
 Research Fellow
Physiology Laboratory
Oxford University
Oxford, United Kingdom

Alexander R. Vaccaro, M.D.
Professor
Department of Orthopedic Surgery
Thomas Jefferson Medical College
Co-Director
Reconstructive Spine Service
The Rothman Institute
Philadelphia, Pennsylvania

Gordon Waddell, C.B.E., D.Sc.
Professor
Orthopaedic Surgeon
The Glasgow Nuffield Hospital
Glasgow, United Kingdom

Karsten Wiechert, M.D.
Staff Surgeon
Spine Center
Orthozentrum Munich
Munich, Germany

S. Tim Yoon, M.D., Ph.D.
Assistant Professor
Department of Orthopedics
Emory University
Chief
Department of Orthopedics
Atlanta VA Medical Center
Decatur, Georgia

Jing Yu, Ph.D.
Research Fellow
Physiology Laboratory
Oxford University
Oxford, United Kingdom

Thomas A. Zdeblick, M.D.
Professor and Chairman
Departments of Orthopedics and Rehabilitation
University of Wisconsin
Madison, Wisconsin

Preface

The human intervertebral disc is a unique structure with very particular characteristics. It is avascular and contains few nerves. Although its biomechanics and biochemistry are still only partly understood, a large number of operative interventions on the disc are being proposed and carried out as it is generally believed to be responsible for the sometimes very disabling condition referred to as "low back pain." Intervertebral disc degeneration seems to evolve naturally from the human spine, and the relationship between degeneration and pain is at best unclear.

In this book, we attempt to demystify this structure by examining it from different viewpoints: descriptive, physiologic, pathologic, diagnostic, clinical, and therapeutic. We analyze in detail the role of the endplate in degenerative disc disease, as well as the biochemical and physiologic changes that occur. We also discuss the role of occupational exposure and lumbar spinal instability in the genesis of disc degeneration.

Iconographic appearance is seen from different angles: standard radiography, computer-assisted tomography scanning, discography, and magnetic resonance imaging—both classic and upright open. Of course, the understanding of the origin of pain in degenerative disc disease is paramount if one intends to install any form of therapy. The original of pain is discussed in general chapters preceding the therapy section.

Conservative treatment includes medical approaches, physical medicine, and revalidation, as well as manipulation. New treatments will most likely be made available in the not-so-distant future as gene therapy research is progressing steadily.

Surgical treatment comprises fusion and, apart from the very many different techniques available, there is an array of biomaterials being researched and produced to decrease morbidity arising from graft harvesting and increase the rate of fusion. Some recently developed intervention modalities, such as intradiscal electrothermal therapy, OptiMesh, and disc replacement, have yet to prove their usefulness; and prospective randomized clinical trials must be undertaken before these techniques are widely adopted. Others prefer dynamic stabilization, several techniques of which are described here.

In the last part of this book, more general topics are put forth—such as the need for central registration, the principles of quality assessment, the value of evidence-based medicine, outcome measures, and controlled randomized trials.

This book is addressed to clinicians and researchers alike, as well as basic scientists, physical therapists, and chiropractors.

Robert Gunzburg, M.D., Ph.D.
Marek Szpalski, M.D.
Gunnar B.J. Andersson, M.D., Ph.D.

1

Is There Such a Thing as Degenerative Disc Disease?

Alf Nachemson

Department of Orthopedics, Göteborg University; Sahlgrenska University Hospital, Göteborg, Sweden; and Department of Orthopedics, Georgetown University, Washington, DC

In this keynote lecture and debate with Dr. Kuslich, a proponent of the view that such a disease exists, I would like to begin with the following statement:

> Yes—when a disc hernia causes sciatica, this is a result of the aging process in the intervertebral disc, and when symptoms of radiculopathy exist with proper confirmatory evidence, then these are a result of changes in the intervertebral disc. However, this is not the case for the remaining 90% of our population of patients with back pain, who never experience radiculopathy but only idiopathic or mechanical low back pain.

During 50 years of clinical and scientific work on this problem, my endeavors have continuously moved upward in the human body: first biomechanical measurements of physiologic loads, then investigations of the chemical and nutritional changes in the nucleus pulposus and annulus fibrosus, investigations of the contents of pain-modulating substances in the cerebrospinal fluid, and lately functional magnetic resonance imaging (fMRI) of the human brain to evaluate abnormal responses in various areas elicited by peripheral pain stimuli.

In addition, I have conducted several prospective randomized trials on possible treatments for low back pain and edited a very well-received book (22) on the entire problem.

WHERE DOES THE PAIN COME FROM?

Numerous structures in the lower back are supplied with nerve endings that can signal pain; the discs, facets, ligaments, fascia, muscles, subcutaneous tissue, cutis, and nerve roots themselves, including the ganglia, all contain unmyelinated C fibers (8).

In addition, psychosocial factors are certainly involved when low back pain becomes prolonged (27).

Miller et al. (19), in 600 autopsy specimens, demonstrated that by the age of 50 years, 90% of people have what they called degenerating (i.e., aging) discs, and Boos and collaborators (6), in their Volvo Award–winning article, clearly demonstrated, on the basis of a large number of microscopic studies, that so-called degeneration of the intervertebral disc cannot be differentiated from aging, which is not in itself a disease.

RADIOGRAPHS

Several studies in which plain radiographs were used (18,21,23,26) have demonstrated very weak evidence for an association between disc degeneration and back pain. Table 1.1

TABLE 1.1. Magnetic resonance imaging studies of structural abnormalities in the cervical and lumbar spine of asymptomatic persons

Study (ref)	Year	Population size	Modality	Abnormal findings
Powell et al. (23b)	1986	n = 302 women	0.15 T	Disc degeneration increase from 6% in <20-y-old women to 79% in >60-y-old women
Weinreb et al. (28)	1989	n = 86 women: 45 pregnant, 41 not pregnant	1.5 T	Disc bulging or herniation in one or more levels 54% in both groups
Boden et al. (4)	1990	n = 57	1.5 T	Individuals <50 y old: 20% disc herniation, 1% spinal stenosis; individuals >60 y old: 35% disc herniation, 21% spinal stenosis
Boden et al. (4a)	1990	n = 63, 20–63 y old	1.5 T	Bulging discs 5%; disc narrowing and degeneration 25% <40 y, 60% >40 y; foraminal stenosis 20%
Tertti et al. (25b)	1991	n = 39 children with low back pain matched for sex, age, and school class	0.02 T	26% disc degeneration, 3% disc protrusion, 26% spinal muscle atrophy, 8% Scheuermann-type changes, 3% transitional vertebra, 3% narrowed disc space
Parkkola et al. (23a)	1993	n = 60 volunteers	0.02 T	3% central spinal stenosis, 15% disc bulging, 72 degenerated discs among 180 analyzed discs (40%)
Jensen et al. (14a)	1994	n = 98 volunteers	1.5 T	52% disc bulging, 27% disc protrusions, 1% disc extrusions, 19% Schmori nodes, 14% annular defects, 8% facet arthropathy
Boos et al. (5)	1995	n = 46 asymptomatic persons matched for age, sex, and risk factor matched with patients selected for discectomy	1.5 T	76% disc herniations (63% protrusions, 13% extrusions), 85% disc degeneration, 22% neural compromise
Buirski and Silberstein (7a)	1993	n = 63; 38 women	1.5 T	39% disc degeneration with protrusion
Matsumoto et al. (18a)	1998	n = 497; 262 women, 235 men; C2–7, 10–70 y old	1.5 T 134 0.5 T 363	Kappa scores for three observers ≈0.6; degeneration, 20 y old 15%; >60 y 88%; foramen stenosis, >40 y 15%; disc protrusion, >40 y 25%; cord compression, 8%
Battié et al. (2)	1995	n = 115 male twin pairs (21% with back pain for last 12 mo)	1.5 T	Two independent observers kappa scores ≈0.8 for signal intensity (degeneration), disc bulging; narrowing common, explained by twinship and early shared environment and upbringing more than physical load
Stadnik et al. (25a)	1998	n = 36	1.5 T, gadolinium enhancement	Bulging discs 81%, disc protrusion 33%, 56% annular tears; of 27 tears, 96% contrast-enhanced
Lane et al. (16a)	1995	n = 30	1.5 T, gadolinium enhancement	Radicular enhancement found in 18 of 30
Lehto et al. (16b)	1994	n = 89, 9–63 y old	0.1 T	Asymptomatic degeneration in cervical discs, common after 30 y of age, 57% in subjects >40 y old
Weishaupt et al. (29)	1998	n = 60, 20–50 y old	1.0 T	Disc bulging 62%, protrusion 67%, HIZ 33%; disc extrusion 18%; sequester or nerve root compromise endplate abnormality uncommon

HIZ, high-intensity zone; T, tesla.

From Nachemson A, Vingård E. Assessment of patients with neck and back pain: a best-evidence synthesis. In: Nachemson AL, Jonsson E, eds. *Neck and back pain: the scientific evidence of causes, diagnosis, and treatment.* Philadelphia: Lippincott Williams & Wilkins, 2000:189–235, with permission.

shows that a significant number of "degenerative disc" findings are also observed in asymptomatic persons, based on computed tomographic (CT) and magnetic resonance imaging (MRI) studies of pain-free, age-matched subjects.

Discograms have been found unreliable (9,10,14,20). In the only examination of non-symptomatic volunteers matched for age, sex, work, and smoking status and compared with patients who had radiculopathy and disc herniation managed surgically, Boos et al. (5) reported that an astounding 76% of the volunteers also had disc herniation, mostly at the midline. When the volunteers, in addition to those described by Boden et al. (4,7,12), were reexamined 5 to 7 years after their first MRI, none gave a history of sciatica, and they reported only a minimal amount of low back pain, such as would be expected from what is known about the occurrence of back pain.

Attempts to diagnose patients with instability have failed (21). Most surgeons and manipulators use their own unreliable definition.

Socioeconomic and psychologic factors certainly influence the duration of symptoms (27). These include family relationships, local culture, social network, job market, employment status, and, most significantly in my opinion, the insurance system—the ease with which remuneration can be obtained, how much, and for how long. The most important psychologic deterrents to the abatement of back pain and return to work are fear of moving and avoidance behavior. In addition, these factors affect the discography examination, making the results unreliable and certainly not useful.

During the last decade, an increasing number of neurophysiologic and neuropsychologic studies have linked the body to the soul (8). In an investigation of the levels of the pain-enhancing factors substance P and nerve growth factor in patients with chronic low back pain lasting longer than 6 months (11), we found that the levels were significantly enhanced in comparison with those in a control population. In fMRI investigations based on the so-called blood oxygen level–dependent (BOLD) effect, whereby neuronal activation induced by local cerebral blood flow and blood oxygenation can be detected indirectly, we observed brain signals in a small preliminary sample of patients with chronic low back pain at a significantly lower level of pain stimuli than in normal controls, supporting the hypothesis of augmented central pain processing in patients with low back pain (13).

That aging and longevity are influenced by genetic factors is well known, and this also applies to aging of the disc, as demonstrated by Battié et al. (2,3) and others (1). In their most recent twin study, they found that disc degeneration did not differ between occupational drivers and twin brothers who did not drive. Their conclusions underscore what I mean when I say that attention should be shifted from degenerative and morphologic changes in the disc and vertebra to other possible explanations for the link between back pain, various occupational situations, MRI and radiology findings, and in particular the reporting of long-standing, severe back problems, which Dr. Kuslich and many other spine surgeons believe they can manage with cages, coagulation, fusion, and lately artificial disc prostheses.

Kuslich et al. (16), on the basis of their 1998 study repeating the earlier experiments of Smyth and Wright (25), claimed that the annulus generates back pain—but this was in patients with radiculopathy who underwent surgery for disc herniation. When the outer part of the annulus was probed, some 30% of the patients experienced pain. We now know that a component of the pain in patients with disc herniation is based on nerve irritation caused by cytokines in disc tissue. Therefore, from that study, it is not possible to infer the existence of such an entity as degenerative disc disease.

Furthermore, Dr. Kuslich's remarkable economic success from the sale of his BAK (Bagby and Kuslich) cages for the surgical treatment of chronic low back pain (15) has not been mirrored by similar success in improving the clinical results (17,24).

REFERENCES

1. Annunen P, Paassilta J, Lohiniva, et al. An allele of COL9A2 associated with intervertebral disc disease. *Science* 1999;285:409–412.
2. Battié MC, Videman T, Gibbons LE, et al. Determinants of lumbar disc degeneration: a study relating lifetime exposures and magnetic resonance image findings in identical twins. *Spine* 1995;20:2601–2612.
3. Battié MC, Videman T, Gibbons LE, et al. Occupational driving and lumbar disc degeneration: a case-control study. *Lancet* 2002;9343:1369–1374
4. Boden SD, Davis DO, Dina TS, et al. Abnormal magnetic-resonance scans of the lumbar spine in asymptomatic subjects: a prospective investigation. *J Bone Joint Surg Am* 1990;72:403–408.
4a. Boden SD, McCowin PR, Davis DO, et al. Abnormal magnetic-resonance scans of the cervical spine in asymptomatic subjects: a prospective investigation. *J Bone Joint Surg Am* 1990;72:1178–1184.
5. Boos N, et al. The diagnostic accuracy of magnetic resonance imaging. Work perception and psychosocial factors in identifying symptomatic disc herniations. *Spine* 1995;20;2613–2625.
6. Boos N, Weissbach S, Rohrbach H, et al. Classification of age-related changes in lumbar intervertebral discs: 2002 Volvo Award in basic science. *Spine* 2002;27:2631–2644.
7. Borenstein DG, O'Mara JW Jr, Boden SD, et al. The value of magnetic resonance imaging of the lumbar spine to predict low-back pain in asymptomatic subjects: a seven-year follow-up study. *J Bone Joint Surg Am* 2001; 83:1306–1311.
7a. Buirski G, Silberstein M. The symptomatic lumbar disc in patients with low-back pain: magnetic resonance imaging appearances in both a symptomatic and control population. *Spine* 1993;18:1808–1811.
8. Carlsson C-A, Nachemson A. Neurophysiology of back pain: current knowledge. In: Nachemson A, Jonsson E. *Neck and back pain. The scientific evidence of causes, diagnosis, and treatment.* Philadelphia: Lippincott Williams & Wilkins, 2000:149–163.
9. Carragee E, Tanner C, Haurana S. The rates of false positive discography in select patients without low back symptoms. *Spine* 2000;25:1373–1381.
10. Carragee E, Tanner C, Norbash A, et al. False positive findings on lumbar discography. *Spine* 1999;24: 2542–2547.
11. Clauw D, Williams D, Lauerman W, et al. Pain sensitivity as a correlate of clinical status in individuals with chronic low back pain. *Spine* 1999; 24:2035–2041.
12. Elfering A, Semmer N, Birkhofer D, et al. Risk factors for lumbar disc degeneration: a 5-year prospective MRI study in asymptomatic individuals. *Spine* 2002;27:125–134.
13. Gracely RH, Giesecke T, Clauw DJ, et al. *Evidence of altered supraspinal pain processing during evoked pressure pain in idiopathic chronic low back pain (ICLBP) patients and fibromyalgia (FMS) patients.* Presented to the American League of Rheumatism, New Orleans, 2002(abst).
14. Holt E. The question of lumbar discography. *J Bone Joint Surg Am* 1968;50:720–726.
14a. Jensen M. Brant-Zawadzki MN, Obuchowski N, et al. Magnetic resonance imaging of the lumbar spine in people without back pain. *N Engl J Med* 1994;331:69–73.
15. Kuslich SD, Ulstrom CL, Griffith SL, et al. The Bagby and Kuslich method of lumbar interbody fusion. History, techniques, and 2-year follow-up results of a United States prospective, multicenter trial. *Spine* 1998;23:1267–1278.
16. Kuslich SD, Ulstrom CL, Michael CJ. The tissue origin of low back pain and sciatica: a report of pain response to tissue stimulation during operations on the lumbar spine using local anesthesia. *Orthop Clin North Am* 1991;22:181–187.
16a. Lane JL, Koeller KK, Atkinson JD. Contrast-enhanced radicular veins on MR of the lumbar spine in an asymptomatic study group. *Am J Neuroradiol* 1995;16:269–273.
16b. Lehto IJ, Tertti MO, Komu ME, et al. Age-related MRI changes at 0.1 T in cervical discs in asymptomatic subjects. *Neuroradiology* 1994;36:49–53.
17. Lonstein JE. Re: Four-year follow-up results of lumbar spine arthrodesis using Bagby and Kuslich lumbar fusion cage. *Spine* 2001;26:1506–1508.
18. Magora A, Schwartz A. Relation between the low back pain syndrome and x-ray findings. I. Degenerative osteoarthritis. *Scand J Rehabil Med* 1976;8:115–125.
18a. Matsumoto M, Fujimura Y, Suzuki N, et al. MRI of cervical intervertebral discs in asymptomatic subjects. *J Bone Joint Surg Br* 1998;80:19–24.
19. Miller J, Schmatz C, Schultz A. Lumbar disc degeneration correlation with and sex and spine level in 600 autopsy specimens. *Spine* 1988;13:173–178.
20. Nachemson A. Lumbar discography—where are we today? *Spine* 1989;14:555–557.

21. Nachemson A. Scientific diagnosis or unproved label for back pain patients? In: Szpalski M, Gunzburg R, Pope MH, eds. *Lumbar segmental instability*. Philadelphia: Lippincott Williams & Wilkins, 1999:297–301.
22. Nachemson A, Jonsson E, eds. *Neck and back pain. The scientific evidence of causes, diagnosis and treatment*. Philadelphia: Lippincott Williams & Wilkins, 2000.
23. Nachemson A, Vingård E. Assessment of patients with neck and back pain: a best-evidence synthesis. In: Nachemson A, Jonsson E, eds. *Neck and back pain: the scientific evidence of causes, diagnosis and treatment*. Philadelphia: Lippincott Williams & Wilkins, 2000:189–235.
23a. Parkkola R, Rytokoski U, Kormano M. Magnetic resonance imaging of the discs and trunk muscles in patients with chronic low back pain and healthy control subjects. *Spine* 1993;18:830–836.
23b. Powell MC, Wilson M, Szypryt P, et al. Prevalence of lumbar disc degeneration observed by magnetic resonance in symptomless women. *Lancet* 1986;13:1366–1367.
24. Slosar PJ. Indications and outcomes of reconstructive surgery in chronic pain of spinal origin. *Spine* 2002;27:2555–2562.
25. Smyth MJ, Wright V. Sciatica and the intervertebral disc. An experimental study. *J Bone Joint Surg Br* 1967;49:502–519.
25a. Stadnik TW, Lee RR, Coen HI, et al. Annular tears and disk herniation: prevalence and contrast enhancement on MR images in the absence of low back pain or sciatica. *Radiology* 1998;206:49–55.
25b. Tertti MO, Salminen JJ, Paajanen HE, et al. Low-back pain and disk degeneration in children: a case-control MR imaging study. *Radiology* 1991;180:503–507.
26. Van Tulder MW, Assendelft WJJ, Koes BW, et al. Spinal radiographic finding and nonspecific low back pain: a systematic review of observational studies. *Spine* 1997;22:427–434.
27. Waddell G, Aylward M, Sawney P. *Back pain, incapacity for work and social security benefits: an international literature review and analysis*. London: The Royal Society of Medicine Press Ltd., 2002.
28. Weinreb JC, Wolbarsht LB, Cohen JM, et al. Prevalence of lumbosacral intervertebral disk abnormalities on MR images in pregnant and asymptomatic nonpregnant women. *Radiology* 1989;170(1 Pt 1):125–128.
29. Weishaupt D, Zenetti M, Hodler J, et al. MR imaging of the lumbar spine: prevalence of intervertebral disk extrusion and sequestration, nerve root compression, end plate abnormalities, and osteoarthritis of the facet joints in asymptomatic volunteers. *Radiology* 1998;209:661–666.

2

Morphologic Changes of Endplates in Degenerative Disc Disease

Robert J. Moore

Department of Pathology, The University of Adelaide; and The Adelaide Centre for Spinal Research, Institute of Medical and Veterinary Science, Adelaide, Australia

The vertebral bodies of the axial skeleton are separated by intervertebral discs, which are highly specialized structures that enable a range of physiologic and mechanical functions associated with motion. The discs have three main structural components—a central nucleus pulposus surrounded by the annulus fibrosus and the endplates, which are located at the cranial and caudal interfaces with the vertebrae. Although the structure and function of the annulus and nucleus are well characterized, much less is known about the endplates. Perhaps this is because their constitution has not yet been consistently defined or because structural changes to the endplates are more subtle than changes to the other disc components and therefore easily overlooked.

In some early anatomic studies, the endplates were described as a transitional zone between the vertebral body and the adjacent disc because they possessed both an osseous and a hyaline cartilage component (19,51). Other authors, however, proposed a more limited situation, describing the endplates as the thin layer of hyaline cartilage interposed between the vertebral body and the disc (40,65). For whatever reason, this latter concept has survived, and they are now more commonly known as the *cartilage endplates*, or simply the *endplates*.

Volumes of literature have been devoted to the normal development of the endplates, which are recognizable from an early embryologic stage and retain their cartilaginous nature during normal maturation while the adjacent vertebrae undergo ossification (57). The cartilaginous component of the mature endplate is essentially an aqueous gel containing large proteoglycan molecules within a dense mesh of collagen fibrils that are aligned along the longitudinal axis (horizontally in humans). Although it has been suggested that a direct physical connection between the endplates and the underlying bone is lacking (24), their juxtaposition almost certainly contributes to the strong bond that is essential for the normal function of the endplate (5). When the epiphyses fuse in the young adult spine, only the outer rim of the endplates is ossified, and a broad central cartilaginous plate is left. The lamellae of the outer annulus attach directly to the adjacent bone, while the fibers of the inner annulus connect the endplates directly with the disc.

The endplates are thin, particularly in the center of the disc, measuring no more than 1 mm at maturity (14), but variation from one side to the other can be considerable (47). In the lower lumbar spine, the endplates are roughly cardioid to elliptic in shape (17). Although this fact in itself may seem to have little relevance, shape is the only one of several parameters investigated by computed tomography–myelography that is claimed to be significantly related to the development of disc herniation (18). The most abundant cell type in the endplate is the chondrocyte, distributed more uniformly than the clearly defined layers of cells within articular cartilage. Otherwise, the endplate bears a close similarity to the articular cartilage of synovial joints.

The biochemical characteristics of the endplates, from normality through the spectrum of degenerative conditions, are well documented (3,6). The two most abundant families of molecules in the disc are the collagens and the proteoglycans, which are found in varying proportions in the annulus, the nucleus, and the endplates. Of the several species of collagen, type X is probably the most important in the endplates because it is a marker of hypertrophic chondrocytes and is thought to be involved in cartilage calcification (1). It has been detected mainly in the central region (27).

Proteoglycan molecules are essential for the maintenance of the water content and overall integrity of the nucleus (32). It is known that altered tissue levels of proteoglycans can adversely influence disc function (62). The proteoglycans of the endplate have not been studied extensively, but it suffices to say that the loss of proteoglycans from the endplate is implicated in the loss of proteoglycans from the nucleus (48). It follows that disc degeneration invariably is preceded by widespread degradation of disc proteoglycans (41). It has long been suspected that alterations to the biochemical composition of the endplate, particularly during the growth phase, may be involved in the development of scoliosis (2,42,46).

Heterozygous inactivation of the Col2a1 gene allele in 1-month-old mice has been shown to lead to a lower glycosaminoglycan concentration in the endplates and thicker, more irregular endplates that become calcified prematurely (50).

The developing discs receive essential nourishment from two sources. From the embryonic stage, a network of blood vessels penetrates the annulus no more deeply than to about one third of its total thickness (56). Most of these vessels do not persist beyond maturity, and by adulthood they can be seen in only the outer two or three lamellae. Blood vessels also penetrate the endplates from the vertebral body margins (57) and arise from ramifications of a large primary nutrient artery on the dorsal surface of each vertebral body. With maturation, however, these small vessels also disappear, leaving only a limited blood supply in the form of capillary buds that perforate the osseous component of the endplate (22). It is curious that mammalian discs have evolved in this way because the central nucleus pulposus in the adult human can be up to 20 mm from the nearest blood vessels and is therefore totally reliant on the diffusion of solutes across the endplates and the annulus for nutrition. No other tissue in the body is so distanced from a blood supply and therefore presumably so susceptible to deterioration.

Extensive *in vitro* study of the transport of solutes and disc nutrition and metabolism performed with small dye molecules has shown that the lateral endplate at the vertebral rim is relatively impermeable compared with the central portion, and even the entire annulus fibrosus (36). The contribution of the periannular blood supply was well accepted, but the permeability of the capillary network immediately beneath the endplate attracted new attention. Quantitative analysis of human autopsy specimens that had been injected with dye solution subsequently confirmed the presence of significantly more marrow contacts along the central endplate adjacent to the nucleus than in the lateral margins (13,31).

Although the significance of these vessels to disc nutrition and cell metabolism was determined, diffusion was shown to be the principal mechanism for transporting small dissolved solutes into the disc (61). Furthermore, the size and ionic charge of the molecules were also shown to govern the rate and extent of diffusion (60,61). Because the high

50. Sahlman J, Inkinen R, Hirvonen T, et al. Premature vertebral endplate ossification and mild disc degeneration in mice after inactivation of one allele belonging to the Col2a1 gene for type II collagen. *Spine* 2001;26:2558–2565.
51. Schmorl G, Junghanns H. *The human spine in health and disease*, 2nd American ed. New York: Grune & Stratton, 1971:158–182.
52. Steffen T, Tsantrizos A, Aebi M. Effect of implant design and endplate preparation on the compressive strength of interbody fusion constructs. *Spine* 2000;25:1077–1084.
53. Steffen T, Tsantrizos A, Fruth I, et al. Cages: designs and concepts. *Eur Spine J* 2000;9[Suppl 1]:S89–S94.
54. Szpalski M, Gunzburg R, Mayer M. Spine arthroplasty: a historical review. *Eur Spine J* 2002;11[Suppl 2]:S65–S84.
55. Tanaka M, Nakahara S, Inoue H. A pathologic study of discs in the elderly. Separation between the cartilaginous endplate and the vertebral body. *Spine* 1993;18:1456–1462.
56. Taylor JR. *Growth and development of the human intervertebral disc* [Thesis]. Edinburgh: University of Edinburgh, 1973.
57. Taylor JR, Twomey LT. Growth of human intervertebral discs and vertebral bodies. *J Anat* 1988;120:49–68.
58. Twomey LT, Taylor JR. Age changes in lumbar vertebrae and intervertebral discs. *Clin Orthop* 1987;224:97–104.
59. Twomey LT, Taylor JR, Furniss B. Age changes in the bone density and structure of the lumbar vertebral column. *J Anat* 1983;136:15–25.
60. Urban JPG, Holm S, Maroudas A. Diffusion of small solutes into the intervertebral disc. An in vivo study. *Biorheology* 1978;15:203–221.
61. Urban JPG, Holm S, Maroudas A, et al. Nutrition of the intervertebral disc. An in vivo study of solute transport. *Clin Orthop* 1977;129:101–114.
62. Urban JP, Maroudas A. Swelling of the intervertebral disc in vitro. *Connect Tissue Res* 1981;9:1–10.
63. Vernon-Roberts B. Age-related and degenerative pathology of intervertebral discs and apophyseal joints. In: Jayson MIV, ed. *The lumbar spine and back pain*, 4th ed. Edinburgh: Churchill Livingstone, 1992:17–41.
64. Vernon-Roberts B, Pirie CJ. Degenerative changes in the intervertebral discs and their sequelae. *Rheum Rehabil* 1977;16:13–21.
65. Walmsley R. The development and growth of the intervertebral disc. *Edinburgh Med J* 1953;60:341–364.
66. Weiler C, Nerlich AG, Zipperer J, et al. SSE Award Competition in Basic Sciences: Expression of major matrix metalloproteinases is associated with intervertebral disc degeneration and resorption. *Eur Spine J* 2002;11:308–320.
67. Zindrick MR, Selby D. Lumbar spinal fusion: different types and indications. In: Wiesel SW, Weinstein JN, Herkowitz H, et al., eds. *The lumbar spine*, 2nd ed. Philadelphia: WB Saunders, 1996.

3

Biochemical Changes in Degenerative Disc Disease

*†Sally Roberts and ‡§Bruce Caterson

*Centre for Science and Technology in Medicine, Keele University, Staffordshire, United Kingdom; †Centre for Spinal Studies, Robert Jones & Agnes Hunt Orthopaedic Hospital, Shropshire, United Kingdom; ‡Cardiff School of Biosciences, Cardiff University; and §Department of Orthopedics and Trauma, University of Wales College of Medicine, Cardiff, United Kingdom

The types of molecules present in the intervertebral disc and the manner in which they are laid down and interconnected directly influence the mechanical properties and physiologic functioning of the tissue. The main components are collagens and proteoglycans, the latter of which attract water to form a gel, which is retained within a fibrous network of collagen and elastin (5,39). In addition to these structural molecules, which make up the bulk of the tissue, an array of many other matrix molecules, such as growth factors, proteases, and cytokines, although occurring in small quantities, nonetheless play a significant role in influencing the physical properties of the tissue through their effects on tissue homeostasis. Each of these is discussed as it occurs in the healthy disc, before the changes known to occur in degenerative disc disease are described.

BIOCHEMISTRY OF THE HEALTHY DISC

Structural Molecules

Collagen

Collagen is the main structural protein in the body and the most common one in the disc, making up approximately 70% of the dry weight in the outer annulus fibrosus and 6% to 25% of the central nucleus pulposus (10). The collagens are a family of proteins, and approximately 80% of the collagen in the disc is either type I (predominantly in the annulus fibrosus) or type II (mostly in the nucleus pulposus) (11). Several other types of collagen exist, but in small quantities—for example, types III, V, VI, IX, X, XII, and XIV. In other cartilaginous tissues, copolymerization between these different collagen types has been clearly demonstrated, with type XI collagen forming a central core within type II fibrils and type IX collagen on the surface and collagen type V or XI distributing together with type I collagen. Similar colocalization is likely in the disc, and evidence has also been found of cross-linking between molecules of collagen types I and II and between molecules of types I and III (9).

The exact function of the different types of collagens in the disc is not known, although possible suggestions are that types III and X may be involved in repair processes (9, 25) and that type VI collagen may bind the cells, by linking with their cell surface integrins, into the extracellular matrix (27). Even though type IX collagen makes up less than 1%

of the total disc collagen (9), it could influence the bulk of it by helping to regulate the size of type II collagen fibers, as occurs in other cartilages (38).

Individual collagen molecules are modified after synthesis and secretion from the cell, with chemical cross-links forming between adjacent collagen molecules. Initially, borohydride-"reducible" cross-links form, but these change with time to "mature," nonreducible hydroxypyridinium cross-links. The concentration of hydroxypyridinium cross-links is higher in human disc collagen than anywhere else in vertebrate connective tissues (10), particularly in the nucleus; a possible explanation for this is the slow turnover of extracellular macromolecules in interstitial disc tissue. Other, nonenzymic collagen cross-links form with increasing age, especially in areas of predominantly low oxygen tension. Pentosidine, for example, is an advanced glycation end-product (AGE) that forms spontaneously from glucose-derived Amadori products and occurs throughout the disc, increasingly so with advancing age (8).

Proteoglycans

Proteoglycans (PGs) have a high anionic charge that, by osmosis, creates a strong swelling pressure, attracting water to form a gel. (Water makes up approximately 75% to 80% of the nucleus pulposus and 65% to 75% of the annulus fibrosus.) The PG concentration is very high in the center of the disc, where the amount of swelling is constrained by tension arising in the collagen fibers in the matrix. This combination provides a composite structure highly suited to carrying and redistributing compressive loads yet allowing movement in all planes. The most common PG in disc is a large, aggregating PG, aggrecan, which consists of up to 100 individual PG monomers connected by a hyaluronan chain, the contact being stabilized by a link protein. The individual PG monomer has a central protein core consisting of as many as 2,000 amino acids; several different structural and functional domains occur along its length. In the newly synthesized PG, three regions are globular: G_1 and G_2 at the N-terminus and G_3 at the C-terminus (Fig. 3.1). Between these, the protein core is linear and comprises three areas, one where keratan sulfate (KS) and two where chondroitin sulfate (CS) repeating sugar chains are attached. In early life, most of these are CS and few KS, but with increasing age, KS chains predominate. It is the negatively charged sulfate and carboxyl groups on these disaccharide

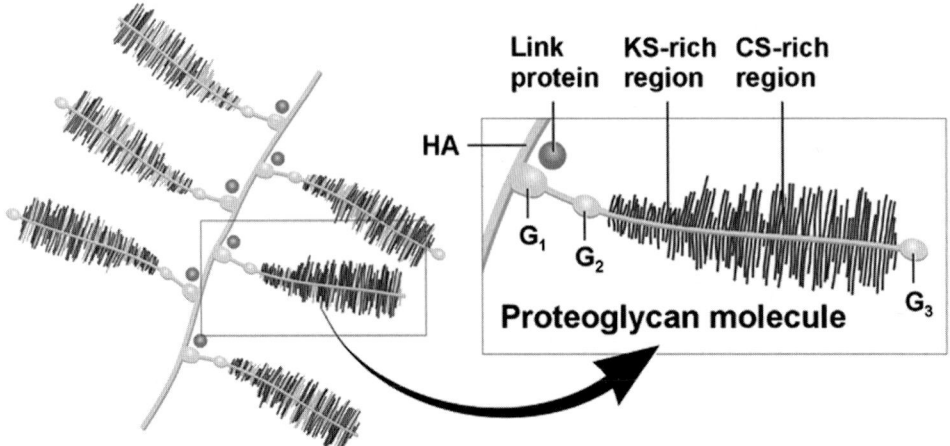

FIG. 3.1. Typical structure of a proteoglycan monomer, up to 100 of which link via hyaluronan *(HA)* to form large aggregates. *CS,* chondroitin sulfate; *KS,* keratan sulfate.

chains that attract cations to neutralize their charge, thereby creating a high ionic concentration and giving the PGs in the disc their high swelling pressure.

Although aggrecan makes up most of the PG in disc, other PG types are also present: one other large, aggregating PG (versican) (32) and several small, low-molecular-weight interstitial PGs (lumican, decorin, and biglycan) (4,15,19). These have a much shorter core protein and few (maybe one or two) glycosaminoglycan (GAG) chains, and they do not form aggregates. Like the several minor collagen types present, these other PGs may contribute significantly to the physiology and functioning of the disc, although they occur only at low concentrations. For example, decorin, like type IX collagen, sits on the fibrillar collagens and controls their diameter, whereas both decorin and biglycan may act within the extracellular matrix to bind and regulate growth factors in the disc and hence influence the physiology and activity of cells. More versican is found in adult disc than in cartilage, and the size of its core protein is more heterogeneous than in articular cartilage (32). This is even more pronounced in the nucleus than in the annulus and increases with age. Unlike the GAG chains on versican in other parts of the body, those on versican in the disc can be KS (32). This may be akin to a higher KS:CS ratio in disc aggrecan than in cartilage aggrecan. Scott (30) suggests that the biosynthesis of KS rather than CS is favored in low oxygen conditions, such as in the deep zone of cartilage in comparison with the surface zone and in the central nucleus of the disc in comparison with the outer annulus. Similarly, an increase in KS:CS production in the human disc occurs at about 3 to 10 years of age, which it is suggested is due to the coincident loss of nutritive pathways when the vascular channels in the adjacent cartilage endplates and outer disc atrophy (30).

Elastin

Elastin has long been demonstrated in the disc and shown biochemically to make up 1% to 2% of the dry weight (22). However, the amino acid composition of disc elastin differs from that of elastin in other tissues, such as nuchal ligament, in that it is enriched in polar amino acids, particularly histidine and lysine (J. Yu, J. Urban, C. Winlove, personal communication, 1999). Once again, however, the relatively small proportion at which elastin occurs may disguise the importance of this molecule and the effect of its presence on the physical properties of the matrix. Elastin may cross-link other structural components within the disc, possibly binding different collagen fibers together or linking collagen and PGs. Elastin, unlike the fibrillar collagens, which have regular tripeptide repeats, is composed of a high proportion of hydrophobic amino acids. However, like collagen molecules, elastin molecules undergo enzymatic modifications that alter the lysine residues that ultimately form labile and then stable cross-links. Hence, in theory, some hydroxypyridinium cross-links could form between the elastin molecules, as well as the collagen molecules, if they were in close proximity.

The organization of elastin fibers appears very structured, and studies of the organization may contribute to our understanding of the mechanical functioning of the disc. For example, although the nucleus matrix is usually described as randomly organized (based on the collagen), elastin appears to be radially organized here (39).

Other Components

Other components, such as the glycoproteins fibronectin (23) and tenascin (12,13), have been identified in the intervertebral disc. Their function in disc is not known, but they may be involved in cell signaling and mechanotransduction, allowing the cell to respond to changes in its environment. For example, fibronectin elsewhere in the body interacts with integrins and influences cellular activity and phenotypic expression. In addition, other matrix proteins may be present that remain to be identified and characterized. For example, chondromodulin and heat shock protein have recently been shown to occur in disc (33,34).

Enzymes, Growth Factors, and Cytokines

Like all other systems, the intervertebral disc must have mechanisms to maintain homeostasis—to synthesize and break down extracellular matrix components continually, albeit slowly. The mean turnover time for the disc PG population in the adult rabbit is estimated to be approximately 300 days and, for collagen in adult dog cartilage, it is estimated to be 120 years (21). Hence, molecules that influence cell metabolism, such as growth factors, cytokines, and proteases, can well be expected to occur in normal disc. Indeed, growth factors including fibroblast growth factor (35) and transforming growth factor-β (20) and the cytokines interleukins-1 and -6 and tumor necrosis factor-α (24) have been demonstrated in human discs. In addition, various proteases are known to occur, including those belonging to the cathepsin family, matrix metalloproteinases (MMPs), and aggrecanases (2,26,28).

ALTERATIONS IN THE PROTEOGLYCAN POPULATION IN DEGENERATIVE DISC DISEASE

The PG population of the disc becomes more heterogenous and fragmented with the degree of degeneration. Changes seen in pathologic degenerative disease are similar to those seen that occur with age, although they may be more extreme. Loss of PG is the most significant biochemical change in degenerate discs, which lose possibly up to 80% of their total GAG content in comparison with apparently "normal" discs of a similar age (Fig. 3.2). However, the structure of newly biosynthesed PGs (at least of large, aggregating PGs) do not differ in pathologically degenerate and normal discs (18). Hence, the mechanism of PG changes in degenerative disc disease is likely to be the same as that in the degeneration of aging. Although disc cells have the capability to synthesize intact, full-length aggrecan, including the region that is able to bind to hyaluronan ("hyaluronan-binding region") (3,18), and hence to form aggregates, only 30% of the disc PGs actually occur as aggregates, even at the age of 20 years (7,17), in comparison with 80% in cartilage (Fig. 3.3). This is believed to be a consequence of enzyme activity cleaving the aggrecan core protein close to the hyaluronan binding region. Both MMPs and aggrecanase can achieve this, and although both have been shown to occur in disc, aggrecanase appears to be relatively less important than in the degradation of articular cartilage (26,31). Perhaps surprisingly, the PGs become more difficult to extract biochemically from the disc with increasing age, probably because of increased interaction with other matrix components, such as collagen (18). Several cross-linking mechanisms may be involved, such as those already described (AGEs and hydroxypyridinium cross-links) and transglutaminases, which are covalent linkages of lysine and glutamine residues, possibly on adjacent matrix molecules.

Less is known of how the small PG population changes during disc degeneration, although some evidence suggests that the amount of decorin and particularly of biglycan is elevated in degenerate human discs in comparison with normal discs (15,16). Studies have shown that the messenger RNA of cells from discs with degenerative disc disease may be elevated for some small PGs but greatly reduced for other matrix molecules that one would expect to be produced in damaged tissue, at least in the early stages, when an attempt at a repair phase could be anticipated (C. Curtis, personal communication, 2002).

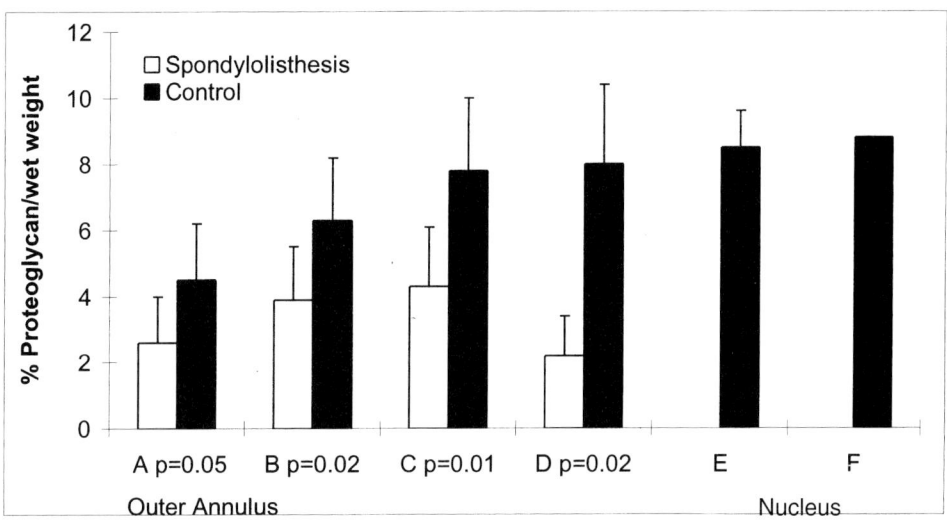

FIG. 3.2. Loss of glycosaminoglycans, mostly from the main proteoglycan of disc, aggrecan, is the most significant biochemical change in degenerative disc disease and other disc disorders, such as spondylolisthesis (shown here), in comparison with "normal" control discs of a similar age. (Adapted from Roberts S, Beard HK, O'Brien JP. Biochemical changes of intervertebral discs in patients with spondylolisthesis or with tears of the posterior annulus fibrosus. *Ann Rheum Dis* 1982;41:78–85.

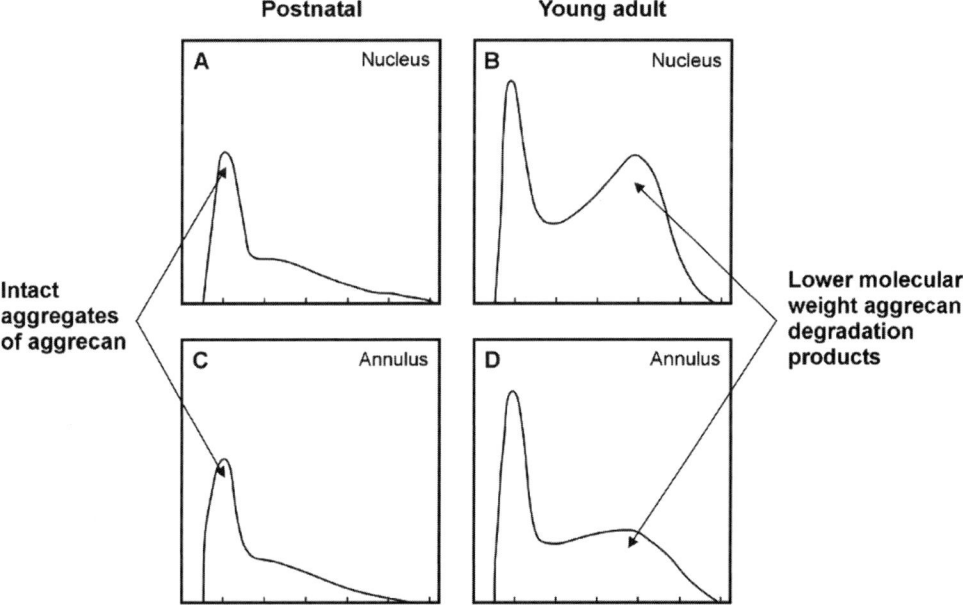

FIG. 3.3. Graphs showing how the aggregation and size of proteoglycans diminish in young adult discs (*B,D*) in comparison with postnatal discs (*A,C*), especially in the nucleus (*B*), where the peak formed by denatured products represents a larger proportion of the total than in the annulus (*D*). (Adapted from Donohue PJ, Jahnke MR, Blaha JD, et al. Characterization of link protein(s) from human intervertebral-disc tissues. *Biochem J* 1998;251:739–747, with permission.)

ALTERATIONS IN COLLAGENS AND OTHER STRUCTURAL COMPONENTS IN DISC DEGENERATION

Although the disc collagens are altered in degenerative disc disease, the alterations are not as obvious as those in the PG population. The absolute quantity of collagen changes little, but the types and distribution of collagens can change. For example, more of types I, III, VI and X collagen is found in degenerate discs (1,25); types III and VI, which are normally pericellular, are deposited more widely throughout the matrix in degenerate discs (27). Type II collagen fibrils show evidence of denaturation and rupturing of the triple helix, which is always greater in disc than, for example, in articular cartilage from the same individual and increases with degeneration (1,14).

No change in the reducible or mature hydroxypyridinium cross-links was observed with disc degeneration. However, an increase in age-related pentosidine cross-links was associated initially with the degree of degeneration, then a decrease in the most severely degenerate discs (8). This finding suggests an increased turnover and synthesis of new collagen molecules without age-accumulated pentosidine cross-links, consistent with an attempted reparative phase in disc degeneration, as has been suggested previously (25).

The quantity or distribution of other components can change in disc degeneration and disease. For example, increased AGEs have been reported in herniated human intervertebral disc (37), and elastin becomes more disorganized with increasing degeneration (J. Yu, personal communication, 2002).

The content of fibronectin increases as degeneration progresses, and it becomes more fragmented (23). The elevated levels of fibronectin may reflect the response of cells to an altered environment. Whatever the cause, the formation of fibronectin fragments feeds into the degenerative cascade because the fragments down-regulate aggrecan synthesis but up-regulate the production of some MMPs, in addition to diminishing cell movement.

The matrix glycoprotein tenascin has a repeated structural domain homologous with that of epidermal growth factor and fibronectin, and elsewhere in the body it modulates cell adhesion, migration, and growth. Tenascin interacts with the CS chains of matrix PGs and the G_3 C-terminal globular domain of large, aggregating PGs, such as versican and aggrecan. It has been reported that tenascin levels are decreased in degenerate discs and that tenascin is restricted to the pericellular matrix in the outer annulus in older, degenerate discs (13). In contrast, tenascin is increased in other arthritic tissues (29).

ENZYMES IN DISC DEGENERATION

Several families of enzymes are capable of breaking down the various matrix molecules of disc, including cathepsins, MMPs and aggrecanases. The activity of cathepsins is maximal in acid conditions; for example, cathepsin D has no activity at a pH above 7.2. In contrast, an approximately neutral pH is optimal for MMPs and aggrecanases. All these enzymes have been identified in disc, with higher levels of MMPs, for example, in more degenerate discs (6). Cathepsins D and L have been found at sites of degeneration in human intervertebral disc (2). Several types of MMPs (MMPs-1, -2, -3, -7, -8, -9, and -13) occur in human discs; they are produced by both the disc cells (Fig. 3.4) and the cells of invading blood vessels (26). Aggrecanases have also been shown to occur in human disc, but their activity is less obvious, at least in more advanced disc degeneration (26,31). Aggrecanase may be more active earlier in the course of disease, as appears to occur in cartilage in osteoarthritis. Two aggrecanases have been described in disc, ADAMTS-4 and ADAMTS-5 (ADAMTS: *a d*isintegrin *a*nd *m*etalloproteinase with

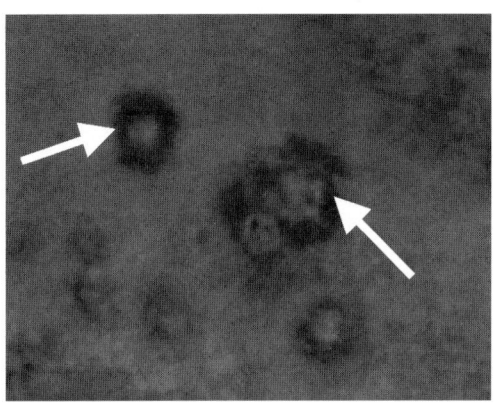 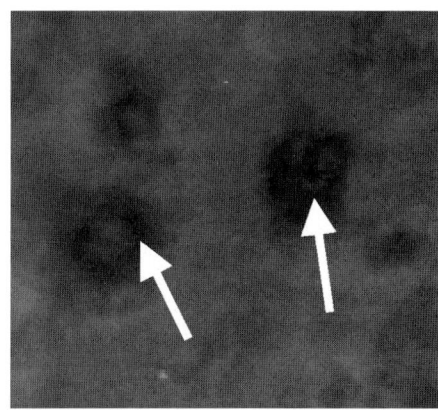

FIG. 3.4. Disc cells can produce enzymes capable of degrading matrix molecules, as shown by *in situ zymography*. A section of disc tissue is placed over fluorescently labeled **(A)** casein and **(B)** gelatin (collagen fragments) and incubated. During this time, the enzymes in and around the disc cells, which contain matrix metalloproteinases, degrade the casein or gelatin, shown by the dark area *(arrows)*.

*t*hrombo*s*pondin motifs), that can act in the interglobular domain between G_1 and G_2 (Fig. 3.1) and at four sites in the CS-2 region of the core protein (28,36). Link protein is resistant to aggrecanases but can be broken down by MMPs and, indeed, appears to be more fragmented in disc than in cartilage, particularly in degenerate tissue (7).

RELEVANCE TO FUTURE THERAPEUTIC DEVELOPMENTS

Understanding the biochemical changes that occur in disc degeneration may lead to the identification of the following: (a) genes that could be targeted, either to increase the production of certain growth factors or cytokines if, for example, they beneficially affected disc cell metabolism, or to switch them off if they promoted further catabolism of the disc matrix and (b) molecules for which antagonists or blocking agents could be designed. For example, if it could be shown that one specific MMP is elevated only in degenerative disc disease but is not involved in normal disc homeostasis, then such as MMP would be an ideal molecule to "inactivate" specifically.

REFERENCES

1. Antoniou J, Goudsouzian NM, Heathfield TF, et al. The human lumbar endplate: evidence of changes in biosynthesis and denaturation of the extracellular matrix with growth, maturation, aging, and degeneration. *Spine* 1996; 21:1153–1161.
2. Ariga K, Yonebnobu K, Nakase T, et al. Localization of cathepsins D, K and L in degenerated human intervertebral discs. *Spine* 2001;26:2666–2672.
3. Bayliss MT, Johnstone B, O'Brien JP. Proteoglycan synthesis in the human intervertebral disc. *Spine* 1988; 13:972–981.
4. Bianco P, Fisher LW, Young MF, et al. Expression and localization of two small proteoglycans biglycan and decorin in developing human skeletal and non-skeletal tissues. *J Histochem Cytochem* 1990;38:1549–1563.
5. Broom ND, Marra DL. New structural concepts of articular cartilage demonstrated with a physical model. *Connect Tissue Res* 1995;14:1–8.
6. Crean JKG, Roberts S, Jaffray DC, et al. Matrix metalloproteinases in the human intervertebral disc: role in disc degeneration and scoliosis. *Spine* 1997;22:2877–2884.
7. Donohue PJ, Jahnke MR, Blaha JD, et al. Characterization of link protein(s) from human intervertebral-disc tissues. *Biochem J* 1998;251:739–747.

8. Duance VC, Crean JKG, Sims TJ, et al. Changes in collagen cross-linking in degenerative disc disease and scoliosis. *Spine* 1998;23:2545–2551.
9. Eyre D, Matsui Y, Wu J-J. Collagen polymorphisms of the intervertebral disc. *Biochem Soc Trans* 2002;30: 844–848.
10. Eyre DR. Collagens of the disc. In: Ghosh P, ed. The biology of the invertebral disc. Boca Raton: CRC Press, 1986;7:171–188.
11. Eyre DR, Muir H. Quantitative analysis of types I and II collagens in human intervertebral discs at various ages. *Biochim Biophys Acta* 1977;492:29–42.
12. Freemont AJ, Watkins A, Le Maitre C, et al. Current understanding of cellular and molecular events in intervertebral disc degeneration: implications for therapy. *J Pathol* 2002;196:374–379.
13. Gruber HE, Ingram JA, Hanley EN. Tenascin in the human intervertebral disc: alterations with aging and disc degeneration. *Biotech Histochem* 2002;77:37–41.
14. Hollander AP, Heathfield TF, Liu J, et al. Enhanced denaturation of the $\alpha 1$ (II) chains of type-II collagen in normal adult human intervertebral discs compared with femoral articular cartilage. *J Orthop Res* 1996;14:61–66.
15. Inkinen R, Lammi MJ, Lehmonen S, et al. Relative increase of biglycan and decorin and altered chondroitin sulfate epitopes in the degenerating human intervertebral disc. *J Rheumatol* 1998;25:506–514.
16. Isogai N, Landis WJ, Kim TH, et al. Formation of phalanges and small joints by tissue-engineering. *J Bone Joint Surg Am* 1999;81:306–316.
17. Jahnke MR, McDevitt CA. Proteoglycans of the human intervertebral disc. *Biochem J* 1988;251:347–356.
18. Johnstone B, Bayliss MT. The large proteoglycans of the human intervertebral disc: changes in their biosynthesis with age, topography, and pathology. *Spine* 1995;20:674–684.
19. Johnstone B, Markopoulos M, Neame P, et al. Identification and characterization of glycanated and non-glycanated forms of biglycan and decorin in the human intervertebral disc. *Biochem J* 1993;292:661–666.
20. Konttinen YT, Kemppinen P, Li TF, et al. Transforming and epidermal growth factors in degenerated intervertebral discs. *J Bone Joint Surg Br* 1999;81:1058–1063.
21. Maroudas A. Metabolism of cartilaginous tissues: a quantitative approach. In: Maroudas A, Holborow EJ, eds. *Studies in joint diseases*. Bath, U.K.: Pitman Press, 1980:59–86.
22. Mikawa Y, Hamagami H, Shikata J, et al. Elastin in the human intervertebral disk. *Arch Orthop Trauma Surg* 1986;105:343–349.
23. Oegema TR, Johnson SL, Aguiar DJ, et al. Fibronectin and its fragments increase with degeneration in the human intervertebral disc. *Spine* 2000;25:2742–2747.
24. Roberts S, McCall IW, Urban JPG, et al. Cytokines, inflammation and neurology in herniated disc patients. *J Bone Joint Surg* 2002;84B (Suppl III):326.
25. Roberts S, Bains MA, Kwan A, et al. Type X collagen in the human intervertebral disc: an indication of repair or remodelling? *Histochem J* 1998;30:89–95.
25a. Roberts S, Beard HK, O'Brien JP. Biochemical changes of intervetebral discs in patients with spondylolisthesis or with tears of the posterior annulus fibrosus. *Ann Rheum Dis* 1982;41:78–85.
26. Roberts S, Caterson B, Menage J, et al. Matrix metalloproteinases and aggrecanase: their role in disorders of the human intervertebral disc. *Spine* 2000;25:3005–3013.
27. Roberts S, Menage J, Duance VC, et al. Collagen types around the cells of the intervertebral disc and cartilage end plate: an immunolocalization study. *Spine* 1991;16:1030–1038.
28. Roughley PJ, Alini M, Antoniou J. The role of proteoglycan in aging, degeneration and repair of the intervertebral disc. *Biochem Soc Trans* 2002;30:869–874.
29. Salter DM. Tenascin is increased in cartilage and synovium from arthritic knees. *Br J Rheumatol* 1993;32:780–786.
30. Scott JE. Oxygen and the connective tissue. *Trends Biochem Sci* 1992;17:340–343.
31. Sztrolovics R, Alini M, Roughley PJ, et al. Aggrecan degradation in human intervertebral disc and articular cartilage. *Biochem J* 1997;326:235–241.
32. Sztrolovics R, Grover J, Cs-Szabo G, et al. The characterization of versican and its message in human articular cartilage and intervertebral disc. *J Orthop Res* 2002;20:257–266.
33. Takao T, Iwaki T. A comparative study of localization of heat shock protein 27 and heat shock protein 72 in the developmental and degenerative intervertebral disc. *Spine* 2002;27:361–368.
34. Takao T, Iwaki T, Kondo J, et al. Immunohistochemistry of chondromodulin-I in the human intervertebral disc with special reference to the degenerative changes. *Histochem J* 2000;32:545–550.
35. Tolenen J, Gronblad M, Virri J, et al. Basic fibroblast growth factor immunoreactivity in blood vessels and cells of disc herniations. *Spine* 1995;20:271–276.
36. Tortorella MD, Burn TC, Pratta MA, et al. Purification and cloning of aggrecanase-1: a member of the ADAMTS family of proteins. *Science* 1999;284:1664–1666.
37. Tsuru M, Nagata K, Jimi A, et al. Effect of AGEs on human disc herniation: intervertebral disc hernia is also effected by AGEs. *Kurume Med J* 2002;49:7–13.
38. Wotton SF, Duance VC, Fryer PR. Type IX collagen: a possible function in articular cartilage. *FEBS Lett* 1988;234:79–82.
39. Yu J, Winlove CP, Roberts S, et al. Elastic fibre organization in the intervertebral discs of the bovine tail. *J Anat* 2002;201:465–475.

4

The Physiology of Intervertebral Disc Degeneration

Susan R. S. Bibby, Jing Yu, and Jill P. G. Urban

Physiology Laboratory, Oxford University, Oxford, United Kingdom

Disc degeneration is characterized by changes in the morphology and composition of the disc and endplate (see Chapters 2 and 3). In this short review, we outline the consequences of the degenerative biochemical and morphologic changes on disc function. Because degeneration ultimately arises from a failure of disc cells to make and maintain the organization and composition of the disc matrix, we also discuss factors that affect cellular activity and viability.

MECHANICAL ROLE OF THE MATRIX

The main functions of the discs are mechanical; the discs serve both to transmit load and to act as the joints of the spinal column. *In vivo*, the discs are always under load, both from body weight and from the activity of the spinal muscles. The magnitude of the load thus varies with every change in posture and activity. Loading the disc increases the hydrostatic pressure in the nucleus. Nachemson and Elfstrom (52) found that even in a relaxed supine subject, the pressure on the lower lumbar discs is 0.1 to 0.2 megapascals (MPa); it rises to about 0.6 to 0.7 MPa in unsupported sitting and to considerably greater values during strenuous activity. More recent studies have shown that in normal discs, the pressure is hydrostatic across all regions apart from the outermost regions of the annulus (50). The load on the spine and, hence, intradiscal pressure tend to follow a cyclic pattern, with pressure lowest during rest at night and increasing fivefold to sixfold during daytime activities (70).

The behavior of the disc in response to these changing loads depends directly on the properties of the disc matrix, in particular on the concentrations and organization of the major structural molecules, collagen and proteoglycans (PGs). These, together with water, constitute about 95% of the matrix (69); the proportions of these constituents varies across the disc, with the annulus containing more collagen and less PG and water than the nucleus.

Mechanical Roles of Collagen and Proteoglycan

Collagen, PGs, and water, through their interactions, form a load-bearing structure. The highly organized network of fibrillar collagens (Fig. 4.1) forms a framework for the disc and anchors it to the bone. The network is inflated by PGs, which with their high

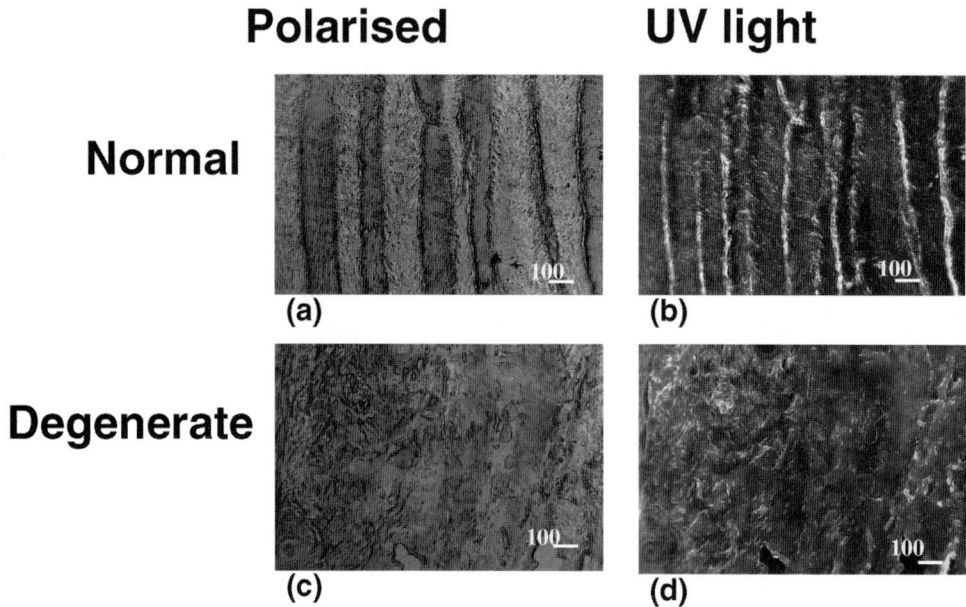

FIG. 4.1. Comparison of the network organization in normal and degenerate discs. Normal (*a,b*) and degenerate (*c,d*) discs visualized by polarized light (*a,c*) and under ultraviolet light (*b,d*).

osmotic pressure tend to imbibe water and maintain tissue hydration. The composite structure is able to carry high loads while still maintaining tissue turgor.

PG osmotic pressure depends directly on PG concentration and is considerable at the concentrations found in resting normal discs (more than 2 atmospheres). It is balanced in the disc *in vivo* by body weight and muscular activity and also by the restraining forces of the collagen network (68). If loads are removed, the discs swell considerably until the osmotic swelling pressure is balanced by the tension of the collagen network. Load is thus an important factor governing disc hydration.

Behavior of the Disc Under Load

With every change in load, the disc deforms, initially through a rearrangement of the collagen network (42). The extent of the deformation varies from disc to disc, but the factors that govern this are not well understood. No consistent pattern associated with age, sex, or degree of degeneration has been found. If the load is maintained, the disc loses height or creeps, and a large part of the creep deformation results from fluid loss (40). Thus, for each applied load, the extent of the initial deformation depends largely on the structure and integrity of the collagen network (29). In contrast, the rate and magnitude of the creep deformation are related more to the osmotic behavior of the PGs (67).

Because the disc is an osmotic system, disc hydration undergoes a diurnal cycle; fluid is expressed when the disc is under high loads during the day's activities and reimbibed under low loads during rest at night (6). Magnetic resonance imaging (MRI) studies indicate that the water content of the disc may vary as much as 25% between morning and evening (6). The average measured loss of height of 6 mm during the day is thought to arise in part from load-induced loss of fluid from the disc (16,56). In contrast, the height of the Skylab astronauts, who were weightless for 85 days, increased about 5 cm (65), in part probably through swelling of their discs under low external loads.

Effect of Degenerative Changes in the Matrix on Disc Function

Collagen Network

In disc degeneration, the collagen network and that of other structural components, such as elastin, become disorganized (Fig. 4.1). Changes in cross-linking and collagen integrity during degeneration have also been noted (14,22). The functional effect of such changes in the collagen network are unknown; however, it is difficult to believe that they do not affect the mechanical behavior of the disc matrix. Changes in the organization of minor components, such as elastin, may be equally important. Elastin fibers are concentrated mainly at the boundaries between lamellae, which indicates that they play a role in load-induced deformation in normal discs (71). If, as suggested, elastin has a role in maintaining lamellar deformation and organization, the loss of such a minor component could have a major effect on disc properties.

Proteoglycan Loss

One of the major compositional changes in disc degeneration is the loss of PG (47). The fall in PG content has a major effect on the load-bearing properties of the disc matrix. With the loss of PG, the osmotic pressure of the disc falls (68), and the disc is less able to maintain hydration under load. The water content of degenerate discs is thus lower than that of normal, age-matched discs (47), and degenerate discs lose height (18) and fluid more rapidly and to a greater extent under load (Fig. 4.2). The degenerate disc is also less stiff and tends to bulge more than a normal disc when loaded. Such major

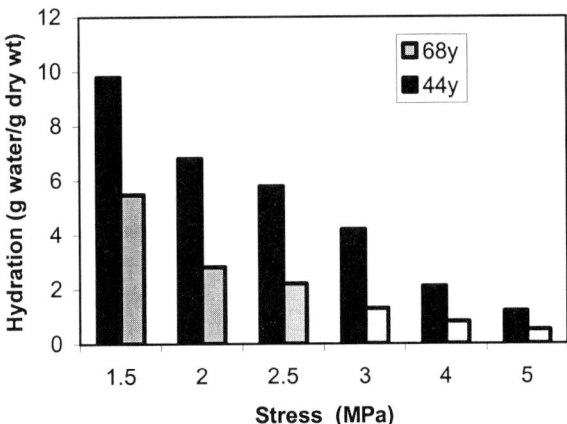

FIG. 4.2. The effect of compressive stress on the hydration of normal and degenerate discs. The equilibrium hydration decreased as compressive stress increased for both normal and degenerate discs; however, under all conditions, the 44-year disc (grade 1/2) was more hydrated than the 68-year disc (grade 3/4) and was able to retain hydration to a greater extent under high loads. (Adapted from Urban JPG, McMullin JF. Swelling pressure of the lumbar intervertebral discs: influence of age, spinal level, composition and degeneration. *Spine* 1988;13:179–187, with permission.)

changes in disc behavior have a strong influence on other spinal structures. For instance, as a result of the rapid loss of height when degenerate discs are loaded, the apophyseal joints may see inappropriate compressive loads, possibly leading to the development of osteoarthritic changes (1). A significant loss of disc height has other effects, such as reducing the tension on spinal ligaments, possibly causing remodeling and thickening; this mechanism may have a part in the development of spinal stenosis.

Loss of Hydrostatic Properties

The loss of PG and matrix disorganization have other important mechanical effects because with the loss of hydration, degenerate discs no longer behave hydrostatically under load (49). Loading may thus lead to inappropriate stress concentrations along the endplate or in the annulus, which could adversely affect matrix structure or cellular activity. The stress concentrations seen in degenerate discs have also been associated with discogenic pain during discography (49).

Loss of Permeability Barrier

The loss of PGs has other consequences. Because of their charge and their "bottle brush structure," which divides the extracellular spaces into small "pores," PGs act as a barrier to the entry of molecules into the disc. Charge affects the concentration of antibiotics; positively charged antibiotics, such as aminoglycosides, reach higher concentrations in the disc than negatively charged antibiotics, such as penicillin (63), and degeneration affects these distributions. Size also influences distribution, and large uncharged molecules, such as serum proteins and cytokines, are virtually excluded from the normal disc matrix. Although this process has not been well investigated, the loss of PGs in degenerate discs could increase the penetration of large molecules, such as growth factor complexes and cytokines into the disc, possibly influencing the development and progression of degeneration. Another important effect of the loss of PGs is the increased vascular and neural ingrowth seen in degenerate discs (see Chapter 3); disc aggrecan has been shown to inhibit neural growth (33).

DISC CELLS

Cells form less than 1% of the disc by volume, but their role is vital because they make and maintain the matrix and thus control disc composition. They synthesize not only the extracellular matrix but also the proteinases responsible for matrix breakdown. In healthy tissue, the rates of production and breakdown are in balance; however, if the rate of synthesis decreases or the rate of breakdown increases, the matrix can start to deteriorate. Matrix degradation ultimately results from failure of the cells to maintain and repair the matrix. This failure could arise from changes in the number or activity of cells.

Cell Types in the Disc

At least three distinct cell phenotypes exist in the annulus of the adult disc (7), all of which differ from the chondrocyte-like cells of the adult nucleus (17). Each cell type produces and maintains a different matrix; the rounded chondrocyte-like cells of the nucleus and inner annulus produce more large PGs than the elongated fibroblast-like cells of the outer annulus, in line with the profiles of PG concentration across the disc (26).

CELL ENERGY METABOLISM AND NUTRITION

Energy Metabolism

The production of energy by disc cells is dominated by anaerobic glycolysis (i.e., the conversion of glucose to lactate), with a net yield of 2 mol of lactate and 2 mol of adenosine triphosphate (ATP), the "energy currency" of the cell, per mole of glucose. Even at high oxygen concentrations, only approximately 20% of the energy of the disc is obtained by oxidative phosphorylation. Disc cells have very few mitochondria (66), which is further evidence that they derive most of their energy from glycolysis alone. At low oxygen concentrations, a positive Pasteur effect has been reported in the disc; oxygen consumption falls and the rate of glycolysis accelerates (23,31), possibly in an attempt to compensate for the reduction in aerobic metabolism. However, overall energy production still decreases because the less efficient (anaerobic) pathways are used; intracellular ATP levels have been shown to fall in disc cells cultured at low oxygen concentrations (58), with a consequent fall in other cellular activities.

Disc Nutrition

The intervertebral disc is the largest avascular tissue in the body; adult lumbar disc cells may be up to 7 or 8 mm away from the closest blood vessels. Cells receive nutrients such as glucose and oxygen, essential for their survival, from blood vessels surrounding the disc; metabolic wastes such as lactic acid are removed by the same blood vessels (Fig. 4.3). There are two main routes of nutrient supply. Capillaries running around the edge of the disc supply the ligaments, soft tissues, and outermost annulus. The rest of the disc

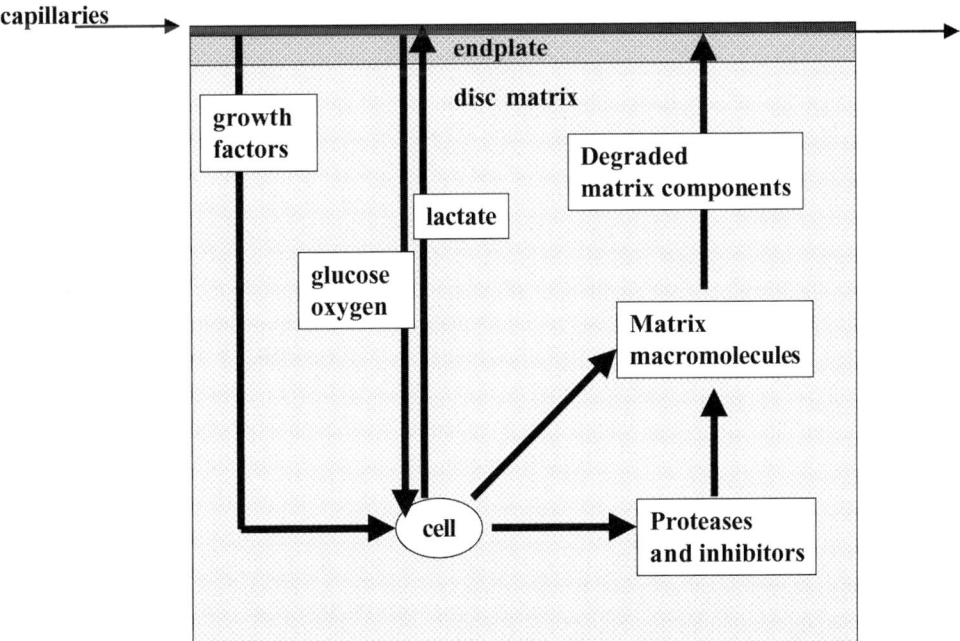

FIG. 4.3. Schematic view of solute transport pathways between the blood supply, cell, and disc matrix.

is supplied by vessels that travel through the vertebral body to terminate at the endplate (12). Nutrients diffuse through the disc to the cells or can be carried by water moving into the disc in response to changing loads; small molecules, such as oxygen, glucose, lactic acid, and amino acids, move through the disc matrix mainly by diffusion (38). Steep gradients result for solutes with rates of diffusion that are slow in comparison with the rates of cellular metabolism, even in normal discs; the glucose and oxygen concentrations in the center of the disc are therefore low, whereas lactic acid levels are high, and the pH is acidic (23).

Disc Degeneration and Nutrient Supply

It has long been thought that loss of nutrient supply is an important cause of disc degeneration. Although the relationship between loss of nutrient supply and disc degeneration has not been measured directly, several studies have shown that a fall in blood supply to the vertebrae (39) or diseases that affect blood flow, such as sickle cell disease (36), are associated with disc degeneration. Similarly, changes in the endplate that restrict solute transport are found in degenerate or scoliotic discs (53,60). It has been suggested that the relationship between smoking and back pain arises from the adverse effect of smoking on nutrient transport (25). Although few direct measurements are available at present, new MRI techniques should eventually be able to provide more information on nutrient supply to degenerate and normal discs (9).

Nutrient levels have been measured in patients' discs during surgical procedures. Oxygen levels (Po_2) in degenerate discs were quite variable and even high in some discs (4). This finding is not surprising because in addition to endplate permeability, oxygen levels in degenerate discs would be affected by the number of viable cells (Po_2 would scarcely fall if most of the cells were dead) and by vascular ingrowth. Lactic acid levels, however, were found to be higher in degenerate than in normal discs; the pH consequently was more acidic, especially in symptomatic (41) or severely degenerate (13) discs.

Cell Viability in the Disc

Cell death has been reported to occur in the human disc at all ages; the percentage of dead cells increases with age, from about 2% in the fetus to more than 50% in adults (66), although some viable cells remain even into old age. It appears that the disc can replace dead cells, or at least attempt to replace them. In discs that are not degenerate, cells have been reported to occur singly, in pairs, and in occasional small clusters; in severely degenerate discs, the number and size of cell clusters increase markedly (21,34).

Whether cell death occurs in the disc by necrosis or apoptosis is debatable. Apoptosis (programmed cell death) has been reported (19,46); however, dead cells in the disc are often noted to be "necrotic" (i.e., "accidental" cell death has taken place) (66). Apoptosis is usually assessed by TUNEL (*t*erminal deoxynucleotidyl transferase–mediated deoxy*u*ridine triphosphate *n*ick *e*nd *l*abeling), which is notoriously prone to yielding false-positive results (2). Cell death can be assessed according to the presence or absence of an intact cell membrane by using membrane-impermeant solutes such as trypan blue, propidium iodide, or ethidium homodimer, which can stain the DNA only of dead cells. Such assays do not differentiate between the types of cell death but may nevertheless pro-

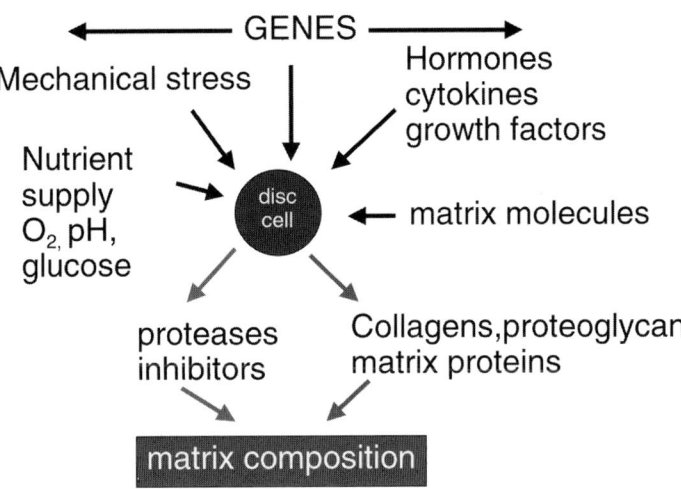

FIG. 4.4. Some factors that regulate matrix turnover.

vide the most valuable information; whatever the mechanism, cell death eventually results in a failure of the cell population to maintain the matrix of the disc. As Aigner wrote (2), "No matter how and why cells die, the result is always the same: the cells disappear."

Influence of Environmental Factors on Cell Death

Both the nutritional/metabolic and the mechanical environment have been shown to be able to induce disc cell death. In a cell culture model of the intervertebral disc, cells far from the nutrient supply died; the percentage of dead cells increased with distance and with cell density (27). A lack of glucose and an acidic pH were identified as critical factors (Fig. 4.4). Mechanical stresses, such as tensile strain, compression, and impact loading of explants, have also been shown to cause cell death *in vivo* and *in vitro* in both the intervertebral disc and articular cartilage (46)

MATRIX SYNTHESIS AND TURNOVER

The disc cells actively synthesize PGs and collagen throughout life (35). The rate of synthesis and the proportions of the different matrix molecules synthesized have been found to vary with age and with degeneration (3). The disc cells also produce proteases, which are able to break down matrix constituents (11,45,59). The type of protease produced and the degree of protease activation also vary with age and pathology. In the normal disc, the rates of matrix synthesis and breakdown are in balance, but in degeneration, breakdown overtakes synthesis, leading to a loss of matrix components with consequent effects on matrix morphology and function.

Factors Affecting Production and Turnover of Matrix

Nutrient Supply

In vitro models have shown that matrix synthesis depends on an adequate supply of oxygen and glucose and on the removal of lactic acid (27,31,54). Cells can survive low oxygen levels for at least 7 days; however, matrix synthesis is low under such conditions. A low pH arising mainly from the accumulation of lactic acid is more dangerous for the disc; matrix synthesis is reduced, protease activity still remains high (58), and prolonged exposure of disc cells to an acidic pH may lead to cell death (Fig. 4.4).

Mechanical Stress

The cells of most tissues are very responsive to mechanical forces *in vitro*, and disc cells are no exception. *In vitro* tests show that matrix and protease production is affected by signals such as the application of hydrostatic pressure and change in osmolality or stretch (28,32,48); physiologic loads in general stimulate the synthesis of both PGs and proteases, whereas high loads inhibit synthesis (10,20,30). The response of disc cells to mechanical stress *in vivo*, however, is complex and difficult to predict because with each change in posture or activity, the cells receive many different mechanical signals, such as a rise in pressure, increase in deformation, and change in osmolality. All these signals vary in duration and magnitude, and how the cells integrate the signals *in vivo* is not clear. The net responses to normal loads may be slight because long-term heavy exercise (running 40 km daily for 15 months) had little effect on cellular activity or the composition of the disc matrix (57). However, degenerative changes were induced by the application of high static compressive loads to an otherwise healthy disc in mice (46), and in both humans and animals, spinal fusion appears to lead to degenerative changes in adjacent discs (15,24). At present, the role of exercise or adverse mechanical stress in the pathogenesis of disc degeneration is unclear.

Injury

Degeneration has been induced by injury to the annulus in animals (44,55). Here, the changes in the disc radiate from the injured site and mimic to some extent the changes seen in degenerate human discs. The pathway is unknown, but typical changes seen in degeneration, such as blood vessel and nerve ingrowth and PG loss, appear to radiate from the lesion (51).

Growth Factors and Cytokines

Disc cells respond to growth factors such as insulinlike growth factor-1, which are responsible for stimulating matrix production (64). The concentration of growth factors and receptors falls in degenerate discs, further decreasing matrix production (43). Discs also respond to cytokines such as interleukin-1 and tumor necrosis factor-α, which both stimulate the activity of matrix metalloproteinases and other agents involved in matrix breakdown and repress the synthesis of matrix macromolecules. The concentration of cytokines increases in herniated tissue (37), possibly because inflammatory cells invade and populate the protruding disc. The cytokines may play a positive role in stimulating resorption of the protrusion; however, they may also set off a degenerative cascade in the disc itself and possibly stimulate pain in the nerve fibers in the outer regions of the disc

(8). *In vitro* work suggests that PG loss induced by cytokines such as interleukin-1 can be reversed by treatment with growth factors (62).

SUMMARY

The integrity of the disc depends on the ability of the disc cells to make and maintain a normal matrix. Degeneration ultimately results when the cells are no longer able to repair and replace damaged matrix, or when they are switched to a pathway in which the production of active proteases overtakes the production of matrix. As shown schematically in Figure 4.4 and discussed above, many factors regulate cellular activity. However, the overriding control is genetic. Genes determine mechanical stress by regulating muscles; they also determine responses to cytokines, cytokine production, the vascularity of the vertebral body, and how the cell integrates the complex signals it receives. It is therefore not surprising that twin studies have demonstrated that the major risk factors for disc degeneration are genetic (5,61).

ACKNOWLEDGMENTS

We thank the Arthritis Research Campaign, the Wellcome Trust, the Cotrel Foundation, and the Engineering and Physical Sciences Research Council for their support.

REFERENCES

1. Adams MA, Dolan P, Porter RW. Diurnal changes in spinal mechanics and their clinical significance. *J Bone Joint Surg Br* 1990;72:266–270.
2. Aigner T. Apoptosis, necrosis, or whatever: how to find out what really happens? *J Pathol* 2002;198:1–4.
3. Antoniou J, Steffen T, Nelson F, et al. The human lumbar intervertebral disc: evidence for changes in the biosynthesis and denaturation of the extracellular matrix with growth, maturation, ageing, and degeneration. *J Clin Invest* 1996;98:996–1003.
4. Bartels EM, Fairbank JCT, Winlove CP, et al. Oxygen and lactate concentrations measured *in vivo* in the intervertebral discs of scoliotic and back pain patients. *Spine* 1998;23:1–8.
5. Battié MC, Videman T, Gibbons LE, et al. 1995 Volvo Award in Clinical Sciences. Determinants of lumbar disc degeneration. A study relating lifetime exposures and magnetic resonance imaging findings in identical twins. *Spine* 1995;20:2601–2612.
6. Boos N, Wallin A, Gbedegbegnon T, et al. Quantitative MR imaging of lumbar intervertebral disks and vertebral bodies: influence of diurnal water content variations. *Radiology* 1993;188:351–354.
7. Bruehlmann SB, Rattner JB, Matyas JR, et al. Regional variations in the cellular matrix of the annulus fibrosus of the intervertebral disc. *J Anat* 2002;201:159–171.
8. Burke JG, Watson RW, McCormack D, et al. Intervertebral discs which cause low back pain secrete high levels of proinflammatory mediators. *J Bone Joint Surg Br* 2002;84:196–201.
9. Bydder GM. New approaches to magnetic resonance imaging of intervertebral discs, tendons, ligaments, and menisci. *Spine* 2002;27:1264–1268.
10. Chen J, Baer AE, Paik PY, et al. Matrix protein gene expression in intervertebral disc cells subjected to altered osmolarity. *Biochem Biophys Res Commun* 2002;293:932–938.
11. Crean JK, Roberts S, Jaffray DC, et al. Matrix metalloproteinases in the human intervertebral disc: role in disc degeneration and scoliosis. *Spine* 1997;22:2877–2884.
12. Crock HV, Goldwasser M, Yoshizawa H. Vascular anatomy related to the intervertebral disc. In: Ghosh P, ed. *Biology of the intervertebral disc*. Boca Raton, FL: CRC Press, 1991:109–133.
13. Diamant B, Karlsson J, Nachemson A. Correlation between lactate levels and pH in discs of patients with lumbar rhizopathies. *Experientia* 1968;24:1195–1196.
14. Duance VC, Crean JK, Sims TJ, et al. Changes in collagen cross-linking in degenerative disc disease and scoliosis. *Spine* 1998;23:2545–2551.
15. Eck JC, Humphreys SC, Hodges SD. Adjacent-segment degeneration after lumbar fusion: a review of clinical, biomechanical, and radiologic studies. *Am J Orthop* 1999;28:336–340.
16. Eklund JA, Corlett EN. Shrinkage as a measure of the effect of load on the spine. *Spine* 1984;189–194.
17. Errington RJ, Puustjarvi K, White IF, et al. Characterisation of cytoplasm-filled processes in cells of the intervertebral disc. *J Anat* 1998;192:369–378.

18. Frobin W, Brinckmann P, Kramer M, et al. Height of lumbar discs measured from radiographs compared with degeneration and height classified from MR images. *Eur Radiol* 2001;11:263–269.
19. Gruber HE, Hanley EN. Analysis of aging and degeneration of the human intervertebral disc—comparison of surgical specimens with normal controls. *Spine* 1998;23:751–757.
20. Handa T, Ishihara H, Ohshima H, et al. Effects of hydrostatic pressure on matrix synthesis and matrix metalloproteinase production in the human lumbar intervertebral disc. *Spine* 1997;22:1085–1091.
21. Hastreiter D, Ozuna RM, Spector M. Regional variations in certain cellular characteristics in human lumbar intervertebral discs, including the presence of alpha-smooth muscle actin. *J Orthop Res* 2001;19:597–604.
22. Hollander AP, Heathfield TF, Liu JJ, et al. Enhanced denaturation of the alpha (II) chains of type-II collagen in normal adult human intervertebral discs compared with femoral articular cartilage. *J Orthop Res* 1996;14:61–66.
23. Holm S, Maroudas A, Urban JP, et al. Nutrition of the intervertebral disc: solute transport and metabolism. *Connect Tissue Res* 1981;8:101–119.
24. Holm S, Nachemson A. Nutritional changes in the canine intervertebral disc after spinal fusion. *Clin Orthop* 1982;169:243–258.
25. Holm S, Nachemson A. Nutrition of the intervertebral disc: acute effects of cigarette smoking. An experimental animal study. *Ups J Med Sci* 1988; 93:91–99.
26. Horner HA, Roberts S, Bielby RC, et al. Cells from different regions of the intervertebral disc: effect of culture system on matrix expression and cell phenotype. *Spine* 2002;27:1018–1028.
27. Horner HA, Urban JP. 2001 Volvo Award in Basic Science Studies. Effect of nutrient supply on the viability of cells from the nucleus pulposus of the intervertebral disc. *Spine* 2001;26:2543–2549.
28. Hutton WC, Elmer WA, Boden SD, et al. The effect of hydrostatic pressure on intervertebral disc metabolism. *Spine* 1999;24:1507–1515.
29. Iatridis JC, Kumar S, Foster RJ, et al. Shear mechanical properties of human lumbar annulus fibrosus. *J Orthop Res* 1999;17:732–737.
30. Ishihara H, McNally DS, Urban JP, et al. Effects of hydrostatic pressure on matrix synthesis in different regions of the intervertebral disk. *J Appl Physiol* 1996;80:839–846.
31. Ishihara H, Urban JP. Effects of low oxygen concentrations and metabolic inhibitors on proteoglycan and protein synthesis rates in the intervertebral disc. *J Orthop Res* 1999;17:829–835.
32. Ishihara H, Warensjo K, Roberts S, et al. Proteoglycan synthesis in the intervertebral disk nucleus: the role of extracellular osmolality. *Am J Physiol* 1997;272:C1499–C1506.
33. Johnson WE, Caterson B, Eisenstein SM, et al. Human intervertebral disc aggrecan inhibits nerve growth *in vitro*. *Arthritis Rheum* 2002;46:2658–2664.
34. Johnson WEB, Eisenstein SM, Roberts S. Cell cluster formation in degenerate lumbar intervertebral discs is associated with increased disc cell proliferation. *Connect Tissue Res* 2001;42:197–207.
35. Johnstone B, Bayliss MT. The large proteoglycans of the human intervertebral disc. Changes in their biosynthesis and structure with age, topography, and pathology. *Spine* 1995;20:674–684.
36. Jones JP, Engleman EP. Osseous avascular necrosis associated with systemic abnormalities. *Arthritis Rheum* 1966;9:728–736.
37. Kang JD, Georgescu HI, McIntyre-Larkin L, et al. Herniated lumbar intervertebral discs spontaneously produced matrix metalloproteinases, nitric oxide, interleukin-6, and prostaglandin E_2. *Spine* 1996;21:271–277.
38. Katz MM, Hargens AR, Garfin SR. Intervertebral disc nutrition. Diffusion versus convection. *Clin Orthop* 1986;243–245.
39. Kauppila LI, McAlindon T, Evans S, et al. Disc degeneration/back pain and calcification of the abdominal aorta. A 25-year follow-up study in Framingham. *Spine* 1997;22:1642–1647.
40. Keller TS, Nathan M. Height change caused by creep in intervertebral discs: a sagittal plane model [In Process Citation]. *J Spinal Disord* 1999;12:313–324.
41. Kitano T, Zerwekh JE, Usui Y, et al. Biochemical changes associated with the symptomatic human intervertebral disk. *Clin Orthop* 1993;372–377.
42. Klein JA, Hukins DW. X-ray diffraction demonstrates reorientation of collagen fibres in the annulus fibrosus during compression of the intervertebral disc. *Biochim Biophys Acta* 1982;717:61–64.
43. Konttinen YT, Kemppinen P, Li TF, et al. Transforming and epidermal growth factors in degenerated intervertebral discs. *J Bone Joint Surg Br* 1999;81:1058–1063.
44. Lipson SJ, Muir H. Experimental intervertebral disc degeneration: morphologic and proteoglycan changes over time. *Arthritis Rheum* 1981;24:12–21.
45. Liu J, Roughley PJ, Mort JS. Identification of human intervertebral disc stromelysin and its involvement in matrix degradation. *J Orthop Res* 1991;9:568–575.
46. Lotz JC, Colliou OK, Chin JR, et al. 1998 Volvo Award in Biomechanical Studies. Compression-induced degeneration of the intervertebral disc: an *in vivo* mouse model and finite-element study. *Spine* 1998;23:2493–2506.
47. Lyons G, Eisenstein SM, Sweet MB. Biochemical changes in intervertebral disc degeneration. *Biochim Biophys Acta* 1981;673:443–453.
48. Matsumoto T, Kawakami M, Kuribayashi K, et al. Cyclic mechanical stretch stress increases the growth rate and collagen synthesis of nucleus pulposus cells *in vitro*. *Spine* 1999;24:315–319.
49. McNally DS, Shackleford IM, Goodship AE, et al. *In vivo* stress measurement can predict pain on discography. *Spine* 1996;21:2580–2587.

50. McNally DS, Adams MA. Internal intervertebral disc mechanics as revealed by stress profilometry. *Spine* 1992;17:66–73.
51. Melrose J, Roberts S, Smith S, et al. Increased nerve and blood vessel ingrowth associated with proteoglycan depletion in an ovine anular lesion model of experimental disc degeneration. *Spine* 2002;27:1278–1285.
52. Nachemson A, Elfstrom G. Intravital dynamic pressure measurements in lumbar discs. A study of common movements, maneuvers and exercises. *Scand J Rehabil Med* 1970;2[Suppl 1]:1–40.
53. Nachemson A, Lewin T, Maroudas A, et al. *In vitro* diffusion of dye through the end-plates and annulus fibrosus of human lumbar intervertebral discs. *Acta Orthop Scand* 1970;41:589–607.
54. Ohshima H, Urban JPG. Effect of lactate concentrations and pH on matrix synthesis rates in the intervertebral disc. *Spine* 1992;17:1079–1082.
55. Osti OL, Vernon-Roberts B, Fraser RD. 1990 Volvo Award in Experimental Studies. Anulus tears and intervertebral disc degeneration: an experimental study using an animal model. *Spine* 1990;15:762–767.
56. Paajanen H, Lehto I, Alanen A, et al. Diurnal fluid changes of lumbar discs measured indirectly by magnetic resonance imaging. *J Orthop Res* 1994;12:509–514.
57. Puustjarvi K, Lammi M, Kiviranta I, et al. Proteoglycan synthesis in canine intervertebral discs after long distance running training. *J Orthop Res* 1993;11:738–746.
58. Razaq MS. *The effect of extracellular pH on metabolism of cartilage cells* [Thesis/Dissertation]. Oxford: University of Oxford, 2002.
59. Roberts S, Caterson B, Menage J, et al. Matrix metalloproteinases and aggrecanase: their role in disorders of the human intervertebral disc. *Spine* 2000;25:3005–3013.
60. Roberts S, Urban JPG, Evans H, et al. Transport properties of the human cartilage endplate in relation to its composition and calcification. *Spine* 1996;21:415–420.
61. Sambrook PN, MacGregor AJ, Spector TD. Genetic influences on cervical and lumbar disc degeneration: a magnetic resonance imaging study in twins. *Arthritis Rheum* 1999;42:366–372.
62. Takegami K, Thonar EJ, An HS, et al. Osteogenic protein-1 enhances matrix replenishment by intervertebral disc cells previously exposed to interleukin-1. *Spine* 2002;27:1318–1325.
63. Thomas RDM, Batten JJ, Want S, et al. A new in-vitro model to investigate antibiotic penetration of the intervertebral disc. *J Bone Joint Surg [Br]* 1995;77:967–970.
64. Thompson JP, Oegema TR, Bradford DS. Stimulation of mature canine intervertebral disc by growth factors. *Spine* 1991;16:253–260.
65. Thornton WE, Moore TP, Pool SL. Fluid shifts in weightlessness. *Aviat Space Environ Med* 1987;58:A86–A90.
66. Trout JJ, Buckwalter JA, Moore KC. Ultrastructure of the human intervertebral disc: II. Cells of the nucleus pulposus. *Anat Rec* 1982;204:307–314.
67. Urban JPG. Factors influencing fluid flow in the intervertebral disc. *Adv Microcirc* 1987;13:160–170.
68. Urban JPG, McMullin JF. Swelling pressure of the lumbar intervertebral discs: influence of age, spinal level, composition and degeneration. *Spine* 1988;13:179–187.
69. Urban JPG, Roberts S. Development and degeneration of the intervertebral discs. *Mol Med Today* 1995;1:329–335.
70. Wilke HJ, Neef P, Caimi M, et al. New *in vivo* measurements of pressures in the intervertebral disc in daily life. *Spine* 1999;24:755–762.
71. Yu J, Petis C, Roberts S, et al. Elastic fibre organization in the intervertebral discs of the bovine tail. *J Anat* 2002;201:465–475.

5

Degenerative Disc Disease and Occupational Exposure

Malcolm H. Pope

Department of Environmental and Occupational Medicine, Aberdeen University; and Department of Biomedical Physics, Aberdeen Royal Infirmary, Aberdeen, United Kingdom

The lifetime prevalence of low back pain (LBP) is nearly 70% in industrialized countries, and herniated nucleus pulposus (HNP) may occur in 25% of those experiencing low back disorders (LBDs) (5). LBD rates vary by industry, occupation, and job (5,11,26,73, 77,80). LBD is multifactorial in origin and may be associated with both work-related and non–work-related factors. These include age, gender, smoking, physical fitness, strength, lumbar mobility, anthropometry, medical history, and structural abnormalities (33). Both work-related and non–work-related psychosocial factors have been associated with LBD.

EPIDEMIOLOGY

This review examines (a) heavy physical work, (b) lifting and forceful movements, (c) awkward postures, (d) whole-body vibration (WBV), and (e) static work postures in relation to LBP, HNP, and degenerative disc disease (DDD). Most studies do not specifically diagnose DDD. Many people who are asymptomatic have DDD (13,76). Savage et al. (76) found a greater prevalence of DDD in the older age group and no relationship between LBP and DDD. The studies addressing HNP may be a better indicator because it is thought that DDD precedes HNP. However, the cross-sectional magnetic resonance imaging (MRI) study of Luoma et al. (59) found an increased risk for LBP with DDD. An increased risk for sciatic pain was found with posterior bulges. Risks for LBP and sciatic pain were related to occupation. Elfering et al. (32) carried out a longitudinal MRI investigation of lumbar DDD in asymptomatic persons. Only a weak correlation was found between progressive DDD and the development of LBP during a 5-year follow-up period. The extent of HNP [odds ratio (OR), 12.63], a lack of sports activities (OR, 2.71), and night shift work (OR, 23.01) were predictors of DDD at follow-up.

All studies are reviewed according to objective criteria (strength of association, temporal relationship, consistency in association, coherence of evidence, and exposure–response relationship).

Heavy Physical Work

Strength of Association

Bigos et al. (11,12) found no association with physical work in a prospective LBP study, but the workers had a low level of exposure. Svensson and Andersson (83) also found that physical work was not related to LBP. Bergenudd and Nilsson (10) reported more LBP in persons engaging in heavier work (OR, 1.8). Others found LBP was associated with a high level of physical effort, with ORs of 1.5 (55), 1.8 (44), 1.2 (36), and 4.0 (23). Heliövaara et al. (35) found that LBP was associated with high physical stress scores (OR, 2.5), whereas Videman et al. (88) found that the prevalence of LBP was higher for heavy work [risk ratio (RR), 1.1] in younger women. Heliövaara et al. (35) found a dose–response relationship for HNP (OR, 1.9) and for LBP and physical stress (OR, 2.5) after adjusting for covariance.

Videman et al. (89) used discography and radiography in a cross-sectional autopsy study. Symptoms and work exposures were determined from next of kin. Those engaging in sedentary or heavy work were at increased risk for symmetric DDD (OR, 24.6 for sedentary work; OR, 2.8, for heavy work). Similar findings were found for endplate defects and facet joint osteoarthrosis. The risk for osteophytes was highest for those in heavy work (OR, 12.1). Those engaging in heavy physical work had an increased risk for DDD in comparison with those engaging in mixed work (OR, 2.8 for symmetric DDD; OR, 12.1 for osteophytes). Savage et al. (76) studied differences in MRI appearance between five different occupations (auto workers, ambulance crews, office staff, hospital porters, and brewery draymen). No differences in MRI appearance were observed between the groups. Yasukawa (97) determined the morphologic changes secondary to aging in the lumbar spine and disc by radiologic follow-up studies carried out during 10 years. Disc narrowing increased with age and was not related to occupation, and disc narrowing differed between the upper and the lower lumbar discs. The growth of osteophytes in the lumbar spine was more progressive in physical laborers but was not related to disc narrowing.

Riihimäki et al. (74) used lateral lumbar radiographs of concrete reinforcement workers and house painters to study mechanical loading in the development of lumbar DDD. Disc space narrowing occurred 10 years and osteophytes 5 years earlier in concrete workers. The RR for the effect of occupation on disc space narrowing was 1.8; adjustments for age, previous back accidents, height, body mass index, and smoking had only minor effects. The RR for osteophytes was 1.5. Previous back accidents showed a significant relationship with LBD. It was concluded that heavy physical work increases lumbar spine degeneration. Materials handling and postural loading are proposed to be important in the development of both DDD and osteophytes.

Temporal Relationship

Most studies had a cross-sectional design and could not directly address temporality. However, Burdorf et al. (24) and Burdorf and Zondervan (23) excluded cases with onset before the current job and found positive relationships between exposure and LBD. Bergenudd and Nilsson (10), Bigos et al. (11,12), and Clemmer et al. (29) used cohort designs in which temporal relationships between outcome and exposure could be determined. In one, no association was observed; in another, a modest increase in risk was seen. In the third, exposure was significantly associated with LBP. For most studies, the data suggest a temporal relationship in which exposure precedes LBP, but not HNP or DDD.

Consistency in Association

Half of the studies examined found no significant association between exposure and outcome. All those that showed significant associations were positive in direction (one OR, 1.2; two ORs, 1.5 to 2; six ORs, 2.2 to 12.1).

Coherence of Evidence

The stresses induced at the low back during manual materials handling (MMH) are due to a combination of the weight lifted and the way it is lifted. The internal reaction forces that equilibrate the body segment weights and external forces are supplied by muscle contraction, ligaments, and body joints. Injury to the supporting tissues can occur when the forces from the load, body position, and movements of the trunk create compressive, shear, or rotational forces that exceed the capacities of the disc and supporting tissues to counteract the load moments.

Exposure–Response Relationships

Only a few studies examined exposure in sufficient detail to assess exposure–response relationships in LBD. Results were mixed. Heliövaara et al. (35) observed an exposure–response relationship between HNP and physical stress score; Videman et al. (88) found a dose–response relationship between LBP prevalence and workload categories in younger nurses, but not in older groups or for HNP in any age group. In a "high-exposure group," duration of employment was associated with LBP (6). Bergenudd and Nilsson (10) and Johansson and Rubenowitz (44) found no relationships between LBDs and their exposure measures. Evidence of exposure–response relationships is equivocal, especially for DDD.

Lifting and Forceful Movements

Strength of Association

Studies with independent lifting exposure measures provide the best contrast among exposure levels and the least misclassification. In such studies, strengths of association for LBD and lifting included a negative relationship (61), no association (24), and positive associations with ORs ranging from 2.2 to 10.0. Magora (1973) found a positive relationship between sudden maximal efforts and LBP (OR, 1.7). Punnett et al. (72) found an OR of 2.16 after adjusting for confounders; Chaffin and Park (28) found an OR of 5 for lifting strength rating (LSR). The LSR is a ratio of the maximum weight lifted to the strength of a strong man in the same position. Marras et al. (64,65) found that the greatest risk for injury was lifting in combination with posture-related risk factors (OR, 10.7). Liles et al. (56) observed an OR of 4.5 for LBP and the highest job severity index (JSI). The JSI is the ratio of job requirements to the lifting capacity of the worker.

Studies in which subjective exposure measures were used found ORs from 0 (44–46,88) to between 1.3 and 5.2 (23,37,47,51,84,92). In the HNP case control study of Kelsey (45,46), cases and controls had similar lifting histories (RR, 0.94). In a second HNP case control study, Kelsey et al. (47) found an association with work-related lifting without twisting only at the highest lifting level (OR, 3.8). A combination of both risk factors at moderate levels yielded an OR of 3.1. The greatest risk was associated with simultaneous lifting and twisting with straight knees (OR, 6.1).

Luoma et al. (58) studied risk factors for lumbar DDD in a cross-sectional study of machine drivers, carpenters, and office workers ages 40 to 45 years. Data on possible risk factors were available from current structured questionnaires and for 4 and 7 years in retrospect. The prevalence of lumbar DDD at L2–3 through L5–S1 was determined with MRI. An increased risk was found for posterior disc bulges among those with increased lifting demands. DDD was not related to occupation but was related to a history of back accidents. Savage et al. (76) found no differences in the MRI appearance of the lumbar spine between occupational groups with different lifting demands.

Temporal Relationship

Two prospective studies found positive associations between exposure and LBD. Of four cross-sectional and case control studies that attempted to address temporality, three found positive relationships between lifting and LBD.

Consistency in Association

Although the studies reviewed used varying designs and methods to assess outcomes and exposure, they were fairly consistent in demonstrating a relationship between lifting and LBD when objective measures of exposure were used to evaluate populations with high exposures. Results were less consistent when subjective measures of exposure were used.

Coherence of Evidence

Studies of worker compensation claims have shown that MMH, including lifting, is associated with 25% to 70% of cases of LBP (30,38,81). According to data from the *Bureau of Labor Statistics 1994 Annual Survey of Occupational Injuries and Illnesses*, the highest rates of time loss injuries due to overexertion are in workers engaged in nursing and personal care (who frequently handle and lift patients).

Compressive, shear, and torsion stress is transmitted through the spinal tissues during lifting (93). It has been suggested that disc compression causes endplate fracture and HNP (27). However, Adams and Hutton (2) described HNP as a hyperflexion injury in combination with compression. Models show that large moments are created in the trunk area during lifting that result in large compressive forces on the spine. In laboratory experiments, dynamic trunk motion components of lifting have been associated with greater spine loading. Increased trunk motion during lifting activities has been associated with increased trunk muscle activity (65). Loading of the spine has become somewhat controversial. Pioneering measurements of intradiscal pressure (IDP) were made by Nachemson during the 1960s (68). Wilke et al. (95) also determined the effect of muscle forces on the IDP. Simulated muscle activity strongly influenced load pressure characteristics, especially for the multifidus. Without active muscle forces, pressure increased proportionally with increasing moment.

Some laboratory studies have shown that lateral shear forces make trunk motions more vulnerable to injury than in a compressive loading situation. *In vitro* evidence also suggests that the viscoelasticity of spinal tissues may cause increased strain during increased speed of motion (65).

Exposure–Response Relationships

Eight studies examined exposure–response relationships in some form. Of these, four found dose–response relationships between LBD and objective measures of lifting (28,56,65,72); another found a dose–response relationship between disorder and sudden maximal efforts (62). Two studies (in which a posture analysis assessment and an MMH index were used) found no dose–response relationship (24,44). Most studies that examined exposure–response relationships and in particular those that used quantitative exposure measures found these trends.

Awkward Postures

Strength of Association

The case control study of Punnett et al. (72) found time in nonneutral postures to be strongly associated with LBDs (OR, 8.09). The OR for lifting was 2.2. Burdorf et al. (24) found the OR for posture index to be 1.23. However, the case control study of HNP performed by Kelsey et al. (47) found that twisting without lifting had an OR of 3.0; in combination, the two had an OR of 3.1. The highest risk was observed for a combination of lifting, twisting, and straight knees (OR, 6.1). In the cross-sectional study of Marras et al. (64,65), LBP was associated with spinal loading during lifting, which included simultaneous exposures to lifting frequency, load weight, trunk lateral velocity, trunk twisting velocity, and trunk sagittal angle. An OR of 10.7 was observed for the highest combination of exposure measures. Univariate ORs were 1.73 for trunk lateral velocity, 1.66 for trunk twisting velocity, and 1.60 for maximum sagittal flexion when the high- and low-risk groups were compared (64).

Magora (61,62) found the highest LBP rate for those who rarely or never bent. The highest LBP rate was in workers who sometimes twist and reach. Johansson and Rubenowitz (44) found extreme work postures to be significantly associated with LBP in blue-collar workers. Riihimäki et al. (75) found exposure to twisted and bent postures was associated with an incidence of HNP only in univariate analysis. In women, bending was associated with a lifetime incidence of LBP only in univariate analysis (RR, 1.3) (83). Masset and Malchaire (66) found that trunk torsion was related to LBP in steelworkers (OR, 1.55). Toroptsova et al. (84) found that LBP in the past year was associated with bending (OR, 1.7). Riihimäki et al. (73) noted a dose–response relationship for HNP and twisted or bent postures (OR, 1.5). Holmström et al. (37) observed that stooping and kneeling were associated with severe LBP, with ORs of 2.6 and 3.5, respectively.

Most studies in which more quantitative exposure assessments were used showed elevated risk estimates for the relationship between LBD and bending, twisting, or awkward postures, with ORs from 1.23 to 8.09. The highest OR, 10.7, was based on combined exposure to lifting and posture risk factors. Most of these were based on multivariate analyses that adjusted for confounders (usually age and gender). The remaining studies found risk estimates ranging from none to a high of 3.5. The cross-sectional study of Luoma et al. (58) found an increased risk for posterior disc bulges among carpenters subject to awkward postures. Savage et al. (76) determined no differences in DDD between occupational groups with different exposure to awkward postures.

Temporal Relationship

One prospective study assessed exposures before LBD and found positive associations in univariate but not multivariate analyses (75). Burdorf et al. (24) excluded cases of LBP with onset before the current job to increase the likelihood that exposure preceded the disorder. No association between exposure and LBD was observed. One case control study examined only exposures experienced in the job just before disorder onset (72). A strong association between exposure to awkward postures and LBP was observed.

Consistency in Association

Although the studies used varying designs, the studies using quantitative exposure measures were fairly consistent in demonstrating a moderate relationship between awkward postures and LBD, but not DDD.

Coherence of Evidence

Most studies that examined the effects of posture also examined the effects of lifting. Therefore, a discussion of coherence of evidence for the former relationship is similar to that found in the section on lifting and forceful movements. Forward flexion can generate compressive forces on the structures of the low back similar to those generated when a heavy object is lifted. Similarly, rapid twisting can generate shear or rotational forces on the low back (65).

Adams and Hutton (3) compared postures that flatten the lumbar spine with postures that preserve the lumbar lordosis. Flexed postures have several advantages: Flexion improves the transport of metabolites in the discs, reduces the stresses on the facets and posterior annulus fibrosus, and gives the spine a high compressive strength. Flexion also has disadvantages: It increases the stress on the anterior annulus fibrosis and increases the hydrostatic pressure in the nucleus pulposus. The disadvantages are not of much significance, and one can conclude that it is mechanically and nutritionally advantageous to flatten the lumbar spine when heavy weights are lifted. However, Magnusson et al. (60) determined that hyperextension gave a significantly increased height recovery in comparison with the prone posture.

Exposure–Response Relationships

Six studies examined dose–response relationships between posture and LBD. In one study, no dose–response relationship was found between LBP and bending and twisting/reaching. In five studies, relationships were found between back injury and spinal loading score, LBP and posture index, HNP and awkward postures, LBP and stooping, and LBP and kneeling. DDD was not examined in these studies.

Whole-Body Vibration

Strength of Association

Studies with quantitative exposure assessments provide the most information on the relationship between WBV and LBD. ORs calculated by measured WBV exposure (usually including magnitude and duration) ranged from 1.4 (20) to 9.5 (16). Analyses conducted by exposure level found stronger relationships. In tractor drivers, ORs for lifetime LBP were 3.79 for total WBV dose, 3.42 for equivalent WBV magnitude, and 4.51 for duration of exposure (21). For LBP in the previous year, ORs were 2.36, 2.29, and 2.74 for the highest levels of the same exposure measures. In urban bus drivers, the highest ORs for LBP were found for the intermediate rather than the highest exposure; ORs were 3.46 for total WBV dose, 3.77 for equivalent WBV magnitude, and 3.08 for total WBV duration (22). The investigation of Bongers et al. (16) of LBP in helicopter pilots found that the highest ORs for LBP were in the highest categories for total flight time (OR, 13.4), total WBV dose (OR, 39.5), and hours of flight time per day (OR, 14.4). A study of tractor drivers found LBP ORs of 2.8 for the highest total WBV dose and 3.6 (95% confidence interval, 1.2 to 11) for the highest duration of exposure category (18). In the same population, the OR for all sick leaves for LBD was 1.47, in a comparison of exposed persons and controls (19). For sick leaves related to DDD, the highest OR was for the highest exposure category (OR, 7.2). The study of Boshuizen et al. (20) of forklift truck and freight container tractor drivers showed no association between LBP and total WBV dose (OR, 0.99) but did show an association for WBV in the preceding 5 years (OR, 2.4). In this study, the increased LBP prevalence in the exposed group was significant only for ages 25 through 34 (OR, 5.6) in multivariate analyses. Magnusson et al. (60) found an OR of 1.79 for LBP in bus and truck drivers in comparison with controls.

Other studies assessed both exposure and LBD by interview or questionnaire. Burdorf and Zondervan (1990) and Toroptsova et al. (84) observed no association between WBV exposure and LBP. The cross-sectional study of Masset and Malchaire (66) found that LBP was associated with vehicle driving (OR, 1.2) in univariate analyses. Similar results were observed in multivariate analyses (OR, 1.2). Riihimäki et al. (73) observed an OR of 1.3 for dockers and earth movers in comparison with controls. No association was seen for annual car driving (OR, 1.1). Walsh et al. (92) found that driving (on job before LBP) was significantly associated with LBP in men (RR, 1.7) in multivariate analyses. Burdorf et al. (24) found that WBV was significantly associated with LBP (OR, 3.1) in multivariate analyses that adjusted for age. Burdorf et al. (25) found an OR of 3.29 for crane operators and of 2.51 for WBV-exposed straddle carrier drivers after adjustments were made for confounders. Skov et al. (79) found that annual driving distance was related to LBP in salespersons (OR, 2.79). Magora (61,62) found that bus drivers had LBP rates similar to those of controls (RR, 1.19).

Prospectively, HNP was associated with WBV in univariate but not multivariate models (75). The case control study of Kelsey (45) found a significant association between HNP and time driving (OR, 2.75) and, more specifically, working as a truck driver (OR, 4.7). In crane operators, the exposed group had ORs of 2.00 and 2.95 for DDD after adjustments for age and shift, respectively (15). An examination of risk estimates for DDD by years of exposure showed the highest OR (5.73) in the highest exposure category. In the study of Johanning (43) of subway train operators, an OR of 3.9 was observed for HNP. The cross-sectional study of Luoma et al. (58) found an increased risk for anterior disc bulges among machine drivers, but decreased signal intensity was not related to occupation. Car driving was also associated with anterior disc bulges. Anterior and posterior disc bulges appear to be related to different types of physical loads.

Most studies in which quantitative exposure assessments were used found positive associations between LBD outcomes and WBV exposures, with ORs ranging from 1.4 to 39 after adjustment for confounders. In the remaining studies, risk estimates varied, including the following: no association (n = 3); ORs of 1.2, 1.7, and 2.8 for driving; an OR of 1.8 for truck or bus driving; an OR of 4.7 for truck driving; an OR of 1.3 for machine operation; ORs of 2.0, 2.95, and 5.73 for crane operation; an OR of 3.1 for WBV; and an OR of 3.9 for subway train operation. Evidence was found, but in fewer studies, for a positive relationship between HNP and DDD. However, Savage et al. (76) determined no differences in the MRI appearance of the lumbar spine between five occupational groups with different exposures to WBV.

In a well-controlled study of lumbar MRI findings in monozygotic twins, lifetime driving had no effect on DDD (7). Videman et al. (91) investigated the effect of rally driving on lumbar DDD in a case control study. The subjects were interviewed and underwent MRI for DDD. No differences in lumbar DDD were noted between the groups. Even extreme vehicular vibration in rally driving does not appear to affect DDD. The study results do not support driving, and its associated WBV, as a significant cause of DDD and question the theory that the higher incidence of back pain among drivers is caused by accelerated DDD.

In a retrospective cohort study, tractor-driving farmers and non–tractor-driving farmers were matched by Kumar et al. (52). Both groups were interviewed for details of WBV exposure and confounders to assess their influence on LBP and DDD. MRI was performed to assess DDD. WBV measurements were performed on tractors. LBP was found in 40% of tractor-driving farmers and 18% of non–tractor-driving farmers. Clinical examination and MRI showed no difference between the two groups. Tractor-driving farmers reported LBP more often than non–tractor-driving farmers, but no significant differences on clinical or MRI evaluation were found.

Temporal Relationship

Bongers et al. (15), Boshuizen et al. (19), and Riihimäki et al. (75) used prospective designs in which temporal relationships between outcome and exposure could be determined. In the studies of Bongers et al. (15) and Boshuizen et al. (19), clear positive relationships between LBD and exposure were found. Most studies were cross-sectional and could not directly address temporality. However, Burdorf et al. (24,25) and Burdorf and Zondervan (23) attempted to clarify relationships by excluding from analysis the cases with disorder onset before the current job. A fourth cross-sectional study truncated self-reported exposures on the birthday preceding disorder onset (92). In these four investigations, positive relationships between LBD and WBV were also observed.

Consistency in Association

Results with regard to the relationship between LBD and WBV were most consistent in the studies in which observational or measurement approaches to exposure assessment were used. The strength of association was more variable in studies in which job titles or questionnaires were used to assess exposures. Studies in which more quantitative exposure measures were used were fairly consistent in showing higher risk estimates.

Hulshof and Veldhuijzen van Zanten (39) concluded that although the earlier studies varied in quality, most showed a strong tendency toward a positive association between WBV exposure and LBP. Seidel and Heide (78) stated that the literature they had reviewed indicated an increased risk for spine disorders after intense long-term exposure to WBV. Bongers and Boshuizen (14) conducted a metaanalysis of studies published through 1990 that examined the relationship between WBV and several LBDs. The overall OR for WBV exposure and degenerative changes of the spine was 1.5; the summary OR for LBP was also 1.5. These conclusions are consistent with the positive associations observed in the evidence reviewed in the preceding sections (although the studies published in the 1990s have tended to report larger ORs).

Coherence of Evidence

Laboratory studies have shown that exposure to WBV causes spine changes that may be related to LBP. These include fatigue of the paraspinal muscles and ligaments, lumbar disc flattening, disc fiber strain, IDP increases, HNP, and microfractures in vertebral endplates. Studies of acute effects have shown that the vertebral endplate is the structure most sensitive to a high level of WBV exposure, followed by the intervertebral disc (94). Experimental investigations have found that a high level of exposure to WBV causes injuries such as degeneration and fracturing of the vertebral endplate. These could then result in disc degeneration. WBV causes creep, an increase in IDP from cyclic compression and fatigue failure. WBV may also change the nutritional balance and lead to DDD. Thus, prolonged WBV exposure may cause spine pathology through mechanical damage, changes in tissue metabolism, or both.

WBV exposure has been shown to cause changes in electromyographic (EMG) activity in muscles of the lower back (94). EMG experiments have found that lower back muscle fatigue increases during WBV exposure in truck driving. Decreased stability of the lower back may result from slower muscle response, possibly increasing the risk for injury to other structures. Laboratory investigations have shown that other work-related factors, including prolonged sitting, lifting, and awkward postures, may act in combination with WBV to cause LBD (31,94).

Exposure–Response Relationships

Most studies in which quantitative exposure assessment was performed found dose–response relationships between WBV and LBD. Bovenzi and Betta (21) observed a dose–response relationship between chronic LBP and total WBV dose, equivalent WBV magnitude, and duration of exposure. Bovenzi and Zadini (22) found increasing trends for nearly all types of LBP by exposure level. Bongers et al. (16) found increased ORs for HNP pain and transient LBP with increasing hours of daily flight time.

In tractor drivers, Boshuizen et al. (19) observed an increased risk of disc disorder with total WBV level. In other studies, Bongers et al. (15) found an increase in risk for DDD with years of exposure to crane operation and Skov et al. (79) found an increase in LBP with annual driving distance. Johanning (43) found no association between years of employment as a subway train operator and LBP symptoms. Most studies that examined LBDs by exposure level found dose–response relationships.

Static Work Postures

Strength of Association

Several studies found no relationship between sitting and LBD (23,37,66,83,84). In a cross-sectional study, the highest LBP rates were found for those rarely sitting and standing (61,62). Walsh et al. (92) found that LBP was associated with lifetime occupational sitting only in women (RR, 1.7). The case control study of Kelsey (46) found that sedentary work (50% of the time at work) was associated with lumbar HNP for those 34 years of age or older (RR, 2.4). In salespersons, a dose–response relationship was observed for sedentary work and LBP (OR, 2.45) (79). The study of Videman et al. (89) of cadavers found that those with a history of either sedentary or heavy work exposure were at increased risk for symmetric DDD (ORs, 24.6 and 2.8, respectively). Similar results were seen for other disc pathologies. Savage et al. (76) determined no differences in the MRI appearance of the lumbar spine between five occupational groups with different exposure to static postures.

Toroptsova et al. (84) found that standing and static work postures were not associated with LBP history. Svensson and Andersson (83) found that standing was associated with a lifetime incidence of LBP in univariate analyses (OR, 1.3), but not in multivariate models. Most studies found static work postures, including standing and sitting, were not a risk for LBD. However, the cadaver study of Videman et al. (89) found a high risk for disc pathology in those with a history of sedentary work. Videman et al. (89) found that the least pathology stemmed from moderate or mixed physical loading, but the least LBP was associated with sedentary work. The L5–S1 disc was the one most frequently affected with degenerative changes. Ambulating women had no lumbar DDD, and sedentary women had a high rate of DDD. The men in the study did not demonstrate a significant difference in the prevalence of DDD.

Temporal Relationship

Most studies were cross-sectional, but two of these attempted to increase the likelihood that exposure preceded disorder by excluding cases with onset before current job and truncating exposures before disorder onset. One found a positive relationship between prolonged sitting and LBP symptoms.

Consistency in Association

The studies showed poor consistency in estimations of the relationship between LBD and static work postures, possibly because of differences in definitions of exposure.

Coherence of Evidence

LBP has been associated with mechanical forces causing an increased load on the lumbar spine (93). Increased loading on the spine causes increased IDP, which, in turn, may be responsible for HNP and DDD. Disc pressure has been found to be substantially greater in unsupported sitting than in standing positions (27). Loading of the spine has become somewhat controversial. Pioneering IDP measurements were made by Nachemson during the 1960s. Since that time, few data have corroborated or disputed those findings. Wilke et al. (96) made *in vivo* measurements of IDP in various activities. It was concluded that the IDP during sitting may be less than that in erect standing and that constantly changing position is important to promote flow of fluid to the disc.

Lumbar spines (L1–S1) were loaded while in simulated flexed and extended seated postures. Time-dependent forces were measured in the anterior column at the L4 and L5 superior endplates and in the facets. The remaining principal joint forces, including ligament, disc shear, and facet impingement forces, were computed. The vertical creep displacement was greater in the extended seated posture, but the escalation of forces was more severe in the flexed posture. The results suggest that flexed postures produce large increases in the tensile forces in the region of the posterior annulus fibrosus. Adams and Hutton (3) compared postures that flatten the lumbar spine with those that preserve the lumbar lordosis. Flexed postures have several advantages, but one can conclude that it is mechanically and nutritionally advantageous to flatten the lumbar spine during sitting.

The results of some epidemiologic studies are consistent with the hypothesis that static work postures may be associated with LBD. Kelsey (45) observed that in addition to sedentary work, amount of time spent sitting on weekends is associated with HNP. The finding that sedentary work is associated with HNP only in older age groups suggests that duration of exposure may be important and that a threshold may exist. Toroptsova et al. (84) observed that LBP is lower in those who engage in sports activity, suggesting that greater muscle strength prevents LBP.

The perception of "sedentary" is subjective, and many jobs may permit considerable movement throughout the day. The cadaver study shows increased DDD with sitting, but the occupational histories may be inaccurate.

Exposure–Response Relationships

Three studies addressed dose–response relationships, two of which did not show any trends. Magora (61,62) found the highest risk for LBP in the lowest exposure categories for sedentary postures, sitting, and standing. Videman et al. (89) found a high rate of lumbar disc pathology in those with histories of sedentary and heavy work, with relationships stronger for sedentary work. A dose–response relationship for LBP symptoms and sedentary work was observed by Skov et al. (79).

BIOLOGIC EVIDENCE

DDD involves structural disruption of the annulus fibrosus and cell-mediated changes throughout the disc and subchondral bone. Disruption of the annulus is related to LBP (17,67), but other degenerative disc changes, such as a dehydrated nucleus pulposus, are not clinically relevant (90) and are signs of aging. DDD can occur when the fatigue damage rate outpaces the adaptive disc remodeling response. Complex changes in cell biology and tissue composition occur in degenerate discs, but animal experiments show that these can follow mechanical interventions (70) and can be explained in terms of disc cell responses to an altered mechanical environment (42). Biologic changes may be consequences rather than causes of structural failure. A genetic predisposition to disc degeneration (8) does not argue against mechanical causes because inheritance may involve small discs and a heavy body.

In skeletal tissues, cells repairing and strengthening the tissue counter microscopic damage. Cells also respond to increased deformation by increasing matrix stiffness; a stiffer matrix deforms less, so deformation returns to normal levels (53). Heavily loaded vertebrae may form marginal osteophytes (90) in an attempt to increase their cross-sectional area and reduce stress. These self-regulating processes are related to the Heuter–Vinkmann law for ligaments (69) and intervertebral discs (71).

Lotz and Chin (57) examined whether disc cell death is correlated with the magnitude and duration of compressive loading. Static compression induces cell death. Cell death, in turn, has been associated with disc degeneration in humans. The percentage of dying cells was proportional to the sum of the logarithmic transformations of the compressive stress and the time of loading. The results of this study demonstrate the feasibility of developing a quantitative correlation between spinal loading and disc degeneration.

Iatridis et al. (41) studied compression-induced changes in the intervertebral disc in a rat tail model loaded with an Ilizarov-type apparatus. Chronically applied compressive forces caused changes in the mechanical properties and composition of the tail discs. Hutton et al. (40) used springs to compress the lumbar intervertebral discs of dogs for 53 weeks, but no obvious signs of DDD could be observed. No disc bulging, fissures, or disc space narrowing was noted. Compression produced microscopic changes and changes in the amounts of proteoglycan and collagen in the nucleus and the inner and outer annulus. Thus, one study supports the concept that high compressive forces cause DDD, and one does not.

The overall process of DDD, called the *degenerative cascade* by Kirkaldy-Willis and Farfan (49), comprises three stages: dysfunction, instability, and stabilization. Initiation occurs in the disc, which cannot regenerate because it has no direct blood supply and the nutrient flow is compromised by endplate pathology. Metabolite transport within the disc is barely adequate, even for the small cell population (63), and proteoglycan synthesis is slow (9). The water content decreases, and the structure of the proteoglycans changes. The result is that the disc loses turgor, height, and elasticity and allows excessive movement of the functional spinal unit. This is the phase of dysfunction, which results in small tears in the disc. Initially, these are circumferential, but with time, the tears can coalesce and become radial. The next step is disc resorption and desiccation. Abnormal movement is allowed by disc degeneration. This is the phase of instability. The final step is osteophyte formation in an attempt to decrease the abnormal movement. This is the phase of stabilization.

During the dysfunctional and unstable phases, radial tears can become large enough to allow the nucleus pulposus to herniate through the tear in the annulus fibrosus into the spinal canal. This usually occurs posterolaterally. Such focal prolapse differs from the generalized bulge that is part of the normal degenerative process. Disc degeneration during dysfunction and instability is associated with an ingrowth of blood vessels and nerve endings. Venous hypertension develops around the endplate. The result is pain from the disc itself, although the exact cause is unclear.

MECHANICAL EVIDENCE

The least equivocal sign of DDD is an HNP confirmed at surgery, and the most common risk factor is repetitive and high mechanical loading (48). Experiments on cadaver spines have shown that excessive loading applied to normal discs can create radial fissures in the posterolateral annulus (3) and posterior HNP (2) and internal disruption of the annulus (1).

The high risk of repetitive loading (47) suggests that fatigue failure may be more important than trauma. In any material, repetitive loading can cause an accumulation of microscopic damage and lead to gross failure. Fatigue damage accumulates when the cyclic force exceeds a threshold value, which for the annulus fibrosus is approximately 45% of the force required to cause sudden failure (34). The more cycles, the lower the force required for failure. A longitudinal study of student nurses found that LBP is most common after 9 to 12 months of active ward training (50).

All skeletal tissues adapt to increased mechanical loads, but they may not adapt fast enough. Workers with demanding jobs may engage in increased repetitive loading and experience fatigue damage. Conversely, a carefully regulated buildup of physical activity during many years may result in a strong spine, such as is found in elite weight lifters, who have dense vertebrae, and physically active persons, who have strong intervertebral discs (71). Discs adapt more slowly than bones, which could explain why former weight lifters have more bulging discs than former elite runners but fewer endplate defects (90).

A cadaver study showed that vertebrae from physically active people appear to strengthen more than the adjacent discs (71).

Muscle contractions during epileptic fits can crush vertebrae (86); thus, any maximum muscular effort could cause failure. Links between DDD and disc pain are not straightforward, and moderate DDD may be more painful than severe DDD because the reduced height in the latter may cause the discs to be shielded by the apophyseal joints (4).

CONCLUSIONS

Epidemiologic studies show that LBDs are associated with heavy physical work. Despite the fact that the studies defined disorders and assessed exposures in many ways, the results of all the studies that found significant associations between exposure and outcome were positive and showed increased risk. The results of a few studies that examined dose–response relationships were equivocal. Epidemiologic studies relating DDD to heavy physical work are few.

Strong evidence indicates that LBDs are associated with lifting and awkward postures. The best studies consistently showed positive relationships and suggested that both factors were important contributors to LBD risk. Epidemiologic studies relating DDD to lifting and awkward postures are few. The relationships are consistent with the results of biomechanical studies of the effects of lifting and dynamic motion on back tissues.

The investigations reviewed provide evidence that LBDs are associated with work-related awkward postures. Results were consistent in showing an increased risk for LBD with exposure. Several studies suggested that both lifting and awkward postures were important contributors to the risk for LBD, but evidence relating risk to DDD is lacking.

Strong evidence indicates a positive association between WBV and LBD. Laboratory studies have found effects of WBV on the vertebrae, intervertebral discs, and supporting musculature. Both experimental and epidemiologic evidence suggests that WBV may act in combination with other work-related factors, such as prolonged sitting, lifting, and awkward postures, to cause an increased risk for LBD. Other driving-related factors, such as postural stress, may deserve more attention. As a whole, the results of these studies provide inadequate evidence for a relationship between static work postures and LBD.

Kelsey and Ostfeld (48), Lawrence (54), and Spangfort (82) report that disc surgery is performed twice as often in men than in women, perhaps because of the increased occupational disc loading of men. Valkenburg and Haanen (85) reported that unskilled men have more than a fourfold increase in symptomatic disc prolapse in comparison with higher-level employees. Confounders can be a problem in these studies. LBD is multifactorial in origin and may be associated with both occupational and non–work-related factors and characteristics. The latter may include demographics, leisure time activities, psychosocial factors, a history of LBD, and structural characteristics of the back (33). The relative contributions of these confounders may be specific to particular anatomic areas and disorders.

Videman and Battié (87) felt that occupational factors explain little of the variability in DDD found in the adult population. Their prior work links familial influences, which reflect the combined effects of genes and early childhood environment. They challenge the dominant role assumed for occupational loading in DDD and associated LBD and suggest a more complex etiology. Yasukawa (97) pointed out that all discs do not narrow at a constant rate with aging; therefore, DDD should not be considered purely a change of aging but should be regarded as partly related to aging.

The biomechanical and biologic evidence links increased DDD with mechanical loading. Possibly, the low metabolic rate of the lumbar vertebrae prevents them from keeping pace with the adaptive remodeling of adjacent tissues. Epidemiologic studies provide scarce evidence.

REFERENCES

1. Adams MA, Dolan P. *Internal disruption of an intervertebral disc can be caused by previous damage to an adjacent vertebral body*. Presented to the International Society for the Study of the Lumbar Spine, Helsinki, Finland, June 1995.
2. Adams MA, Hutton WC. Prolapsed intervertebral disc: a hyperflexion injury. 1981 Volvo Award in Basic Science. *Spine* 1982;7:184–191.
3. Adams MA, Hutton WC. Gradual disc prolapse. *Spine* 1985;10:524–531.
4. Adams MA, McNally DS, Dolan P. "Stress" distributions inside intervertebral discs. The effects of age and degeneration. *J Bone Joint Surg Br* 1996;78:965–972.
5. Andersson GBJ. Epidemiologic aspects of low back pain in industry. *Spine* 1981;6:53–60.
6. Åstrand NE. Medical, psychological, and social factors associated with back abnormalities and self-reported back pain: a cross-sectional study of male employees in a Swedish pulp and paper industry. *Br J Ind Med* 1987; 44:327–336.
7. Battié MC, Videman T, Gibbons LE, et al. 1995 Volvo Award in Clinical Sciences. Determinants of lumbar disc degeneration. A study relating lifetime exposures and magnetic resonance imaging findings in identical twins. *Spine* 1995;20:2601–2612.
8. Battié M, Videman, Raininko T. *The effects of different lifetime occupational loading patterns on lumbar spine. An MRI study of male identical twins*. Presented to the International Society for the Study of the Lumbar Spine, Seattle, 1994.
9. Bayliss MT. Proteoglycan synthesis in the human intervertebral disc. Variation with age, region and pathology. *Spine* 1988;13:972–981.
10. Bergenudd H, Nilsson B. Back pain in middle age. Occupational workload and psychologic factors: an epidemiologic survey. *Spine* 1988;13:58–60.
11. Bigos SJ, Spengler DM, Martin NA, et al. Back injuries in industry: a retrospective study. II. Injury factors. *Spine* 1986;11:246–251.
12. Bigos SJ, Spengler DM, Martin NA, et al. Back injuries in industry: a retrospective study. III. Employee-related factors. *Spine* 1986;11:252–256.
13. Boden SD, Wiesel SW. Lumbar spine imaging: role in clinical decision making. *J Am Acad Orthop Surg* 1996;4: 238–248.
14. Bongers PM, Boshuizen HC. *Back disorders and whole-body vibration at work* [Dissertation]. Amsterdam, the Netherlands: University of Amsterdam, 1990.
15. Bongers PM, Boshuizen HC, Hulshof CTJ, et al. Back disorders in crane operators exposed to whole-body vibration. *Int Arch Occup Environ Health* 1988;60:129–137.
16. Bongers PM, Hulshof CTJ, Dijkstra L, et al. Back pain and exposure to whole-body vibration in helicopter pilots. *Ergonomics* 1990;33:1007–1026.
17. Boos N, Rieder R, Schade V, et al. 1995 Volvo Award in Clinical Sciences. The diagnostic accuracy of magnetic resonance imaging, work perception, and psychosocial factors in identifying symptomatic disc herniations. *Spine* 1995;20:2613–2625.
18. Boshuizen HC, Bongers PM, Hulshof CTJ. Self-reported back pain in tractor drivers exposed to whole-body vibration. *Int Arch Occup Environ Health* 1990;62:109–115.
19. Boshuizen HC, Hulshof CTJ, Bongers PM. Long-term sick leave and disability pensioning due to back disorders of tractor drivers exposed to whole-body vibration. *Int Arch Occup Environ Health* 1990;62:117–122.
20. Boshuizen HC, Bongers PM, Hulshof CTJ. Self-reported back pain in fork-lift truck and freight-container tractor drivers exposed to whole-body vibration. *Spine* 1992;17:59–65.
21. Bovenzi M, Betta A. Low-back disorders in agricultural tractor drivers exposed to whole-body vibration and postural stress. *Appl Ergonomics* 1994;25:231–241.
22. Bovenzi M, Zadini A. Self-reported low back symptoms in urban bus drivers exposed to whole-body vibration. *Spine* 1992;17:1048–1059.
23. Burdorf A, Zondervan H. An epidemiological study of low-back pain in crane operators. *Ergonomics* 1990; 33:981–987.
24. Burdorf A, Govaert G, Elders L. Postural load and back pain of workers in the manufacturing of prefabricated concrete elements. *Ergonomics* 1991;34:909–918.
25. Burdorf A, Naaktgeboren B, deGroot HC. Occupational risk factors for low back pain among sedentary workers. *J Occup Med* 1993;35:1213–1220.

26. California Workers' Compensation Institute. *Report on CTDs*. San Francisco: California Workers' Compensation Institute, 1993.
27. Chaffin DB, Andersson GBJ. *Occupational biomechanics*. New York: John Wiley & Sons, 1984:15–25.
28. Chaffin DB, Park KS. A longitudinal study of low-back pain as associated with occupational weight lifting factors. *Am Ind Hyg Assoc J* 1973;34:513–525.
29. Clemmer DI, Mohr DL, Mercer DJ. Low-back injuries in a heavy industry: I. Worker and workplace factors. *Spine* 1991;16:824–830.
30. Cust G, Pearson JCG, Mair A. The prevalence of low back pain in nurses. *Int Nurs Rev* 1972;19:169–179.
31. Dupuis H. Medical and occupational preconditions for vibration-induced spinal disorders: occupational disease No. 2110 in Germany. *Int Arch Occup Environ Health* 1994;66:303–308.
32. Elfering A, Semmer N, Birkhofer D, et al. Risk factors for lumbar disc degeneration: a 5-year prospective MRI study in asymptomatic individuals. *Spine* 2002;27:125–134.
33. Garg A, Moore SJ. Epidemiology of low-back pain in industry. *Occup Med State of the Art Rev* 1992;7:593–608.
34. Green TP, et al. Tensile properties of the annulus fibrosus. Part 2. Ultimate tensile strength and fatigue in life. *Eur Spine J* 1993;2:209–214.
35. Heliövaara M, Mäkelä M, Knekt P, et al. Determinants of sciatica and low back pain. *Spine* 1991;16:608–614.
36. Hildebrandt VH. Back pain in the working population: prevalence rates in Dutch trades and professions. *Ergonomics* 1995;38:1283–1298.
37. Holmström E. *Musculoskeletal disorders in construction workers*. Lund, Sweden: Lund University, Department of Physical Therapy, 1992:1–175.
38. Horal J. The clinical appearance of low back disorders in the city of Gothenburg, Sweden. *Acta Orthop Scand Suppl* 1969;118:7–37.
39. Hulshof C, Veldhuijzen van Zanten B. Whole-body vibration and low-back pain: a review of epidemiologic studies. *Int Arch Occup Environ Health* 1987;59:205–220.
40. Hutton WC, Ganey TM, Elmer WA, et al. Does long-term compressive loading on the intervertebral disc cause degeneration? *Spine* 2000;25:2993–3004.
41. Iatridis JC, Mente PL, Stokes IA, et al. Compression-induced changes in intervertebral disc properties in a rat tail model. *Spine* 1999;24:996–1002.
42. Ishihara H, et al. Effects of hydrostatic pressure on matrix synthesis in different regions of the intervertebral disc. *J Appl Physiol* 1996;80: 839–846.
43. Johanning E. Back disorders and health problems among subway train operators exposed to whole-body vibration. *Scand J Work Environ Health* 1991;17:414–419.
44. Johansson JA, Rubenowitz S. Risk indicators in the psychosocial and physical work environment for work-related neck, shoulder and low back symptoms: a study among blue and white collar workers in eight companies. *Scand J Rehabil Med* 1994;26:131–142.
45. Kelsey JL. An epidemiological study of acute herniated lumbar intervertebral disc. *Rheumatol Rehabil* 1975; 14:144.
46. Kelsey JL. An epidemiological study of the relationship between occupations and acute herniated lumbar intervertebral discs. *Int J Epidemiol* 1975;4:197–205.
47. Kelsey JL, Githens PB, White AA, et al. An epidemiologic study of lifting and twisting on the job and risk for acute prolapsed lumbar intervertebral disc. *J Orthop Res* 1984;2:61–66.
48. Kelsey JL, Ostfeld AM. Demographic characteristics of persons with acute herniated lumbar intervertebral disc. *J Chronic Dis* 1975;28:37.
49. Kirkaldy-Willis WH, Farfan HF. Instability of the lumbar spine. *Clin Orthop* 1982;165,110–123.
50. Klaber Moffett JA, Hughes GI, Griffiths P. A longitudinal study of low back pain in student nurses. *Int J Nurs Stud* 1993;30:197–212.
51. Knibbe JJ, Friele RD. Prevalence of back pain and characteristics of the physical workload of community nurses. *Ergonomics* 1996;39:186–198.
52. Kumar A, Varghese M, Mohan D, et al. Effect of whole-body vibration on the low back. A study of tractor-driving farmers in north India. *Spine* 1999;24:2506–2515.
53. Lanyon LE, Goodship AE, Pye CJ, et al. Mechanically adaptive bone remodelling. *J Biomech* 1982;15: 141–154.
54. Lawrence JS. Disc degeneration: its frequency and relationship to symptoms. *Ann J Rheum Dis* 1969;28: 121–138.
55. Leigh JP, Sheetz RM. Prevalence of back pain among full-time United States workers. *Br J Ind Med* 1989;46: 651–657.
56. Liles DH, Deivanayagam S, Ayoub MM, et al. A job severity index for the evaluation and control of lifting injury. *Hum Factors* 1984;26:683–693.
57. Lotz JC, Chin JR. Intervertebral disc cell death is dependent on the magnitude and duration of spinal loading. *Spine* 2000;25:1477–1483.
58. Luoma K, Riihimäki H, Luukkonen R, et al. Low back pain in relation to lumbar disc degeneration. *Spine* 2000; 25:487–492.
59. Luoma K, Riihimäki H, Raininko R, et al. Lumbar disc degeneration in relation to occupation. *Scand J Work Environ Health* 1998;24:358–366.
60. Magnusson ML, Pope MH. Body height changes with hyperextension. *Clin Biomech* 1996;11:236–238.

61. Magora A. Investigation of the relation between low back pain and occupation. III. Physical requirements: sitting, standing, and weight lifting. *Ind Med* 1972;41:5–9.
62. Magora A. Investigation of the relation between low back pain and occupation. IV. Physical requirements: bending, rotation, reaching, and sudden maximal effort. *Scand J Rehabil Med* 1973;5:191–196.
63. Maroudas A, et al. Factors involved in the nutrition of the human lumbar intervertebral disc: cellularity and diffusion of glucose in vitro. *J Anat* 1975;120:113–118
64. Marras WS, Lavender SA, Leurgans SE, et al. The role of dynamic three-dimensional trunk motion in occupationally-related low back disorders: the effects of workplace factors, trunk position, and trunk motion characteristics on risk of injury. *Spine* 1993;18:617–628.
65. Marras WS, Lavender SA, Leurgans SE, et al. Biomechanical risk factors for occupationally-related low back disorders. *Ergonomics* 1995;38:377–410.
66. Masset D, Malchaire J. Low back pain: epidemiologic aspects and work-related factors in the steel industry. *Spine* 1994;19:143–146.
67. Moneta GB, Videman T, Kaivanto K, et al. Reported pain during lumbar discography as a function of anular ruptures and disc degeneration. A re-analysis of 833 discograms. *Spine* 1994;19:1968–1974.
68. Nachemson AL. Lumbar intradiscal pressure. *Acta Orthop Scand Suppl* 1960;43:1–104.
69. Neumann P, Keller T, Ekstrom L, et al. Structural properties of the anterior longitudinal ligament. Correlation with lumbar bone mineral content. *Spine* 1993;18:637–645.
70. Osti OL, Vernon-Roberts B, Fraser RD. 1990 Volvo Award in Experimental Studies. Anulus tears and intervertebral disc degeneration. An experimental study using an animal model. *Spine* 1990;15:762–767.
71. Porter RW, Adams MA, Hutton WC. Physical activity and the strength of the lumbar spine. *Spine* 1989;14:201–203.
72. Punnett L, Fine LJ, Keyserling WM, et al. Back disorders and nonneutral trunk postures of automobile assembly workers. *Scand J Work Environ Health* 1991;17:337–346.
73. Riihimäki H, Mattsson T, Zitting A, et al. Radiographically detectable degenerative changes of the lumbar spine among concrete reinforcement workers and house painters. *Spine* 1990;15:114–119.
74. Riihimäki H, Tola S, Videman T, et al. Low-back pain and occupation: a cross-sectional questionnaire study of men in machine operating, dynamic physical work, and sedentary work. *Spine* 1989;14:204–209.
75. Riihimäki H, Viikari-Juntura E, Moneta G, et al. Incidence of sciatic pain among men in machine operating, dynamic physical work and sedentary work. *Spine* 1994;19:138–142.
76. Savage RA, Whitehouse GH, Roberts N. The relationship between the magnetic resonance imaging appearance of the lumbar spine and low back pain, age and occupation in males. *Eur Spine J* 1997;6:106–114.
77. Schibye B, Skov T, Ekner D, et al. Musculoskeletal symptoms among sewing machine operators. *Scand J Work Environ Health* 1995;21:427–434.
78. Seidel H, Heide R. Long-term effects of whole-body vibration: a critical survey of the literature. *Int Arch Occup Environ Health* 1986;58:1–26.
79. Skov T, Borg V, Orhede E. Psychosocial and physical risk factors for musculoskeletal disorders of the neck, shoulders, and lower back in sales people. *Occup Environ Med* 1996;53:351–356.
80. Skovron ML, Szpalski M, Nordin M, et al. Sociocultural factors and back pain: a population-based study in Belgian adults. *Spine* 1994;19:129–137.
81. Snook SH, Ciriello VM. The design of manual handling tasks: revised tables of maximum acceptable weights and forces. *Ergonomics* 1991;34:1197–1213.
82. Spangfort EV. The lumbar disc herniation: A computer-aided analysis of 2,504 operations. *Acta Orthop Scand Suppl* 1972;142:1–95.
83. Svensson H, Andersson GBJ. The relationship of low-back pain, work history and work environment, and stress: a retrospective cross-sectional study of 38- to 64-year old women. *Spine* 1989;14:517–522.
84. Toroptsova NV, Benevolenskaya LI, Karyakin AN, et al. Cross-sectional study of low back pain among workers at an industrial enterprise in Russia. *Spine* 1995;20:328–332.
85. Valkenburg HA, Haanen HCM. The epidemiology of low back pain. In: White AA III, Gordon SL, eds. *Symposium on idiopathic low back pain*. St. Louis: Mosby–Year Book, 1982:9–22.
86. Vascancelos D. Compression fractures of the vertebra during major epileptic seizures. *Epilepsia* 1973;14:323–328.
87. Videman T, Battié MC. The influence of occupation on lumbar degeneration. *Spine* 1999;24:1164–1168.
88. Videman T, Nurminen T, Tola S, et al. Low-back pain in nurses and some loading factors of work. *Spine* 1984;9:400–404.
89. Videman T, Nurminen M, Troup JD. Lumbar spinal pathology in cadaveric material in relation to history of back pain, occupation and physical loading. *Spine* 1990;15:728–740.
90. Videman T, Sarna S, Battié MC, et al. The long-term effects of physical loading and exercise lifestyles on back-related symptoms, disability and spinal pathology among men. *Spine* 1995;20:699–709.
91. Videman T, Simonen R, Usenius J, et al. The long-term effects of rally driving on spinal pathology. *Clin Biomech* 2000;15:83–86.
92. Walsh K, Varnes N, Osmond C, et al. Occupational causes of low back pain. *Scand J Work Environ Health* 1989;15:54–59.
93. Waters TR, Putz-Anderson V, Garg A, et al. Revised NIOSH equation for the design and evaluation of manual lifting tasks. *Ergonomics* 1993;36:749–776.

94. Wickström BO, Kjellberg A, Landström U. Health effects of long-term occupational exposure to whole-body vibration: a review. *Int J Ind Ergonomics* 1994;14:273–292.
95. Wilke HJ, Neef P, Caimi M, et al. New in vivo measurements of pressures in the intervertebral disc in daily life. *Spine* 1999;24:755–762.
96. Wilke HJ, Wolf S, Claes LE, et al. Influence of varying muscle forces on lumbar intradiscal pressure: an in vitro study. *J Biomech* 1996;29:549–555.
97. Yasukawa Y. Age changes in the lumbar spine: radiological follow-up studies over more than ten years. *Nippon Seikeigeka Gakkai Zasshi* 1994;68:854–863.

6
Disc Degeneration and Segmental Instability

Tommy Hansson

Faculty of Medicine, Sahlgrenska Academy; and Department of Orthopedics, Sahlgren University Hospital, Göteborg, Sweden

Several pathomechanical consequences of severe disc degeneration are well established. However, several conditions related to disc degeneration are still controversial or less well defined. Segmental instability is one such entity, long discussed but still questioned as an objective (i.e., possible to define and diagnose properly) and therefore specific cause of back pain.

This chapter presents and discusses the results of experimental studies performed in an *in vivo* pig model, in addition to those of experimental and clinical studies carried out in healthy volunteers and patients. To be able to study segmental instability resulting from disc degeneration in an *in vivo* experimental model, several prerequisites must be fulfilled.

Because the problem to be studied is a consequence of disc degeneration, an appropriate way to create disc degeneration must be found. Presently, several chemical or mechanical methods are available for experimentally inducing disc degeneration *in vivo*. A method mimicking human disc pathology as closely as possible should be used. Another question that arises when an experimental model is used *in vivo* is how to impose realistic and adequate loading on the degenerate disc.

The next problem in the study of segmental instability is to find a method for measuring instability—that is, the pathologic motion possible in the degenerate intervertebral joint.

The last, but not the least, problem is identical for all types of experimental models. The experimentally obtained results must be validated in humans. Otherwise, the experimental results will remain as such and be of little or no use to patients with back pain.

Segmental instability of the human spine has long been considered an objective and specific reason for low back pain. Despite the fact that both definitions and detailed explanatory pathomechanical models have been proposed, many more questions than answers still remain in the ongoing "instability" debate.

For long, it has been assumed that certain pathologic conditions in the human lumbar spine manifest as abnormal motion between the separate vertebrae. Also, it has been assumed that radiographic techniques can be used to diagnose and measure such pathologic motion (10,12).

Proof of instability has been sought especially as an excessive anteroposterior translation in the sagittal plane, seen predominantly on flexion–extension radiographs. Although many have tried with radiographic studies, no one has conclusively been able to relate abnormal motion to a specific back problem. There are several explanations for this:

- Accurate and standardized measurement techniques are lacking.
- Normal motion is not adequately defined.
- Motion varies widely between different subjects and different spinal levels.
- Perhaps most importantly, if cine radiography not is used, radiography is a static measurement device.

For that reason, plain x-ray techniques can reveal only abnormal motions occurring at the endpoints of, for example, a flexion–extension motion.

Movements such as flexion–extension in the lumbar spine are directed by an intrinsic neuromuscular system that involves passive structures (e.g., intervertebral discs, ligaments, bones) and active structures (e.g., muscles and their tendons inclusive). A disorder or injury may disturb the neuromuscular balance and cause dysfunction, pain, or both. In subjects with a healthy back, flexion–extension is a pain-free movement accomplished by appropriately timed excitation of all the involved muscles.

Several studies have demonstrated a spontaneous reduction in the myoelectric activity of the erector spinae muscles during the deeper part of flexion of the lumbar spine (2), referred to as a *flexion–relaxation phenomenon*. It has been suggested that muscular activity is shut off by signals from receptors in the spinal ligaments stimulated through stretching of the ligaments during deep trunk flexion (11). The results of more recent studies indicate that this explanation of the decrease in muscular activity occurring during deep flexion of the lumbar spine is the most plausible one (5).

Among the many structures stretched during deep flexion are the facet joint capsules, which are known to contain proprioceptors (2). Experimental studies in our pig model have also demonstrated that stretching of the joint capsules elicits inhibitory responses in the lumbar paraspinal muscles (1).

It is reasonable to assume that structures such as the discs, posterior ligaments, and fascia, in addition to stretched but electrically silent muscles, provide stability during the flexion–relaxation period (2). Furthermore, it has been shown that the more lateral lumbar muscles (quadratus lumborum and iliocostalis) are activated, whereas the more medial muscles (multifidus) are inactivated during deep and progressive flexion (1). In other words, the spine is guarded not only by passive structures during deep flexion but also by muscles, although more laterally located than previously thought.

The absence of flexion–relaxation is a common finding in patients with chronic low back pain. Because continuous back muscle activity during deep trunk flexion has been found to be closely correlated with ongoing pain, the presence of this phenomenon can be used as an indicator of pain. It seems reasonable to assume that the absence of flexion–relaxation is an indicator of current back pain, irrespective of whether the problem is acute, subacute, or chronic in nature.

EXPERIMENTAL DISC DEGENERATION

Pigs 6 to 8 months old were used as the animal models. All experiments were performed on anesthetized animals. Disc degeneration was induced by making a 15-mm-deep incision with a No. 11 scalpel blade into the anterolateral part of the annulus fibrosus of the L3–4 disc. Three months later, when pronounced disc degeneration had developed, loading exper-

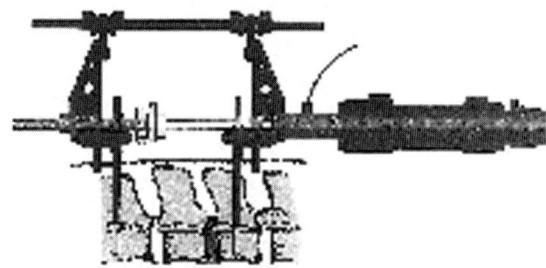

FIG. 6.1. The degenerate disc is loaded *in vivo* with a servohydraulic testing device; this allows testing under either force or displacement control at frequencies of up to more than 30 Hz.

iments were performed. The properties of the degenerate disc were compared with those of nondegenerate discs at the same level, L3–4, from other animals.

For loading the intact and degenerate discs *in vivo*, a specially developed miniature servohydraulic testing device was used (3). It allows loading under force or displacement control at frequencies up to higher than 30 Hz.

The loading device is rigidly fixed to the spine through four intrapedicular screws inserted into each pedicle of the L3 and L4 vertebrae. The screw is driven into the vertebral body and close to its anterior cortex (Fig. 6.1).

The compression induced by the device is an arch-type movement rather than a straight axial motion. When small motions are used, as in these experiments, the differences in loading direction are negligible from a mechanical standpoint. No other coupled forces are induced by the device, which means that the vertebrae are free to rotate, shear, and bend (3,4).

In comparison with the intact L3–4 disc, the degenerate disc was considerably stiffer when loaded once or repeatedly, indicating the profoundly changed properties of a degenerate disc.

Kinematics of the Intervertebral Joint

To measure motion in the vertebral joint, a special device, the intervertebral motion device (IMD), was developed. This device is rigidly fixed to the vertebrae through metal pins inserted approximately 20 mm into the spinous processes of two adjacent vertebrae (8) (Fig. 6.2). The IMD consists of a linkage transducer system that allows dynamic measurement of the sagittal plane. The system is highly repeatable and has an accuracy [root mean square (RMS) error] of 0.4 degrees and 0.14 mm for rotation and translation movements, respectively. Three displacement transducers detect motion occurring between the pins during flexion–extension (Fig. 6.3).

When the IMD is used to measure motions in a human spinal segment, a goniometer is usually used simultaneously to measure total trunk flexion–extension.

Intervertebral Motion Patterns

Pilot studies with the IMD in patients with assumed segmental instability indicated that total flexion–extension motion in the tested intervertebral joint was usually very small (e.g., axial translation was much greater and discriminative). This finding made us believe that the *pattern of motion* was of greater interest than just the achieved angle at the end of a motion.

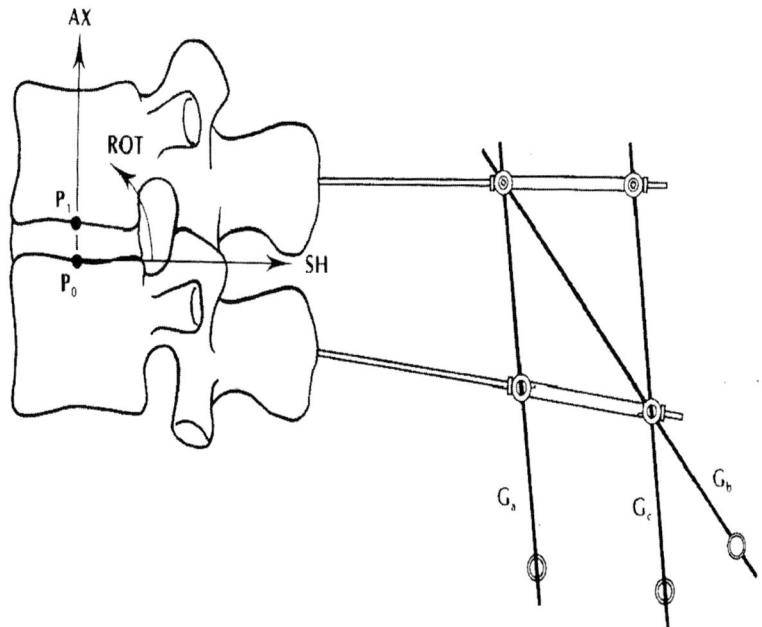

FIG. 6.2. A schematic view of the intervertebral motion device used to measure the dynamic motions between separate vertebrae *in vivo*.

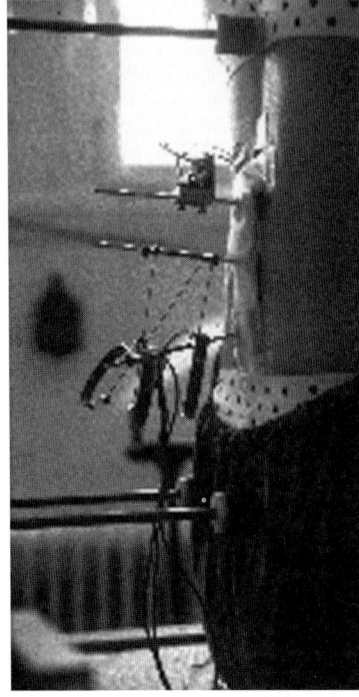

FIG. 6.3. The intervertebral motion device fixed to the spinous processes of L3 and L4 in a patient.

Experimental Injuries and Pattern of Motion in the Intervertebral Joint

To understand better the *pattern of motion* we found in subjects with assumed segmental instability, we had to use an experimental model that simulated the alterations in segmental kinematics that we had detected in the degenerate human intervertebral joint (7). Once again, the pig model was used. With the animal lying prone, one of the following types of injury was created in the L3–4 disc or facet joints.

1. *Disc annulus lesion.* From a left-sided retroperitoneal approach, we used a scalpel blade to make an approximately 12-mm stab incision into the middle part of the anterior annulus fibrosus without penetrating the nucleus.
2. *Disc nucleus lesion.* A 15-mm stab incision was made through the middle part of the anterior annulus of the disc, parallel to the endplates, that penetrated the nucleus pulposus.
3. *Facet capsule lesion.* Using a dorsal approach, we made bilateral central incisions through the collagen capsule of the facet joints into the synovial joint.
4. *Facet joint slit lesion.* We made 2-mm-wide slits bilaterally along the facet joints, removing on both sides the cartilage that covers the surfaces of the articular processes.
5. *Facet joint wedge lesion.* Portions of the superior and inferior articular processes were removed bilaterally to create a wedge gap approximately 3 to 4 mm wide across the joint.
6. *Sham lesion.* The animals in the sham group (n =10) underwent the same standard surgical procedures as the other animals, but without injuries to the L3–4 intervertebral joint (6,7).

Three months after injury, the animals were once again anesthetized and placed on a special table allowing flexion–extension motions of the spinal levels studied. The IMD was applied over the L3–4 level to determine the pattern of motion. The effects of muscular contraction were also examined through bipolar electrodes placed bilaterally around the multifidus and longissimus thoracis at the L2 and L5 vertebral levels. An intense contraction along the paraspinal muscles was achieved by stimulating repetitive pulses with square voltage (6,7). A goniometer placed to the animal measured the global flexion–extension angle.

The kinematic behavior of the spinal motion segment can differ in the loading and unloading phases (e.g., going into and returning from full flexion). In Figure 6.4, such behavior is shown for axial translation in a flexion–extension motion cycle. In this study, we referred to such behavior as *hysteresis*. It is manifested as an opening in the curve throughout the motion cycle (Fig. 6.4).

Depending on the type of injury, the degenerative changes in the disc and facet joints varied. The kinematic behavior differed between injury types but was highly reproducible within each group. The type of injury affects the pattern of motion.

These studies showed that degenerative changes in the lumbar spine similar to those seen in humans develop within 3 months after a disc injury has been created. A pattern of motion typical of injury could be seen when a dynamic measuring technique (IMD) was used. It was also evident that the maximum range of motion is a more sensitive parameter of alterations in segmental kinematics than is the end range of motion. Axial translation—not, as supposed, sagittal rotation or shear translation—was the translation direction that showed the most change after experimental injuries and disc degeneration had been created. The disc annulus lesion, facet joint wedge lesion, and facet capsule lesion were, in that order, the injuries that most influenced axial translation. The ability of the

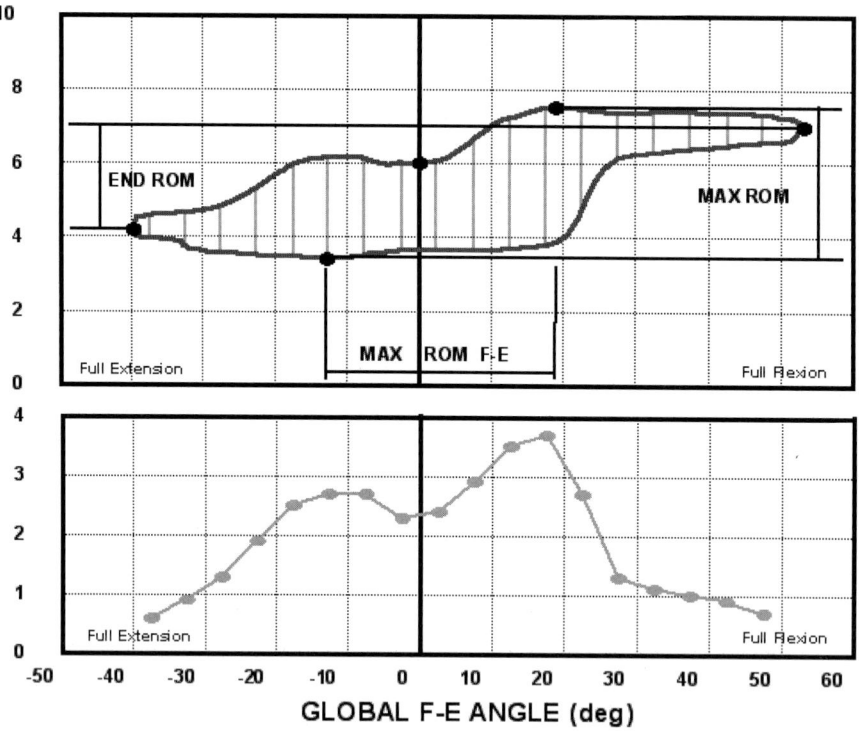

FIG. 6.4. The motion pattern (axial translation) between two vertebrae in the pig spine. The separation of the two curves (*curve in bottom graph*) marks the "hysteresis"—that is, the difference (axial translation) that occurs between flexion and extension of the spine.

paraspinal muscles to provide stability in a chronically changed motion segment was seriously reduced (7).

PATTERN OF MOTION IN PATIENTS WITH ASSUMED SEGMENTAL INSTABILITY

The pattern of motion, muscular activity, and overall trunk motion were determined during dynamic flexion–extension in seven patients with chronic low back pain. Their pain was supposedly caused by changes that might affect the stability of at least one intervertebral joint in the lumbar spine. The supposed diagnosis of segmental instability was based on a history of pain, the clinical findings, and pronounced radiographic changes in at least one of the following intervertebral joints: L2–3, L3–4, L4–5, or L5–S1. The history of pain included sudden episodes of stabbing pain, especially during certain movements of the spine and typically when the spine was not "guarded." The patients also had difficulty flexing the lumbar spine or rising from a flexed position. In all the patients, at least two of the four following radiographic criteria were identified at the suspected level:

1. Anteroposterior translation of more than 3 mm on lateral view static standing radiographs
2. Angulated disc space collapse accompanied by translation of the affected vertebra on flexion–extension radiographs

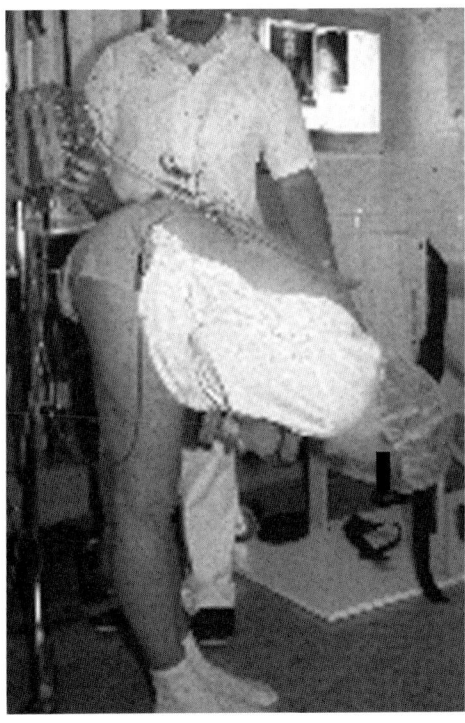

FIG. 6.5. Testing trunk motion and pattern of motion in a patient with suspected "instability" at level L3–4.

3. Pronounced disc space narrowing (decrease of disc height of more than 50% in comparison with the nearest disc of normal height)
4. Apparent traction spurs on both sides of the disc

In all but one patient, just one intervertebral joint was supposedly unstable. In the other patient, two segments were possibly unstable. Both levels were studied in this patient (9).

The suspected levels were three L2–3, two L3–4, and three L4–5. Two adjacent motion segments were studied in half of the controls.

By means of continuous measuring techniques, the muscular behavior could be precisely defined in relation to segmental motion throughout the flexion–extension movement that the subjects performed (Fig. 6.5). An identical protocol was used in six volunteers (control group) without back problems, at least not recently.

The group of patients consisted of four men and three women (mean age, 51.4 years; range, 46 to 56 years). The control group comprised three men and three women (mean age, 40.5 years; range, 38 to 48 years) (9).

Intervertebral Motion Device in Humans

Steinmann pins (2.6 mm in diameter) were rigidly fixed under surgical conditions to the neighboring spinous processes on the actual vertebral level. The IMD was then secured to the pins (Fig. 6.3). In the subjects in whom two segments were tested, the caudal motion segment was tested first (9).

The trunk flexion–extension angle was simultaneously measured during the flexion–extension protocol with a potentiometric goniometer attached to the side of the subject's upper right arm.

During testing, the subject was instructed to hold the arms and hands firmly against the chest and to maintain a constant position during flexion–extension.

Electromyographic Recording

The electromyographic (EMG) activity of the lumbar erector spinae muscles was recorded during flexion–extension from two sets of surface electrodes placed bilaterally at the L3–4 interspace and 3 cm lateral to the spinous process. Signals from the lumbar part of the longissimus thoracis lumbar fibers were recorded.

Flexion–Extension Movement

When performing the flexion–extension protocol, the subjects were asked to maintain sagittal plane symmetry of the body. Beginning from an erect standing posture, the subject bent forward as deeply as possible. The direction of movement was then reversed so that the subject passed through the neutral position and continued until maximum extension was reached, finally returning to the neutral position.

Kinematics in the Experimental Clinical Study

For all three kinematic variables (sagittal rotation, axial translation, and shear translation), the range of motion was significantly *less*, by at least 50%, among the patients than among the controls. The controls also flexed and extended their trunk more than the patients did. As in the animal models, the maximum range of motion did not necessarily occur at the endpoints, which is why the maximum range was not always equal to the end range of motion. This was especially pronounced for axial translation and more for the patients than for the controls.

Many differences in the pattern of motion were observed between the patients and the controls. Overall, the patients displayed *less* intervertebral motion than the controls did, especially in flexion. Even the axial translation motion was less in the patients (9).

Electromyographic Behavior

In the controls, the EMG activity increased to a maximum during forward flexion. After the maximum, a progressive decrease in myoelectric activity occurred to full trunk flexion (i.e., flexion–relaxation phenomenon). From full flexion, the EMG activity increased dramatically to a maximum and then decreased to practically no activity in full extension (Fig. 6.6).

In the patients, the EMG activity increased, but not as much or to a peak value as in the controls. This meant that no flexion–relaxation occurred. From full flexion, the pattern in the patients was similar to that in the controls.

In this study, intervertebral motion was significantly less, by at least 50%, in the patients with chronic low back pain of an assumed specific type, segmental instability. Trunk flexion and extension were also significantly reduced in the patients. In the control group, flexion–relaxation was demonstrated by a 78% increase in EMG activity. On the other hand, most of the patients demonstrated absolutely no flexion–relaxation. Flexion–relaxation in the controls occurred in those in whom intervertebral rotation had reached a stage of completion before maximum trunk flexion was achieved (9).

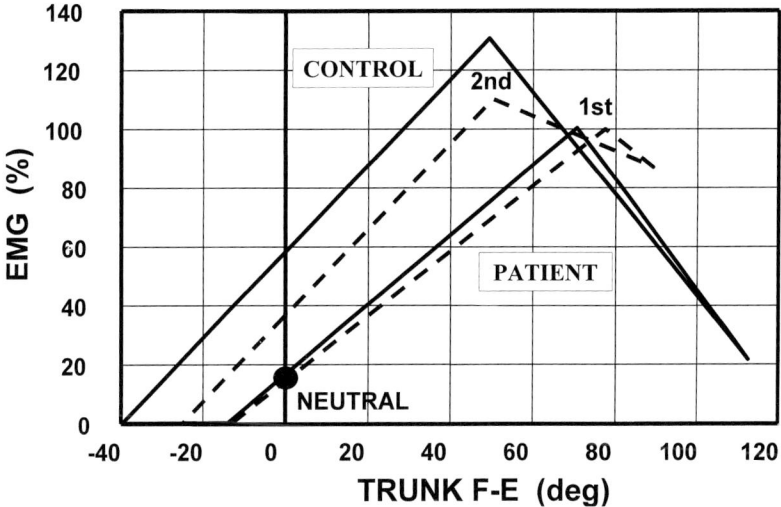

FIG. 6.6. Electromyographic (EMG) activity in patients and controls. Muscular activity remains higher in the patients than in the controls during flexion of the trunk.

CONCLUSIONS

These studies of experimental and clinical segmental instability yielded several unexpected results.

- Dynamic measurements demonstrated that the pattern of motion revealed more and other motions than have been found with static techniques.
- Specific experimental injuries to the intervertebral joint mimicking severe disc degeneration created a specific pattern of motion.
- Patients with "clinical segmental instability" demonstrated less motion than controls with healthy backs in all directions of recorded motions.
- The patients showed no flexion–relaxation.

Our results suggest that long-standing back muscle activity is more likely to be a cause of pain than increased motion.

REFERENCES

1. Andersson EA, Oddsson LI, Grundstrom H, et al. EMG activities of the quadratus lumborum and erector spinae muscles during flexion-relaxation and other motor tasks. *Clin Biomech* 1996;11:392–400.
2. Cavanaugh JM, Ozaktay AC, Yamashita HT, et al. Lumbar facet pain: biomechanics, neuroanatomy and neurophysiology. *J Biomech* 1996;29:1117–1129.
3. Hult E, Ekstrom L, Holm S, et al. HYOMEX: a miniature universal testing machine for *in vivo* biomechanical studies. *J Med Eng Technol* 1994;18:169–172.
4. Hult E, Ekstrom L, Kaigle A, et al. *In vivo* measurement of spinal column viscoelasticity—an animal model. *Proc Inst Mech Eng [H]* 1995;209:105–110; discussion 35.
5. Indahl A, Kaigle A, Reikeras O, et al. Electromyographic response of the porcine multifidus musculature after nerve stimulation. *Spine* 1995;20:2652–2658.
6. Kaigle AM, Holm SH, Hansson TH. Experimental instability in the lumbar spine. *Spine* 1995;20:421–430.
7. Kaigle AM, Holm SH, Hansson TH. 1997 Volvo Award in Biomechanical Studies. Kinematic behavior of the porcine lumbar spine: a chronic lesion model. *Spine* 1997;22:2796–2806.
8. Kaigle AM, Pope MH, Fleming BC, et al. A method for the intravital measurement of interspinous kinematics. *J Biomech* 1992;25:451–456.

9. Kaigle AM, Wessberg P, Hansson TH. Muscular and kinematic behavior of the lumbar spine during flexion-extension. *J Spinal Disord* 1998;11:163–174.
10. Kalebo P, Kadziolka R, Sward L. Compression-traction radiography of lumbar segmental instability. *Spine* 1990;15:351–355.
11. Sihvonen T, Partanen J, Hanninen O, et al. Electric behavior of low back muscles during lumbar pelvic rhythm in low back pain patients and healthy controls. *Arch Phys Med Rehabil* 1991;72:1080–1087.
12. Soini J, Antti-Poika I, Tallroth K, et al. Disc degeneration and angular movement of the lumbar spine: comparative study using plain and flexion-extension radiography and discography. *J Spinal Disord* 1991;4:183–187.

7

Internal Disc Disruption

Henry V. Crock

Department of Orthopedic Surgery, Imperial College of Science and Medicine, Hammersmith Hospital; and Spinal Disorders Unit, Cromwell Hospital, London, United Kingdom

During the last decade of the 20th century, extraordinary advances were made in the imaging technologies—magnetic resonance imaging (MRI), computed tomography (CT), and positron emission tomography (PET)—applied to the investigation of spinal disorders (4,14,17,21) (Fig. 7.1). Also, during this period, the production of new instruments and implants for spinal surgery increased dramatically, leading to the introduction of bewildering arrays of devices for use in spinal fixation. This surge in the production of instruments and implants heralded an era of mechanization of spinal surgery and fueled investment activities among venture capitalists. Toward the end of the century, minimally invasive surgical techniques involving the wider use of surgical microscopes, endoscopes, lasers, and heated wires for intradiscal electrotherapy were introduced (22).

While the accuracy of the diagnosis of disc prolapse increased, the range of surgical techniques used to treat this condition expanded to include percutaneous discectomy, microdiscectomy, and a variety of intradiscal enzyme injections; however, little consensus was reached regarding the indications for using the newly available methods (3,20). By contrast, clinical attitudes toward disc disorders other than disc prolapse changed very little as most practitioners continued to recognize only two entities—disc prolapses and disc degeneration.

Disc degeneration used to be defined by changes seen on plain radiographs of the spine: osteophyte formation on the margins of the vertebral bodies adjacent to the intervertebral discs, variations in the height of the disc space, and narrowing of the facet joints with associated osteophyte formation. The management of patients with disc degeneration remained largely influenced by long-established conventions holding that conservative treatment was usually effective and that surgery might be required only for the few patients with radiologic evidence of spinal instability or spinal stenosis.

Since MRI has been applied to the investigation of spinal disorders, a group of patients has been identified whose plain radiographic findings are normal but whose MR images show changes in the discs themselves, with loss of signal from the nucleus pulposus on T2-weighted sequences. The images are usually reported, in summary, as showing "disc degeneration."

The classification of disc degeneration has thereby been arbitrarily extended, with the implication that this MRI finding represents an early stage of disc pathology that will progress to the familiar features of disc degeneration seen on plain radiographs. Disc pro-

---

The copyright for this chapter is owned by the author.

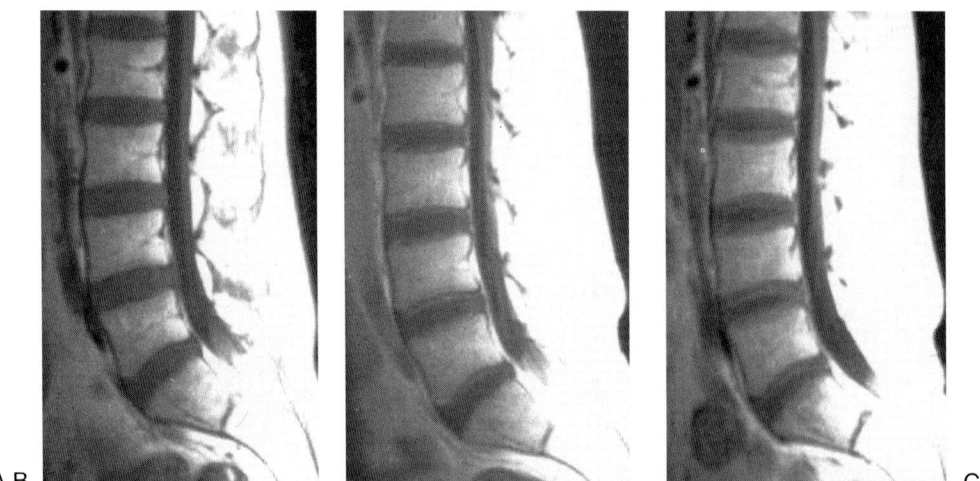

FIG. 7.1. Magnetic resonance images demonstrating the movement of solutes across the vertebral endplate capillary beds into the intervertebral discs in the lumbar spine in a normal subject precontrast **(A)**, 1 hour postcontrast **(B)**, and 4 hours postcontrast **(C)**. (From Bydder G. New approaches to magnetic resonance imaging of the intervertebral discs, tendons, ligaments and menisci. *Spine* 2002;27:1264–1268, with permission.)

lapse fits neatly into this scheme because it is the first of the mechanical disorders that may been seen in the natural course of the degenerative process. However, not all patients with "disc degeneration" identified by MRI progress to the traditionally predicted conditions of disc prolapse, vertebral instability, and spinal stenosis (18).

Two other clinically recognizable disc disorders are found among patients with spinal and limb pain. The first of these is internal disc disruption (IDD). The second is isolated disc resorption (IDR), in which changes on both MR images and plain radiographs include loss of disc height at a single level, sclerosis of the adjacent vertebral bodies, minimal osteophyte formation, a vacuum sign in the disc space, and bilateral facet joint subluxation (14). In IDR, the appearance of the other discs may remain normal on plain radiographs, even into the patient's late middle age. These two disorders produce distinctive syndromes that can be identified on clinical grounds and confirmed with appropriate investigations (7).

BACKGROUND

IDD is a condition marked by alterations in the internal structure and metabolic functions of one or more discs. The term *internal disc disruption* was first introduced in an article titled "A Reappraisal of Intervertebral Disc Lesions," published in the *Medical Journal of Australia* in 1970. Ideas about IDD grew, based on the retrospective analysis of the records of hundreds of patients treated during a period of 10 years who continued to experience disabling symptoms of spinal and limb pain following operations for suspected disc prolapse performed by a number of surgeons in Australia (7). One group of patients with similar features in their histories, investigations, and responses to surgery stood out; in nearly all of them, a specific episode of spinal trauma had preceded the onset of pain. Constitutional features of profound loss of energy and loss of body weight were prominent, and psychologic disturbances were common. Their problems had all been exacerbated by operations to remove suspected disc prolapses; some left the hospital complaining of worse pain than before the surgery, whereas others relapsed within a short time after surgery and a few underwent more than one similar procedure that rendered them progressively more disabled.

Preoperative investigations in this group relied on myelography before CT became widely used and long before MRI became available. Their myelograms, viewed retrospectively, often provided inconclusive evidence of disc prolapse. The value and importance of the use of discography in the further investigation of these disabled patients soon became apparent (16).

EVOLUTION OF THE SYNDROME

The clinical syndrome associated with this disorder usually follows trauma inflicted on the disc, either as the result of sudden and unexpected weight lifting or by forces transmitted through the disc or discs during high-speed accidents. It occurs commonly in heavy workers who have accidentally or suddenly lifted weights of up to 200 kg. For example, a meat worker may slip while carrying a heavy forequarter of beef, so that his or her lumbar spine is subjected to a massive compression load of short duration. Likewise, low back pain often develops in nurses after they accidentally assume unexpected loads while lifting disabled or unconscious patients. Therefore, the first essential in recognizing IDD is to obtain an accurate history of the mechanism of injury. Patients often fail to give an account of the mechanism of their injury, being more concerned with describing the severity of their back pain, which has the character of a deep-seated ache.

Limb pain of acute onset may be the initial complaint of patients with disc prolapse, whereas in those with IDD the pain develops more slowly, and they find it difficult to describe its character. Descriptions of pain deep inside the limb, with an intolerable aching quality, are common and contrast with descriptions of the intense, fluctuating, sharp pain of sciatica or brachial neuralgia secondary to disc prolapse, and of the slowly spreading, cramplike leg pain of spinal stenosis.

Patients with IDD also frequently describe feelings of heaviness and impending weakness in the affected limbs. The back pain becomes worse during several months after its onset; it is aggravated by activities of bending or lifting and by vigorous exercises prescribed by physical therapists. Profound loss of energy occurs, sometimes associated with significant loss of body weight, along with a range of psychologic disturbances.

MECHANISMS OF SYMPTOM PRODUCTION

The interpretation of the clinical characteristics of IDD is based on the theory that toxic catabolites pass out of the affected disc or discs via the vascular system of the vertebral bodies and perineural veins (8–11). These products of disc degeneration have two effects: first, adverse reactions in the regional nerves in and around the discs and in the spinal canal, and second, constitutional disturbances possibly mediated by the immune system. In adults, capillary beds in the vertebral endplate cartilages drain into a complex horizontal subarticular system of collecting veins in the vertebral bodies (11), which in turn drain into the main veins of the vertebral body and into the internal vertebral venous plexus in the spinal canal (Figs. 7.2, 7.3). Fluids moving into and out of a normal intervertebral disc flow through this complex vertebral vascular system, which accounts for the diurnal variations in the height of the intervertebral discs. The catabolic products of IDD act as nociceptors on the intradiscal nerve fibers and on the spinal nerves, which are

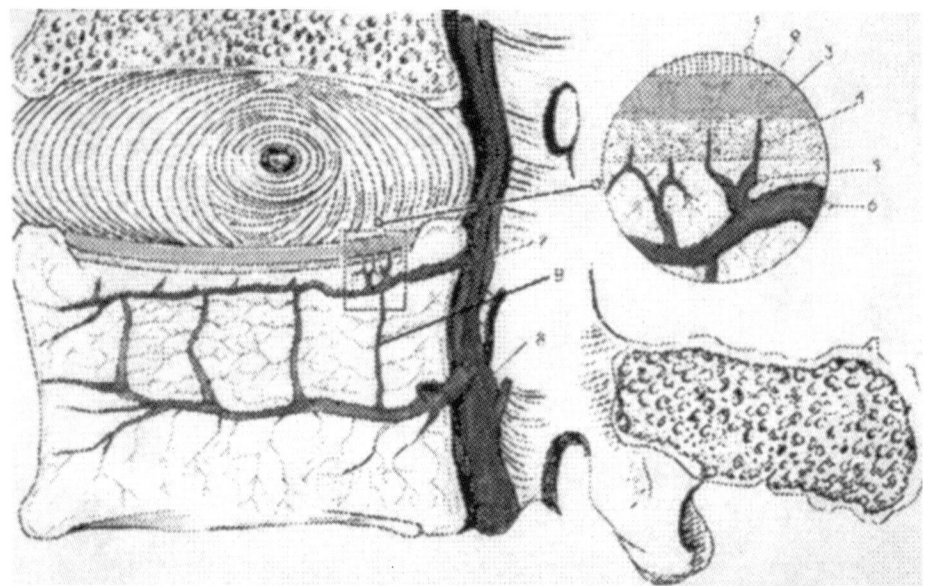

FIG. 7.2. A schematic drawing to show the spatial relationships of the veins of a typical vertebral body. *1*, intervertebral disc; *2*, capillary bed in vertebral endplate cartilage; *3*, subchondral postcapillary venous network on the vertebral endplate; *4*, vertebral endplate perforated by short vertebral venous tributaries; *5*, vertical tributaries from the subchondral postcapillary venous network draining to the horizontal subarticular collecting vein; *6*, horizontal subarticular collecting vein; *7*, horizontal subarticular collecting vein joining the anterior internal vertebral venous plexus; *8*, basilar–vertebral vein joining the anterior internal venous plexus; *9*, vertical tributary of the basilar–vertebral system of veins.

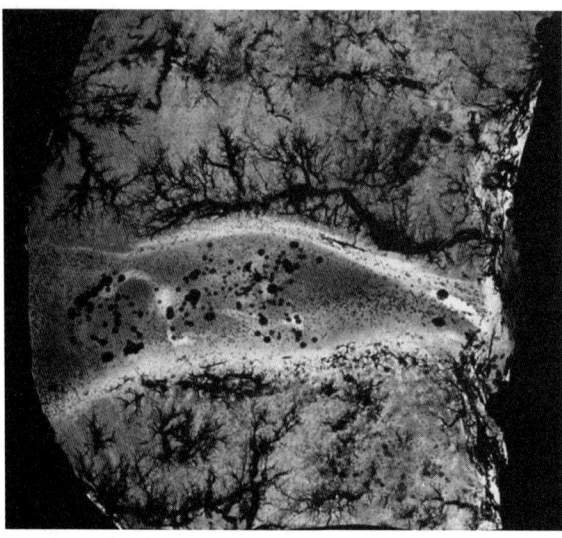

FIG. 7.3. A thin sagittal section from the lumbosacral junction of a 67-year-old woman showing the veins of the vertebral bodies. The Batson plexus can be seen in both vertebrae at the top and bottom of the specimen. The horizontal subarticular collecting vein can be seen coursing along the lower vertebral endplate of L5.

surrounded by the thin-walled veins of the internal vertebral venous plexus, causing spinal and limb pain.

Characteristically, the pain produced by IDD is made worse by activities that force more irritant fluid out of the affected disc or discs. Brickley-Parsons and Glimcher (2) have shown that the chemistry of collagen in the intervertebral discs is actively influenced by overall compressive loading.

Physical exercise may exacerbate spinal pain in patients with symptoms arising from spondylolisthesis or spinal osteoarthritis, but rest usually relieves the pain rapidly. Spinal supports often effectively control the spinal pain of these patients.

By contrast, patients with IDD react quite differently. Their pain resolves only slowly with rest and is often troublesome, even in bed. They rarely tolerate spinal bracing, perhaps because lumbar spinal supports increase the abdominal pressure and change the venous blood flow to the spine. This adverse reaction to lumbar bracing should be taken as an indication for spinal fusion in patients with IDD.

NEUROLOGIC SIGNS

Abnormal neurologic signs in the limbs are uncommon, although weakness, clumsiness, and sympathetic nervous system disturbances, such as a feeling of heat in the limb, are frequent. Because patients with IDD present with normal plain radiographs, normal CT scans, and no abnormal neurologic signs, these findings are often erroneously considered as absolute contraindications to surgical treatment.

PSYCHOLOGIC FACTORS

Some degree of psychologic disturbance is an accepted part of the clinical syndromes associated with a range of spinal disorders. In persons with IDD, this frequently assumes major importance. The diagnosis of the cause of their problems is often long delayed. As they pass through the hands of numerous doctors and paramedical practitioners, they soon realize that their symptoms are a mystery not only to themselves but also to their doctors and therapists. In many cases, after a so-called thorough investigation, when no cause has been found to explain the bizarre, persistent spinal and limb pain, it is concluded that the symptoms are "all in the patient's mind." This attitude leads to antagonism between the patient, relatives, and treating physician. The patients feel that their problems are being taken too lightly and that even their relatives have turned against them under the influence of the doctor's advice. Psychosexual difficulties may arise, leading to serious marital problems. Financial difficulties, resulting from an inability to work, add to their concerns, and eventually the whole fabric of their lives begins to disintegrate.

Mental depression is more often associated with IDD than with any of the other chronically painful spinal disorders. Acute psychotic disturbances, with mental confusion and aggressive violent behavior displayed following disc excision and anterior interbody fusion, have been reported in some cases (23).

The psychologic testing of patients with spinal and limb pain is an essential part of the preoperative studies that should be performed to establish a diagnosis and plan surgical treatment. In particular, observations of behavior during the course of physical examinations can be important in determining a patient's likely response to surgery (24).

In patients with IDD, psychologic factors must be considered in the context of the syndrome as a whole, with the sure knowledge that even major behavioral disturbances can be reversed after appropriate surgery. Without such an approach, these disabled patients may be denied access to the surgery that, in the present state of knowledge and practice, is most likely to cure them.

CHANGES IN BODY WEIGHT

Patients with lumbar disc prolapse are usually otherwise well, as are patients with many of the degenerative forms of spinal disorders that cause chronic back and limb pain, in whom weight loss does not occur. On the other hand, patients with infectious diseases and neoplasms of the spine are often obviously ill and exhibit weight loss.

Because mechanical and degenerative interpretations of disc disorders have so influenced the conventions of history taking, it is unusual to question patients with spinal pain about their body weight. Consequently, patients with IDD, despite numerous consultations with different doctors, may never have been asked about changes in their body weight. Vital clinical information will therefore have been overlooked.

In cases of IDD, weight loss ranging from a few to as many as 20 kg may occur within the first 3 to 4 months following the injury and onset of pain. Less often, patients will report a marked increase in their weight, which they usually relate to decreased physical activity.

LOSS OF ENERGY

Patients with this disc disorder nearly always experience profound fatigue after physical activities, which aggravate their spinal and limb pain. Parents of young adolescents with IDD often draw attention to this aspect of their child's symptoms.

INVESTIGATIONS

Plain Radiography

Investigations with plain radiography, myelography, epidurography, spinal venography, and ultrasonography are of no value in establishing this diagnosis.

Computed Tomography

CT performed after discography demonstrates an abnormal spread of dye in the disrupted disc in three planes and may serve to confirm the diagnosis of IDD.

Discography

In the past, discography has been the key investigation in the diagnosis of IDD (Fig. 7.4). Indications for the use of discography have been clearly defined by the North American Spine Society (19). Discography remains important where more than one lesion is demonstrated by MRI or when disagreement arises in the interpretation of the MRI findings. Ideally, discography should be performed by the patient's surgeon or by a radiologist who is familiar with the surgeon's notions of IDD and the indications for its treatment.

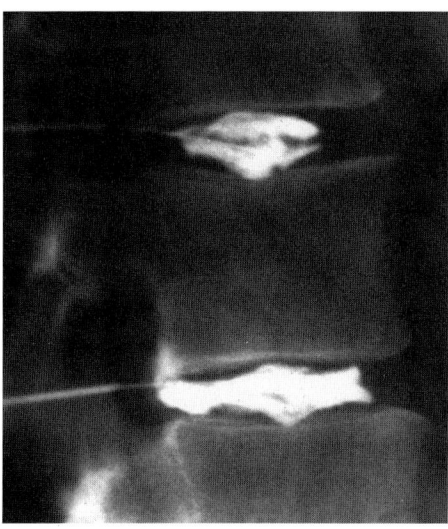

FIG. 7.4. A lateral radiograph of the lumbar spine of a 42-year-old truck driver, injured after heavy lifting, showing a normal disc at L1–2 and internal disc disruption at L2–3.

Discography reports should include three sets of information, as follows:

1. The *volume of dye* injected. Normal lumbar disc nuclei accept between 1.0 and 1.5 mL of dye; volumes in excess indicate IDD.
2. The *spread of dye* in the disc space as shown on anteroposterior and lateral x-ray films and on axial CT images.
3. The *character of pain* induced by the injection. The injection of dye into normal discs causes no pain. Patients with IDD experience pain within seconds after the start of the injection, well before a disrupted disc has been filled with 3 to 5 mL of dye. They describe the induced pain as being similar to their "usual pain" but often claim that it is more severe (25).

Discography may be followed by discitis. Discitis in a normal disc takes the form of localized vertebral endplate erosions on either side of the nucleus and causes excruciating spinal pain developing within 6 to 12 weeks after discography. In such cases, the injection of dexamethasone into the disc rapidly controls the pain (8).

Discitis in disrupted discs is more serious and may lead to vertebral osteomyelitis and epidural abscess formation. The incidence of this complication can be reduced by using stilleted needles; a 19-gauge needle is used to penetrate the skin, and a 22-gauge needle is passed through the "guide" needle to penetrate the disc. Another way to prevent discitis is to mix the radiopaque dye with a small volume of a broad-spectrum antibiotic before injecting it into the disc (12).

Magnetic Resonance Imaging

MRI has become the most important diagnostic test for IDD, largely replacing discography. MRI reports still often refer only to space-occupying defects in the spinal canal secondary to disc prolapse or to the loss of nuclear signal, described as "degenerative disc disease." In patients with IDD, changes are noted in the signals generated from the intervertebral discs and sometimes from within the adjacent vertebral bodies. Surgeons themselves should be confident in diagnosing IDD by MRI because this syndrome is not widely reported by radiologists. An exchange of ideas between spinal surgeons and radiologists is essential for the full value of MRI to become more widely realized in the diagnosis of IDD. Ideally, radiologists in training should spend some time in spinal clinics and in operating rooms with spinal surgeons to acquire first-hand knowledge of the range of clinical problems and the pathology seen at operation, so that they will be able to extend the usefulness of the imaging techniques at their disposal and provide more accurate reports to their colleagues.

SITES OF LESIONS

IDD occurs most commonly in the lower lumbar intervertebral discs, often at a single level. Upper lumbar lesions are rare but should be suspected in patients who experience high lumbar pain associated with abdominal discomfort

In the neck, the lesions generally occur at C5–6 or C6–7, although discs at higher levels are occasionally affected. IDD in the cervical spine may be the result of various mechanisms of injury, including whiplash. The symptom complex usually includes disabling occipitofrontal headache in addition to neck and arm pain and lethargy.

TREATMENT

Disc excision and anterior interbody spinal fusion are indicated for those patients with IDD who have become seriously disabled and who have failed to respond to routine conservative treatments administered during many months.

RESULTS

The overall results of the surgical procedure as the first operative intervention in patients with IDD are good in more than 80% of cases in which one disc is involved and in about 70% of cases with multiple-level involvement. Fujimaki et al. (13) analyzed the results in 75 male and 75 female patients who had undergone interbody fusion operations at 188 disc spaces. The age range of the patients was 19 to 62 years (mean, 41.6 years). Eighty-four of the patients had undergone this procedure as the first and only spinal operation, a second group of 38 patients had undergone previous spinal operations, and a third group of 28 patients had undergone supplementary operations for spinal canal decompression after interbody fusions. Most of the procedures for single-level fusions were at L5–S1, whereas most of the double-level fusions were at L4–5 and L5–S1.

The overall rate of radiologic fusion was 96%. Table 7.1 lists the results as measured by return to work.

Blumenthal et al. (1) studied 34 patients with no prior surgery who fulfilled the authors' criteria for IDD. Twenty-one (62%) of the patients were male, and the age range was 15 to 66 years (average, 36 years). The duration of symptoms ranged from 3 months to 10 years (average, 29.4 months). The levels fused were 19 (53%) at L5–S1, 11 (32%) at L4–5, and 5 (15%) at either L3–4 or L2–3.

The average duration of follow-up was 29 months. A successful result was defined by return to work or normal activities with no requirement for medication or just the occasional use of a nonsteroidal antiinflammatory agent. A satisfactory clinical outcome was achieved in 25 (74%) of the 34 patients, with an average time lost from work of 6.1 months.

TABLE 7.1. *Summary of findings*

Group	Occupation	No.	Time off (mo)	Resumed same occupation	Other occupation	Did not return to work
1	Nonsedentary	49	11.8	39	7	3
	Home duties	18	3.3	16	1	1
	Sedentary	17	7.4	17	0	0
	Total group 1	84				
2	Nonsedentary	23	24.0	14	6	3
	Home duties	7	5.6	6	0	1
	Sedentary	8	6.5	7	0	1
	Total group 2	38				
3	Nonsedentary	19	16.5	10	3	6
	Home duties	5	11.5	3	1	1
	Sedentary	4	12.5	2	0	2
	Total group 3	28				

From Fujimaki A, Crock HV, Bedbrook GM. The results of 150 anterior lumbar interbody fusion operations performed by two surgeons in Australia. *Clin Orthop* 1982;165:161–167, with permission.

The rate of fusion varied at different levels and was lower in patients who smoked. The rate of fusion was 55% at L4–5, reaching 100% at upper lumbar levels and 80% at L5–S1. Overall, the rate of union was 82% for nonsmokers and 63% for smokers. Clinical success did not correlate strictly with radiologic evidence of fusion or nonunion. In patients with a successful result, the union rate was 73%, whereas for those with nonunion, the success rate was 62.5%

Allograft was used in all but seven patients, although the rate of nonunion in the small number of patients with autograft was the same as in those treated by allograft. The reported complications in the first series were minimal and attributed to the extraperitoneal approach. Deep vein thrombosis occurred in 3%; infections and retrograde ejaculation were not quantified. Blumenthal et al. (1) reported one case of graft extrusion and one case of retrograde ejaculation.

These two series show that clinical success, measured by return to work, can be achieved in a significant number of patients who have IDD with the use of appropriate techniques of anterior interbody fusion (5,6,8,13,15) (Fig. 7.5).

REHABILITATION

Rehabilitation after anterior spinal fusion commences with mobilization a few days after surgery. The use of a bed that can be tilted to the vertical allows patients to stand comfortably within 24 hours after surgery and take a few steps away from the bed within 36 hours. Patients and their relatives should be informed of the likely time schedule of recovery. Even in an uncomplicated case, with fusion at a single level and performed within a relatively short time (4 to 6 months) after the onset of symptoms, full recovery is likely to take 6 to 9 months; a patient with multiple-level fusions may require 12 to 18 months. Only in exceptional cases can a patient return to work before 6 months from the time of operation.

Many of these patients have been injured at work and are pursuing claims for compensation. Follow-up medical examinations are usually carried out at the request of insurance companies by doctors who do not always contact the patient's treating team. The patients may be forced to perform spinal movements beyond the limits already achieved through

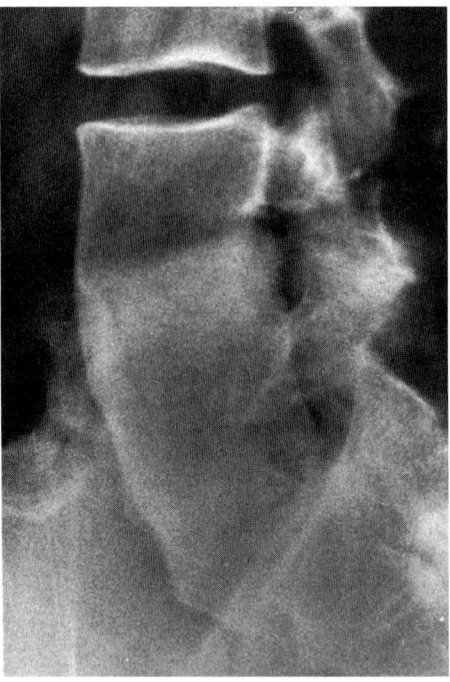

FIG. 7.5. A lateral radiograph showing L4–5 and L5–S1 interbody fusions (autogenous bone grafts) in a 48-year-old man 5 years after surgery.

carefully supervised physical therapy and may emerge from the encounter in severe pain and thoroughly demoralized. Their rehabilitation will thereby be set back many months.

CONCLUSIONS

Starting in the mid-1950s, general surgeons and cardiac surgeons, in pursuing their goal of performing organ transplants, established working relationships with scientists expert in physiology, pharmacology, and immunology, and with specialist physicians and radiologists and specially trained administrators. As a result, one of the great revolutions in patient care in the history of medicine—successful organ transplantation—has taken place.

Faced with the management of the widespread problem of spinal pain, spinal surgeons have yet to achieve the levels of successful treatment that their colleagues have reached with organ transplants. The blueprint for the path ahead that is most likely to lead to major improvements in the care of patients with spinal disorders of discal origin is available in the archives of the publications on organ transplantation.

Meanwhile, we should not forget the clinicians and surgeons of the past who made progress in treating serious diseases long before their scientific bases were identified. Kocher, for example, was awarded the Nobel Prize for Medicine in 1909 for his work on thyroid surgery. It was not until 5 years later that Kendall discovered thyroxin.

REFERENCES

1. Blumenthal SL, Baker J, Dossett A, et al. The role of anterior lumbar fusion for internal disc disruption. *Spine* 1988;13:566–569.
2. Brickley-Parsons D, Glimcher MJ. Is the chemistry of collagen in intervertebral discs an expression of Wolff's law? *Spine* 1984;9:148–163.

3. Brown MD. *Intradiscal therapy*. Chicago: Year Book, 1983:173.
4. Bydder G. New approaches to magnetic resonance imaging of the intervertebral discs, tendons, ligaments and menisci. *Spine* 2002;27:1264–1268.
5. Cauthen JC, ed. *Lumbar spine surgery*. Baltimore: Williams & Wilkins, 1983:225.
6. Cloward RB. Lesions of the intervertebral discs and their treatment by interbody fusion methods. *Clin Orthop* 1963;27:51–77.
7. Crock HV. A reappraisal of intervertebral disc lesions. *Med J Aust* 1970;1:983–989.
8. Crock HV, Bedbrook G. *Practice of spinal surgery*. New York: Springer-Verlag, 1983:319.
9. Crock HV, Goldwasser M, Yoshizawa H. Vascular anatomy related to the intervertebral disc. In: Ghosh P. ed. *The biology of the intervertebral disc*, vol 1. Boca Raton, FL: CRC Press, 1988:109–133
10. Crock HV, Yoshizawa H. *The blood supply of the vertebral column and spinal cord in man*. New York: Springer-Verlag, 1977:129.
11. Crock HV, Yoshizawa H, Kame SK. Observations on the venous drainage of the human vertebral body. *J Bone Joint Surg Br* 1973;55:528–533.
12. Fraser RD, Osti OL, Vernon-Roberts B. Discitis after discography. *J Bone Joint Surg Br* 1987;69:26–35.
13. Fujimaki A, Crock HV, Bedbrook GM. The results of 150 anterior lumbar interbody fusion operations performed by two surgeons in Australia. *Clin Orthop* 1982;165:161–167.
14. Jason MIV, ed. *The lumbar spine and back pain*. Edinburgh: Churchill Livingstone, 1987:463.
15. Lin P, Gill K, eds. *Lumbar interbody fusion*. Rockville, MD: Aspen Publishers, 1989:70.
16. Lindblom K. Diagnostic puncture of intervertebral disks in sciatica. *Acta Orthop Scand* 1948;17:231–239.
17. Modic MT, Masaryk TJ, Ross JS. *Magnetic resonance imaging of the spine*. Chicago: Year Book, 1989:280.
18. Morgan FP, King T. Primary instability of lumbar vertebrae as a common cause of low back pain. *J Bone Joint Surg Br* 1957;39:6–22.
19. North American Spine Society. Position statement on discography. *Spine* 1988;13:13–43.
20. Onik G, Helms CA, eds. *Automated lumbar discectomy*. San Francisco: Radiology Research and Education Foundation, 1988:111.
21. Rothman SLG, Glenn WV Jr. *Multiplanar CT of the spine*. Baltimore: University Park Press, 1985:520.
22. Saal JS, Saal JA. Management of chronic discogenic low back pain with a thermal intradiscal catheter. A preliminary report. *Spine* 2000; 25:382–388.
23. Stevenson HG. Back injury and depression. A medico-legal problem. *Med J Aust* 1970;1:1300–1302.
24. Waddell G, McCulloch JA, Kummel E, et al. Non-organic physical signs in low back pain. *Spine* 1980;5: 117–125.
25. Weinstein J, Claverie W, Gibson S. The pain of discography. *Spine* 1988;13:1344–1348.

8

Imaging of Degenerative Disc Disease

Jean-Louis Dietemann

Department of Radiology, University Louis Pasteur; Department of Radiology, University Hospital of Strasbourg, Strasbourg, France

Degenerative disc disease (DDD) comprises two interrelated but different processes: intervertebral osteochondrosis (affecting primarily the nucleus pulposus) and spondylosis deformans (affecting primarily the annulus fibrosus) (3,16,21). Intervertebral osteochondrosis is related to progressive dehydration, particularly in the nucleus pulposus, secondary to the degradation of proteoglycans and the development of a cleft within the annulus, leading to a loss of height of the intervertebral disc with bulging of the outer fibers of the annulus fibrosus. Simultaneously, degeneration involves the adjacent endplates, with thinning and rupture of the cartilaginous endplate and alteration of the subchondral bone. Spondylosis deformans is related to an initial alteration within the annulus fibrosus. Rupture of the peripheral fibers of the annulus fibrosus, including the Sharpey fibers, allows anterior displacement of disc material, inducing displacement and stretching of the anterior longitudinal ligament; the initial development of osteophytes is located at the site of the vertebral attachment of the ligament and progresses to the level of the edge of the vertebral body (16).

DDD is usually associated with apophyseal joint osteoarthritis, uncovertebral arthrosis, spondylolisthesis, retrolisthesis, and instability leading to central canal, radicular canal, and foraminal stenosis. Plain films clearly identify DDD; however, computed tomography (CT), magnetic resonance imaging (MRI), and sometimes myelography are required for the evaluation of nerve root and spinal cord compression. In rare cases, DDD may be difficult to differentiate from infectious discitis or rheumatoid arthritis.

PLAIN FILMS

Lateral, frontal, and oblique plain films demonstrate disc space narrowing, vacuum phenomenon (Knuttson phenomenon), reactive sclerosis of the vertebral bodies, Schmorl nodes, and osteophytes (anterior and lateral in the lumbar and thoracic spine, anterior and posterior with uncovertebral hypertrophy in the cervical spine) (Fig. 8.1); DDD is located mainly in the lower lumbar and middle cervical spine. In contrast, degenerative disc calcification and Schmorl nodes are located in the lower thoracic and upper lumbar spine. The height of the disc space increases progressively between L1 and L5; normal height of the L5–S1 disc space ranges between 4 and 5 mm; in cases of sacralization of L5, the disc space appears reduced but without dehydration on T2-weighted MRI. Loss of signal on T2-weighted images involving the nucleus pulposus precedes disc height decrease as observed on plain radiographs (9).

Intradiscal gas (nitrogen) is identified in 20% of elderly patients and is accentuated in spinal extension and reduced in spinal flexion; negative intradiscal pressure explains the gas formation (3). Osteophytes differ from traction spurs located 2 mm above the vertebral body edge, indicative of instability (12) (Fig. 8.1).

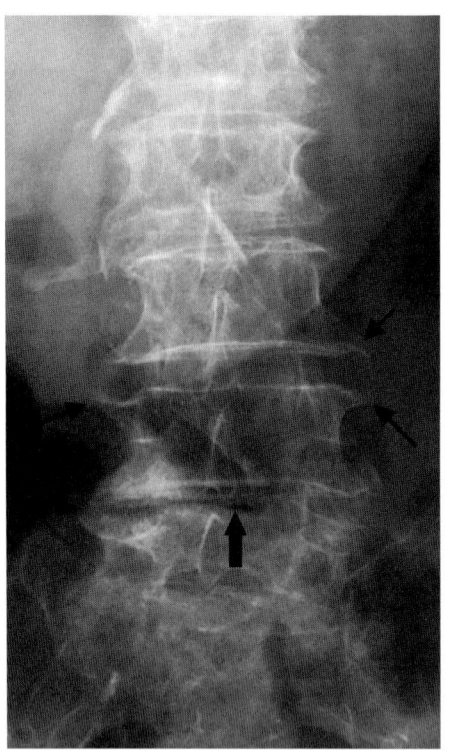 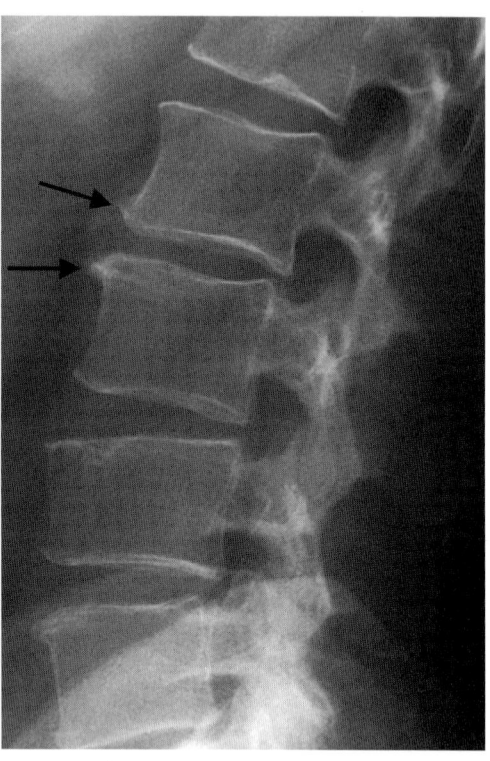

FIG. 8.1. A,B: Frontal **(A)** and lateral lumbar **(B)** plain radiographs of degenerative disc disease. Osteophytes *(arrows)* and vacuum phenomenon *(large arrow)* are noted on the frontal view **(A)**. Traction spurs *(arrows)* are demonstrated on the lateral view **(B)**.

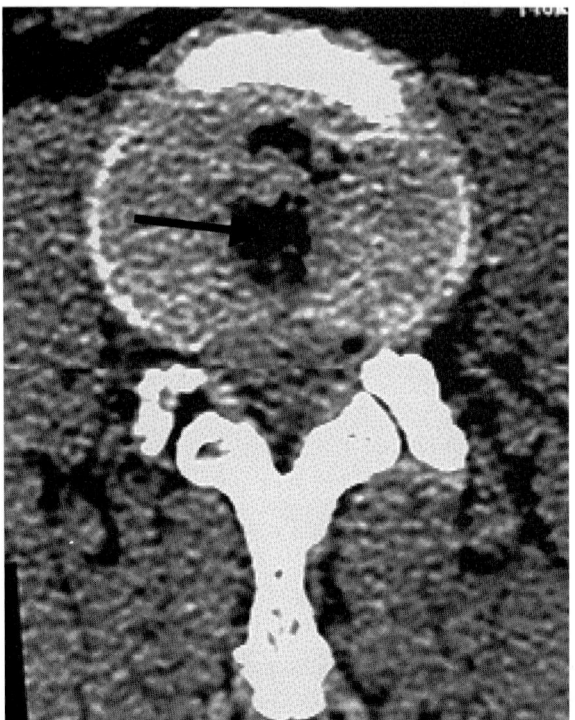 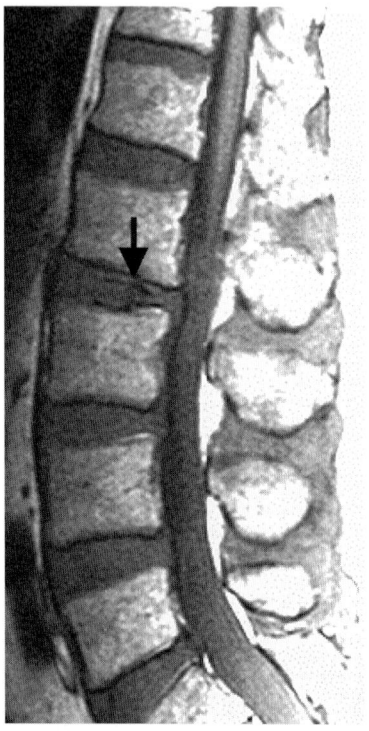

FIG. 8.2. A,B: Vacuum phenomenon *(arrows)* demonstrated on axial computed tomographic scan **(A)** and sagittal T1-weighted lumbar magnetic resonance image **(B)**.

COMPUTED TOMOGRAPHY

High-resolution multislice CT is more sensitive for demonstrating vacuum phenomenon, disc calcification, and subchondral osteosclerosis, particularly on sagittal and frontal re-formations (Fig. 8.2). The diffuse bulging disc is clearly demonstrated on axial scans and sagittal re-formations (Fig. 8.3). Spondylolysis deformans with degen-

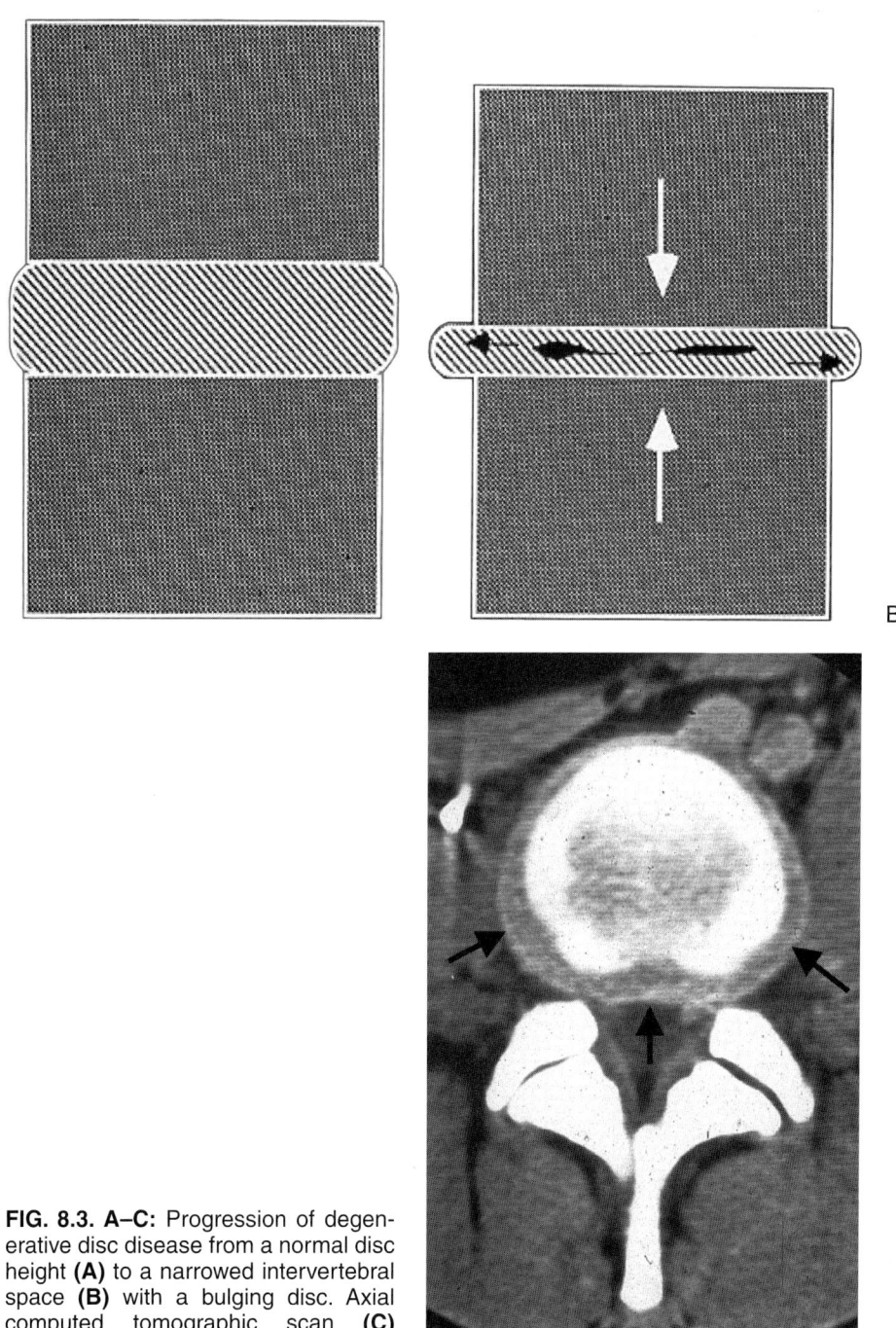

FIG. 8.3. A–C: Progression of degenerative disc disease from a normal disc height **(A)** to a narrowed intervertebral space **(B)** with a bulging disc. Axial computed tomographic scan **(C)** demonstrates bulging disc *(arrows)*.

erative lumbar scoliosis leads to transverse displacements, spondylolisthesis, retrolisthesis, and anterior and anterolateral protrusion of disc material and osteophytes. Anterior and lateral osteophytes do not cause nerve root compression (Fig. 8.4). Large lateral osteophytes are observed in patients with lumbar scoliosis. Only posterolateral and uncovertebral osteophytes may compress nerve roots. Disc calcifications related to DDD are usually located in the annulus fibrosus (Figs. 8.5, 8.6). The differential diagnosis of degenerative disc calcifications includes acromegaly, amyloidosis, alkaptonuria, hemochromatosis, hyperparathyroidism, and calcium pyrophosphate dihydrate crystal deposition disease (3). Weakening of the endplate and subchondral bone related to osteochondrosis leads to cartilaginous Schmorl nodes, which appear as a round radiolucent lesion with a rim of bone sclerosis on CT (Fig. 8.7); gas may be present within the lesion.

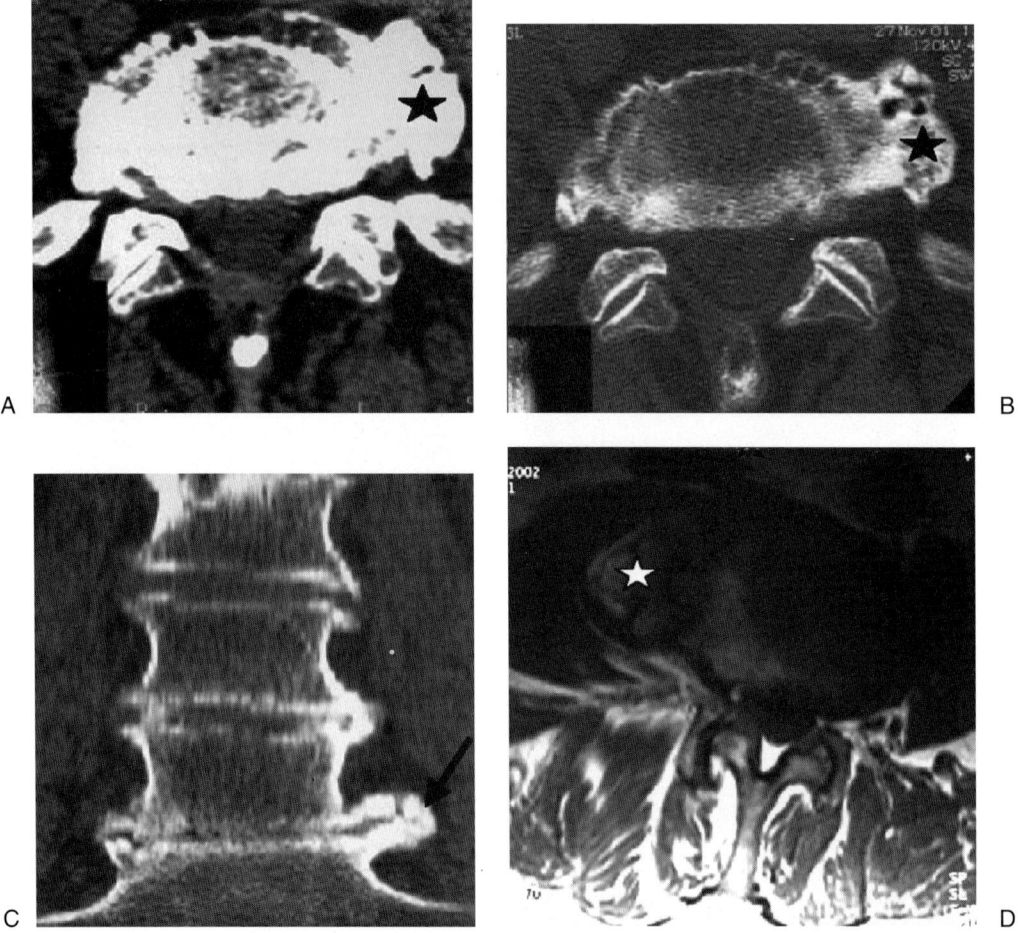

FIG. 8.4. A–D: Large lateral osteophytes *(stars)* of the lower lumbar spine demonstrated on computed tomographic scan **(A–C)** and axial T1-weighted magnetic resonance image **(D)**.

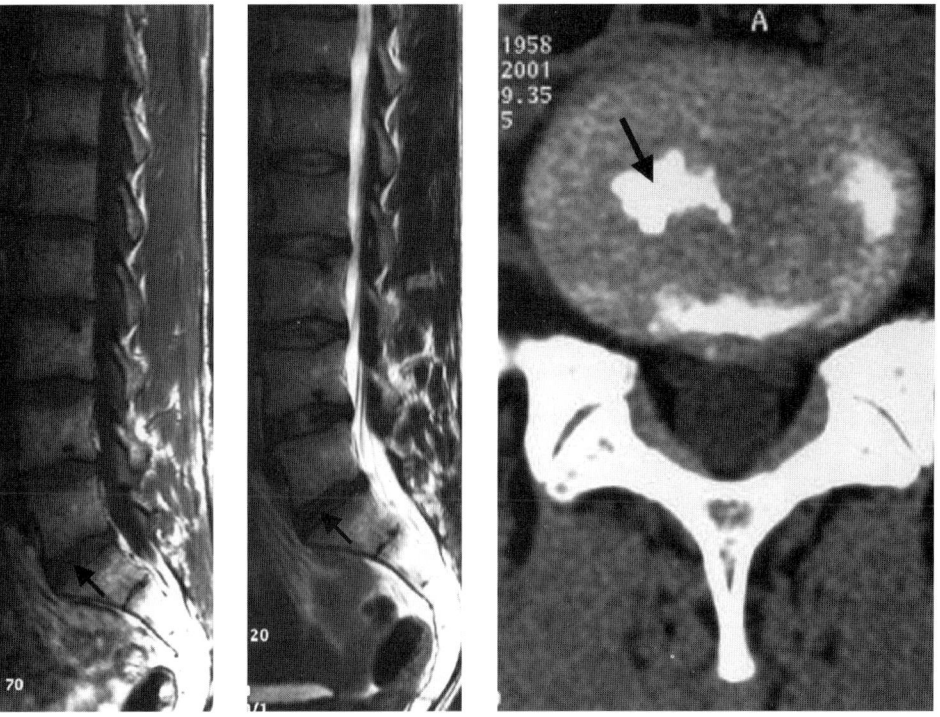

FIG. 8.5. A–C: Calcification of the L5–S1 disc. T1-weighted **(A)** and T2-weighted **(B)** sagittal magnetic resonance images show the calcification as a hypointense intradiscal zone *(arrows)*. The calcifications appear clearly on the axial computed tomographic scan **(C)** *(arrows)*.

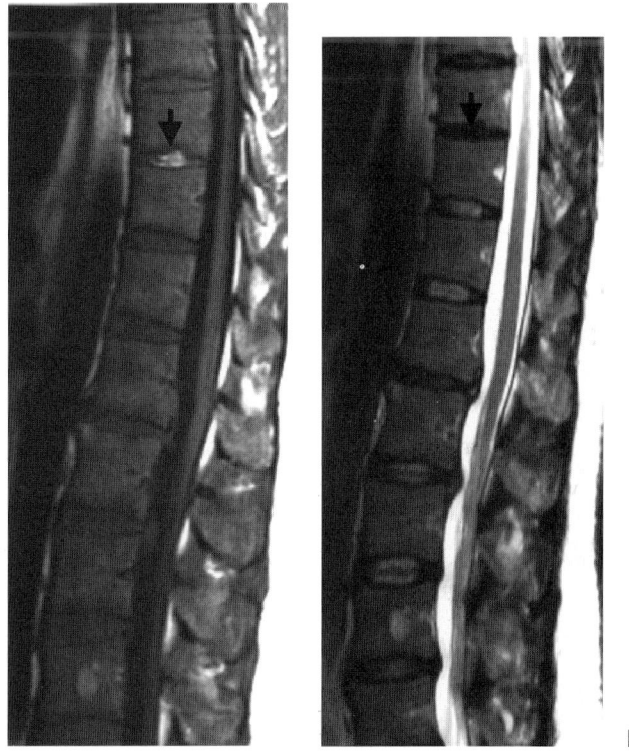

FIG. 8.6. A,B: Hyperintense discal calcification on T1-weighted magnetic resonance image **(A)** *(arrow)*; the same calcified disc appears hypointense on T2-weighted image **(B)** *(arrow)*.

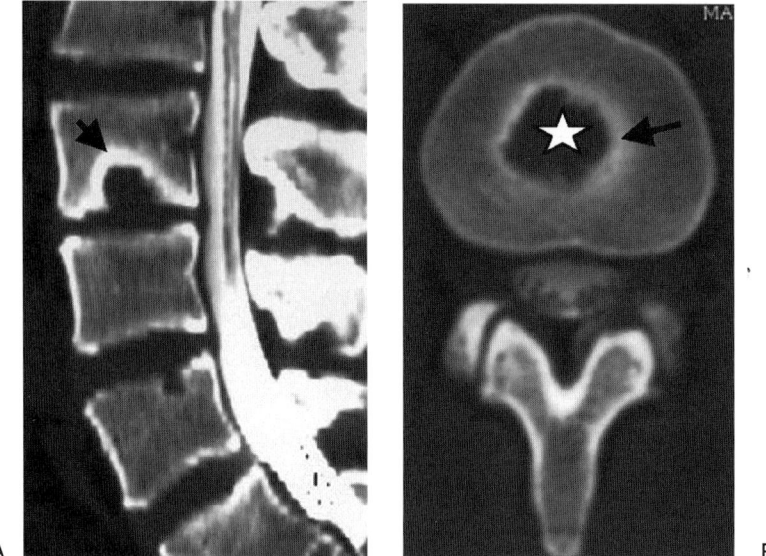

FIG. 8.7. A,B: Cartilaginous Schmorl node appearing on computed tomographic sagittal **(A)** and axial **(B)** scans as a radiolucent area *(star)* with a rim of bone sclerosis *(arrow)*.

MAGNETIC RESONANCE IMAGING

MRI of the spine includes always sagittal spin echo T1-weighted images and sagittal fast (turbo) spin echo T2-weighted images. Sagittal fast spin echo–proton density and T2-weighted images are used to evaluate disc dehydration; gradient echo sequences are less sensitive for the evaluation of disc dehydration. Axial T1- or T2-weighted imaging usually completes the lumbar spine evaluation; axial gradient echo T2-weighted images are used in the cervical region, particularly to differentiate disc herniation (high signal intensity) from osteophytes (low signal intensity) (17) (Fig. 8.8). Short time inversion recov-

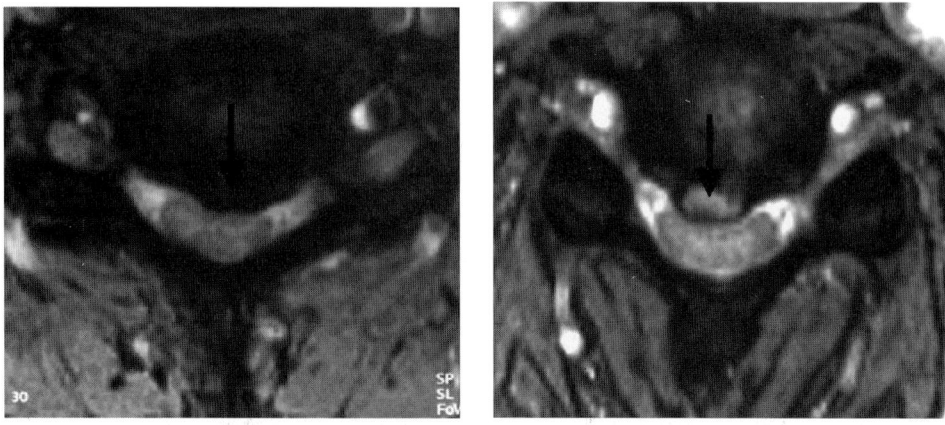

FIG. 8.8. A,B: On axial T2-weighted gradient echo image, the osteophyte **(A)** appears hypointense *(arrow)*, and the herniated disc **(B)** appears hyperintense *(arrow)*.

ery (STIR) sequences are useful for the visualization of bone marrow edema. Enhancement in the subchondral region is related to fibrovascular bone marrow; the differential diagnosis between Modic type I bone marrow changes and discitis may be difficult on postcontrast MR images (Fig. 8.9). Fluorodeoxyglucose (FDG) positron emission tomography appears to be a useful modality for the differentiation of degenerative and infectious endplate abnormalities (19).

On T1-weighted MRI, the signal of the normal intervertebral disc is lower than that of the vertebral body; on T2-weighted MRI, the signal intensity of the disc is higher than that of the vertebral body. According to Pfirrmann et al. (15), disc degeneration can be graded (Fig. 8.10). In normal young patients, the high signal on T2-weighted images appears homogeneous in the central area of the disc; the peripheral annulus has a low signal on T2-weighted images (grade 1). Loss of signal intensity in the nucleus pulposus on T2-weighted images closely correlates with disc dehydration related to alteration of the proteoglycans; gradient echo images are more sensitive to the presence of water, and the loss of signal intensity is more apparent on T2-weighted spin echo images. During the second decade of life, a horizontal linear hypointense band appears within the nucleus pulposus on T2-weighted images because of the development of collagen fibers within the nucleus pulposus (grade 2). Later, a diffuse signal loss appearing on T2-weighted images is associated with mild narrowing of the intervertebral space (grade 3). At this stage, posterior radial tears may be detected as an area of high signal intensity on T2-weighted images in the posterior and peripheral annulus; enhancement is possible after the intravenous administration of gadolinium (Fig. 8.11). A black disc with significant narrowing of the disc space (grade 4) or with

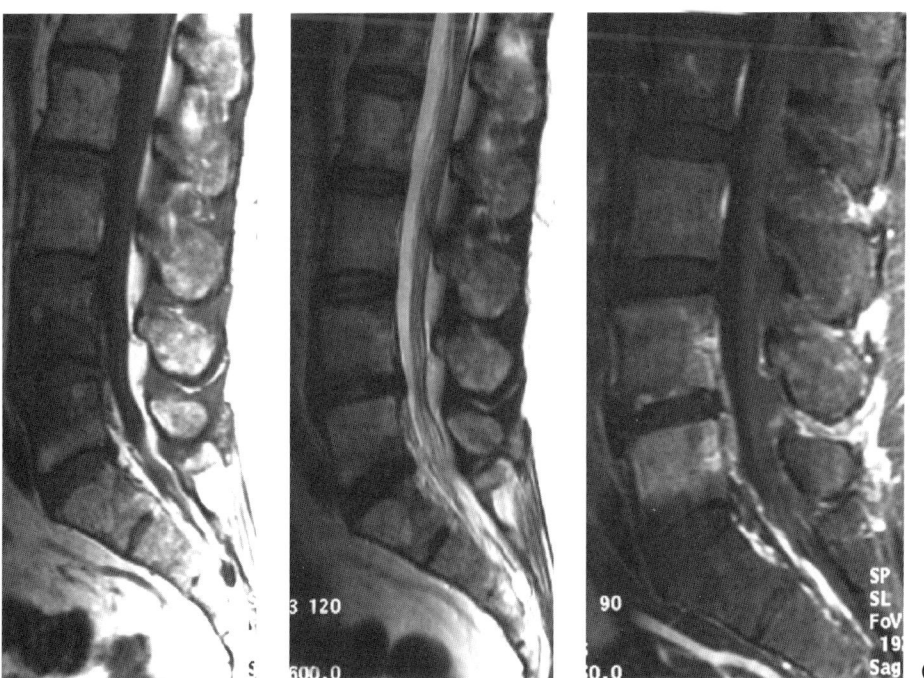

FIG. 8.9. A–C: Modic type I changes involving the L4–5 level. The differential diagnosis with discitis may be difficult with large signal modifications.

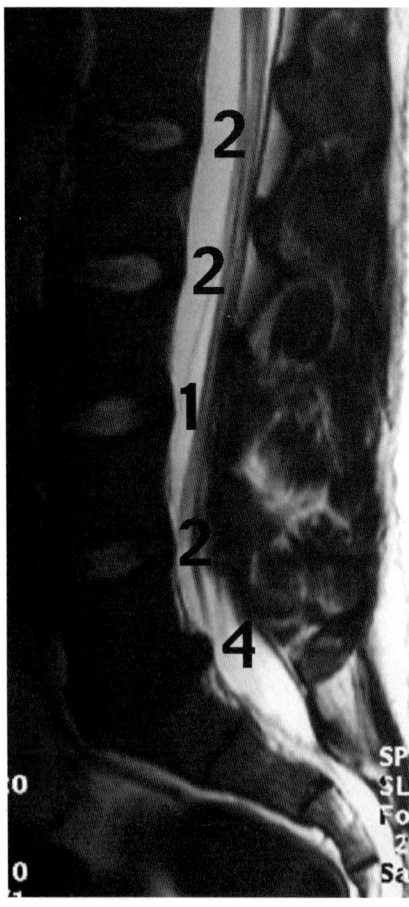

FIG. 8.10. Different grades of disc degeneration, as described by Pfirrmann et al. (15).

a collapsed disc space (grade 5) corresponds to severe disc degeneration. Intradiscal gas appears hypointense on T1- and T2-weighted images; the vacuum phenomenon is more effectively detected with plain radiographs and CT (10). Intradiscal calcifications may also appear hypointense on T1- and T2-weighted images; however, discal calcifications may appear hyperintense on T1-weighted images in DDD (2).

According to Modic et al. (13), three types of signal intensity changes involving the bone marrow of the adjacent vertebral body may be associated with DDD (Figs. 8.9, 8.12–8.15). Type I bone marrow changes are visualized as low signal intensity on T1-weighted images and high signal intensity on T2-weighted images with enhancement after the administration of gadolinium chelates. The replacement of normal bone marrow by fibrovascular marrow explains both the low signal on T1-weighted images and high signal on T2-weighted images, related to an increase in free water, and the enhancement after gadolinium chelate injection, related to hypervascularity (13) (Figs. 8.9, 8.12). Modic type I changes are noted in 4% of patients with back pain and are probably closely correlated with back pain (14,20). A positive pain provocation test is not clearly correlated with Modic type I endplate changes (18,22). Similar changes are observed after surgery or chemonucleolysis for disc herniation. Type I changes may regress or progress to type II changes after several years (Fig. 8.14).

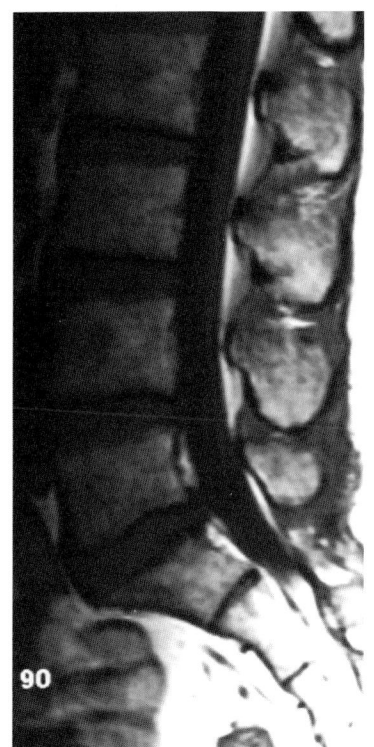
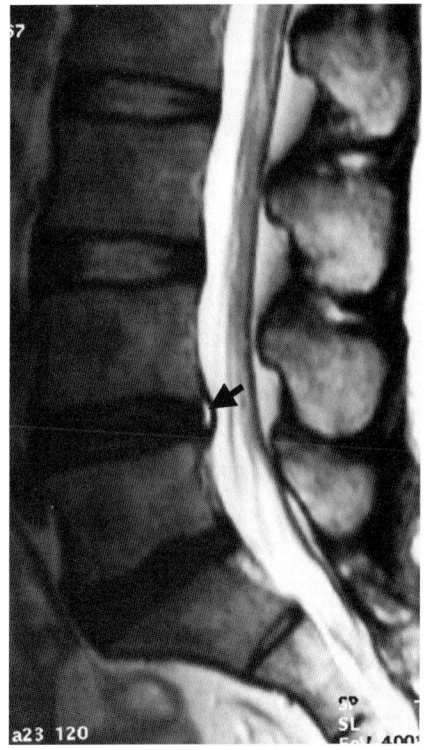
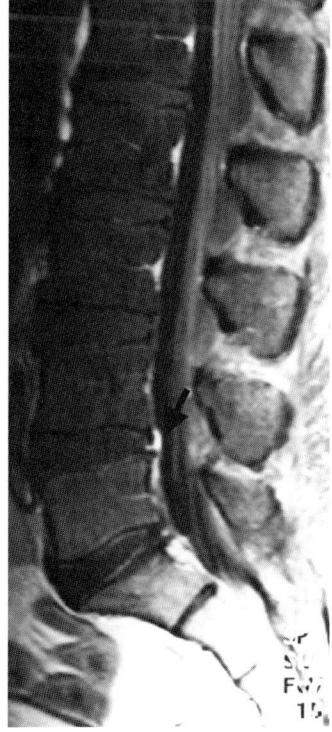

FIG. 8.11. A–C: Posterior high-intensity zone on T2-weighted image **(B)** with enhancement on postcontrast T1-weighted image **(C)** *(arrows)*; no abnormality is seen on T1-weighted image **(A)**.

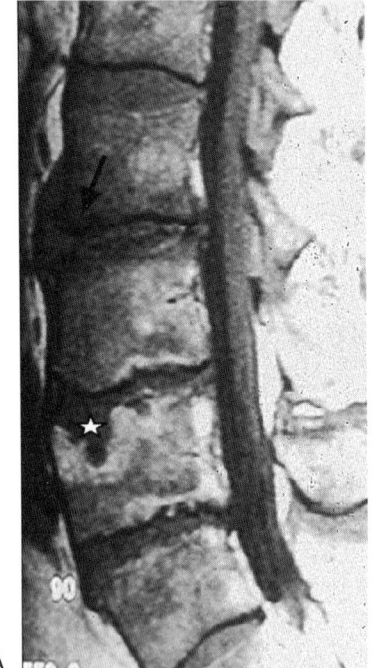
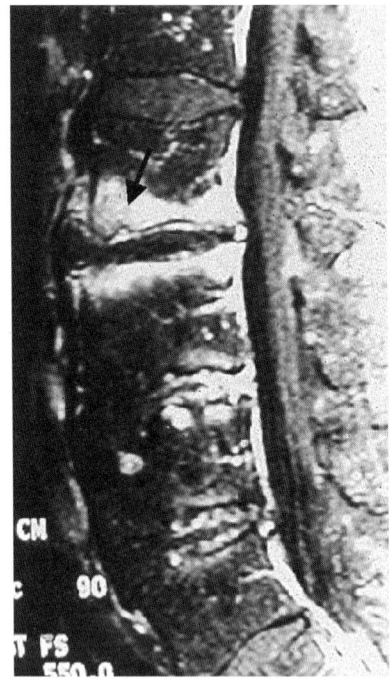
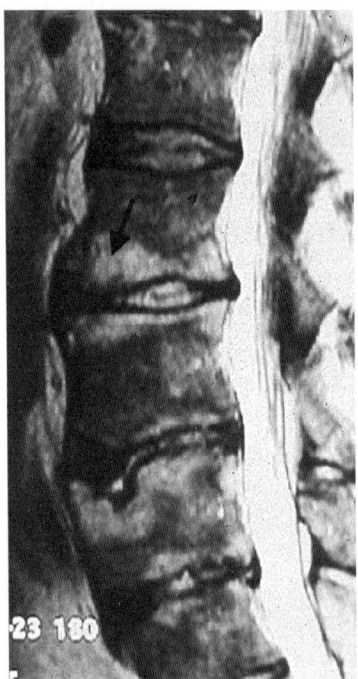

FIG. 8.12. A–C: Modic type I changes with hypointensity on T1-weighted image **(A)**, enhancement on postcontrast T1-weighted image **(B)**, and hyperintensity on T2-weighted image **(C)** of the subchondral bone *(arrows)* of the L2–3 level. Modic type II changes surrounding a cartilaginous Schmorl node *(star)* with hyperintensity on T1-weighted image **(A)**, no enhancement and disappearance of the hyperintensity on postcontrast T1-weighted image with fat saturation **(B)**, and hyperintensity on T2-weighted image **(C)** of the subchondral bone at the L3–4 level.

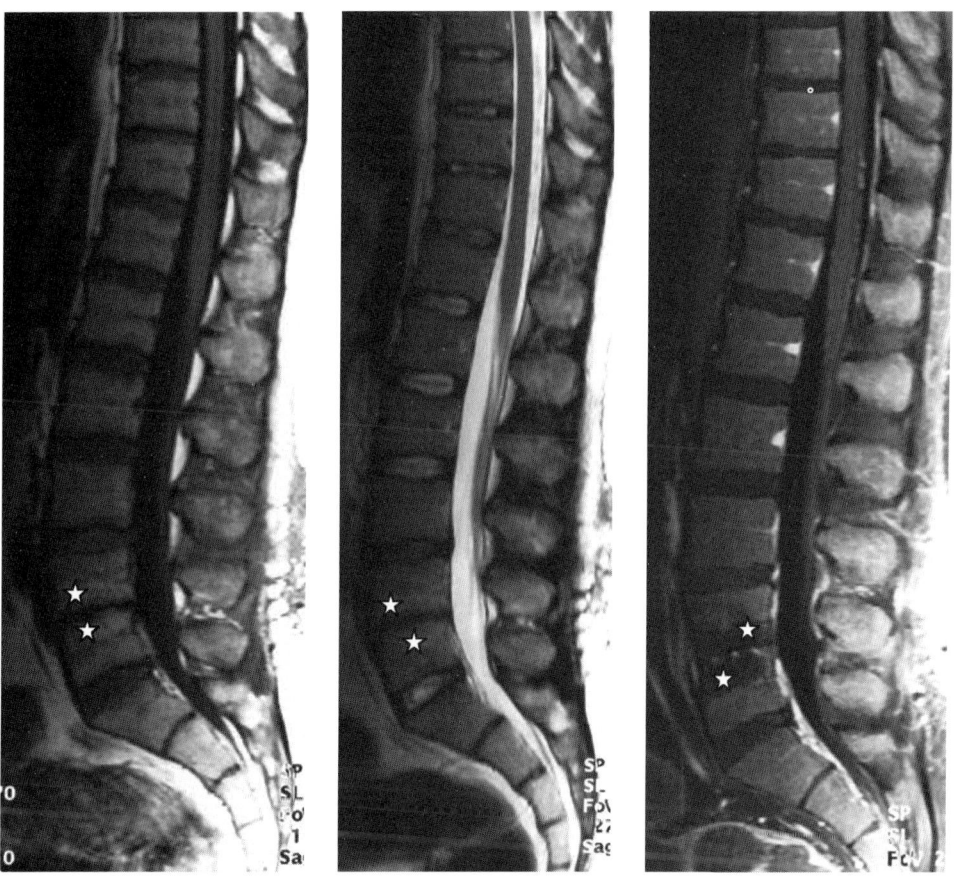

FIG. 8.13. A–C: Modic type II changes with hyperintensity on T1-weighted image **(A)**, absence of enhancement and disappearance of the hyperintensity on postcontrast T1-weighted image with fat saturation pulse **(B)**, and hyperintensity on T2-weighted image **(C)** of the subchondral bone at the L4–5 level *(stars)*.

Type II bone marrow changes are visualized as high signal intensity on T1- and T2-weighted images without enhancement; the type II changes represent fatty marrow and are observed in 16% of patients presenting with back pain (13) (Figs. 8.13, 8.14).

Type III changes are visualized as low signal intensity on T1- and T2-weighted images without enhancement and represent hyperostosis (6,13) (Fig. 8.15).

The signal of cartilaginous Schmorl nodes is similar to that of the corresponding intervertebral disc on T1-weighted images; the nodes appear slightly hyperintense on T2-weighted images and often enhance after contrast infusion. During acute and subacute stages, surrounding edema and inflammatory changes are noted (low signal intensity on T1-weighted images, high signal intensity on T2-weighted images, and postcontrast enhancement).

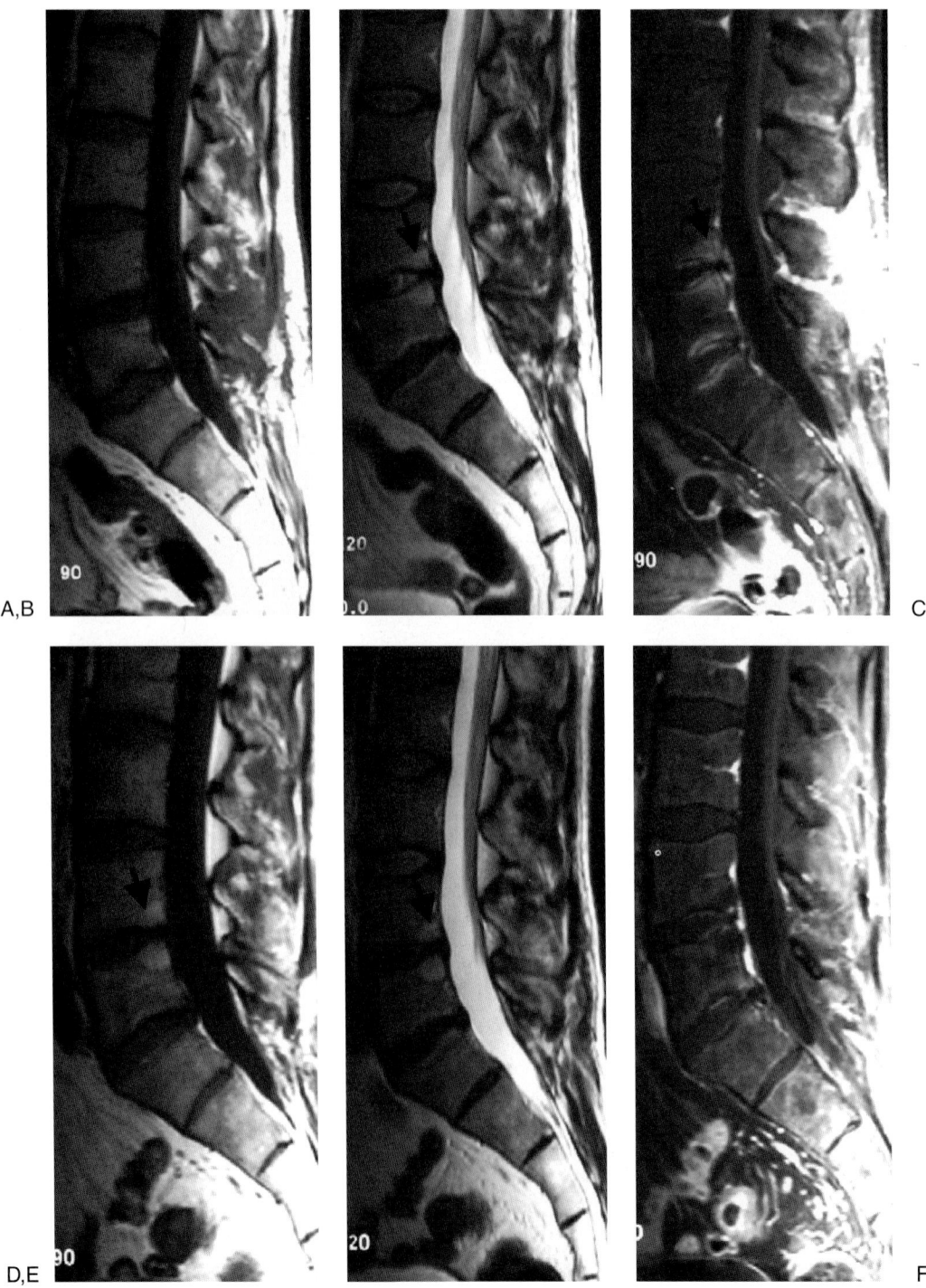

FIG. 8.14. A–F: Modic type I changes with hypointensity on T1-weighted image **(A)**, enhancement on postcontrast T1-weighted image **(B)**, and hyperintensity on T2-weighted image **(C)** involving the posterior subchondral bone *(arrows)* of the L4–5 level. On the control magnetic resonance images obtained 1 year later **(D–F)**, Modic type II changes are seen at the same level.

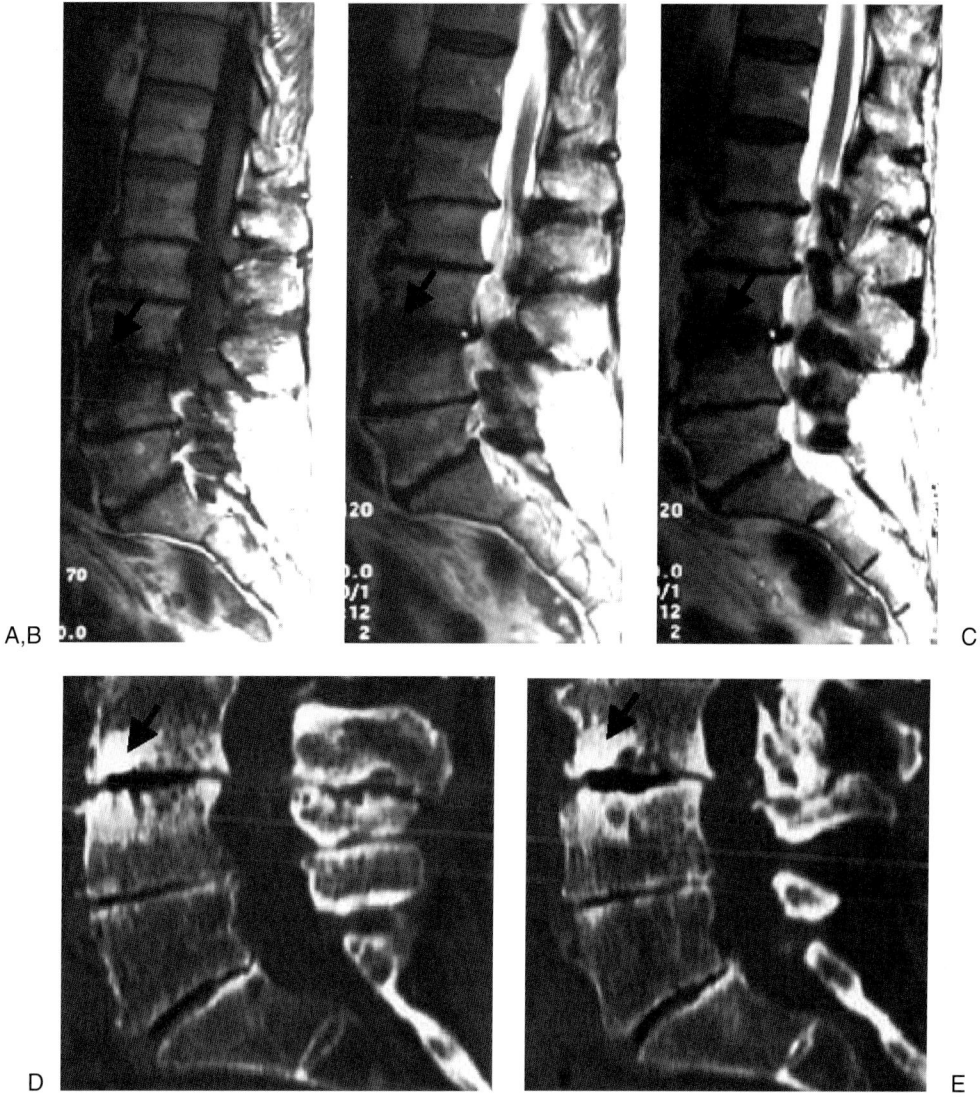

FIG. 8.15. A–E: Modic type III changes with hypointensity on T1-weighted image **(A)** and T2-weighted images **(C,D)** and bone sclerosis on sagittal computed tomographic re-formations **(E)** *(arrows)* involving the subchondral bone at the L3–4 level.

Lumbar Magnetic Resonance Imaging Findings in Asymptomatic Subjects

MRI demonstrates degenerative lumbar disc disease in 90% to 100% of asymptomatic subjects older than 50 years. A posterior high-intensity zone is present on T2-weighted images in 20% to 50% of persons after the age of 50 (5,11). Bulging disc and disc herniation are observed in 20% of cases. Subchondral endplate modifications with Modic type I and type II changes are noted in 7% and 17%, respectively, of asymptomatic persons (11).

Imaging Findings and Correlation with Clinical Symptoms

Patients with low back pain and hypermobility present mainly with Modic type I changes (20). Discordant correlations between provocative discography and vertebral endplate signal changes have been published. Sandhu et al. (18) found no significant relationship; Weishaupt et al. (22) found that moderate and severe endplate abnormalities appear useful in predicting painful disc derangement in patients with low back pain; Braithwaite et al. (4) concluded that Modic changes appear to be a relatively specific but insensitive sign of a painful lumbar disc in patients with discogenic low back pain.

The high-intensity zone in the posterior median annulus fibrosus seen on T2-weighted images and associated with a small area of contrast enhancement on postcontrast (gadolinium) T1-weighted images is the result of an annular tear and is observed in 30% to 60% of patients undergoing MRI for back pain (1,5). The appearance of a high-intensity zone does not reliably indicate the presence of symptomatic internal disc disruption (5) (Fig. 8.10).

Imaging of Associated Spinal Lesions

MRI and CT may demonstrate disc herniation, degenerative changes in the facet joints, ligamentous degeneration, alignment abnormalities (segmental instability, degenerative spondylolisthesis, degenerative retrolisthesis), spinal canal (central and lateral) stenosis, and foraminal stenosis (7,8). Dynamic plain films and dynamic myelography may confirm segmental instability.

REFERENCES

1. Aprill C, Bogduk N. High-intensity zone: a diagnostic sign of painful lumbar disc on magnetic resonance imaging. *Br J Radiol* 1992;65:361–369.
2. Bangert BA, Modic MT, Ross JS, et al. Hyperintense disks on T1-weighted MR images: correlation with calcification. *Radiology* 1995;195:437–443.
3. Boutin RD, Spaeth HJ, Resnick D. Degenerative diseases of the spine. In: Orrison WW Jr, ed. *Neuroimaging*, vol 2. Philadelphia: WB Saunders, 2000:1302–1333.
4. Braithwaite I, White J, Saifuddin A, et al. Vertebral endplate (Modic) changes on lumbar spine MRI: correlation with pain reproduction at lumbar discography. *Eur Spine J* 1998;7:363–368.
5. Carragee EJ, Paragioudakis SJ, Khurana S. 2000 Volvo Award in Clinical Studies. Lumbar high-intensity zone and discography in subjects without low back problems. *Spine* 2000;25:2987–2992.
6. De Roos A, Kressel H, Spritzer C, et al. MR imaging of marrow changes adjacent to endplates in degenerative lumbar disk disease. *AJR Am J Roentgenol* 1987;149:531–534.
7. Dietemann JL. *Imagerie du rachis lombaire*. Paris: Masson, 1994.
8. Dietemann JL, Dosch JC, Steib JP. *Imagerie des spondylolisthésis*. Paris: Masson, 1995.
9. Frobin W, Brinckmann P, Kramer M, et al. Height of lumbar discs measured from radiographs compared with degeneration and height classified from MR images. *Eur Radiol* 2001;11:263–269.
10. Grenier N, Grossman RI, Schiebler ML, et al. Degenerative lumbar disk disease: pitfalls and usefulness of MR imaging in detection of vacuum phenomenon. *Radiology* 1987;164:861–865.
11. Malghem J, Cotten A, Laredo JD, et al. IRM du rachis lombaire asymptômatique. Etude multicentrique du GETROA: résultats préliminaires. In: Morvan G, Deburge A, Bard H, et al., eds. *Le rachis lombaire dégénératif*. Montpellier: Sauramps Médical, 1998:127–140.
12. McCulloch JA, Transfeldt EE. *Macnab's backache*, 3rd ed. Baltimore: Williams & Wilkins, 1997.
13. Modic MT, Masaryk TJ, Ross JS, et al. Imaging of degenerative disk disease. *Radiology* 1988;168:177–186.
14. Modic MT, Steinberg PM, Ross JS, et al. Degenerative disk disease: assessment of changes in vertebral body marrow with MR imaging. *Radiology* 1988;166:193–199.
15. Pfirrmann CWA, Metzdorf A, Zanetti M, et al. Magnetic resonance classification of lumbar intervertebral disc degeneration. *Spine* 2001;26:1873–1878.
16. Resnick D, Niwayama G. Degenerative disease of the spine. In: Resnick D, ed. *Diagnosis of bone and joint disorders*, vol 3. Philadelphia: WB Saunders, 1995:1372–1462.
17. Ross JS, Tkach J, VanDyke C, et al. Clinical MR imaging of degenerative spinal disease: pulse sequences, gradient-echo, techniques and contrast agents. *J Magn Reson Imaging* 1991;1:29–37.

18. Sandhu HS, Sanchez-Caso LP, Parvataneni HK, et al. Association between findings of provocative discography and vertebral endplate signal changes as seen on MRI. *J Spinal Disord* 2000;13:438–443.
19. Stumpe KD, Zanetti M, Weishaupt D, et al. FDG positron emission tomography for differentiation of degenerative and infectious endplate abnormalities in the lumbar spine detected on MR imaging. *AJR Am J Roentgenol* 2002;179:1151–1157.
20. Toyone T, Takahashi K, Kitahara H, et al. Vertebral bone marrow changes in degenerative lumbar disc disease. An MRI study of 74 patients with low back pain. *J Bone Joint Surg Br* 1994;76:757–764.
21. Vande Berg B, Lecouvet F, Theate Y, et al. Imagerie radiologique de la pathologie dégénérative du disque intervertébral: corrélations anatomiques. In: Morvan G, Deburge A, Bard H, et al., eds. *Le rachis lombaire dégénératif*. Montpellier: Sauramps Médical, 1998:115–126.
22. Weishaupt D, Zanetti M, Hodler J, et al. Painful lumbar disk derangement: relevance of endplate abnormalities at MR imaging. *Radiology* 2001;218:420–427.

9

Behavior of the Disc in Upright Magnetic Resonance Imaging

*‡Francis W. Smith, §J. Randy Jinkins, and †¶Malcolm H. Pope

*Departments of *Radiology and †Environmental and Occupational Medicine, University of Aberdeen; ‡MRI Center, Woodend Hospital, Aberdeen, United Kingdom; §Fonar Corporation, Mellville, New York; and ¶Department of Biomedical Physics, Aberdeen Royal Infirmary, Aberdeen, United Kingdom*

A long evolutionary history characterizes *Homo sapiens* in terms of an upright posture and a bipedal mode of locomotion. For example, in the chimpanzee, the center of gravity of the body lies anterior to the lumbar spine and hip, and in the human, it lies above the hip joints. The chimpanzee has limited hip extension and cannot extend the hip to place the femur perpendicular to the ground. It has been suggested that the adaptation of the human to the upright stance is what has been the underlying cause of low back pain. However, no evidence is available to support this view. For example, Putz and Muller-Gerbl (15) stated that the increase in degenerative diseases of the vertebral column is attributable to an inadequate adaptation to upright posture. Their analysis of motion segments demonstrated no qualitative differences in the design features of the vertebrae in the larger mammals and humans that result in higher overall stresses. They concluded that the human vertebral column seems to be an optimized compromise of evolution.

However, there is no doubt that posture does affect the anatomic relationships in the lumbar spine and the stresses in the constituent tissues. Beattie et al. (2) performed magnetic resonance imaging (MRI) in healthy subjects in flexed and extended positions. They found that the distance from the posterior margin of the nucleus pulposus to the posterior margins of the adjacent vertebral bodies was greater in the extended than in the flexed position. They also established that the nucleus pulposus of the degenerate disc does not move in the same way as that of a normal disc.

Weishaupt et al. (19) obtained MR images of patients seated with their backs in flexion and in extension. Nerve root contact without deviation was noted in 22% of the subjects while they were supine, in 41% while seated in a flexed position, and in 30% while seated in an extended position. In comparison with the nerve root deviation in the supine position, the deviation decreased in the seated flexion position and increased in the seated extension position. Positional pain score differences were also significantly related to changes in foraminal size. It was concluded that positional MRI demonstrates minor neurologic compromise more frequently than conventional MRI.

Zamani et al. (21) used a superconducting open configuration MR system to image the spine in the erect position. They found an increased disc bulge in 27% of the discs with extension and in 40% of those with desiccation. They also found that central canal size (50%) and foraminal size (27%) decreased with extension, especially at levels with disc desiccation. They did note, however, that the images obtained with their open configuration MRI unit were of inferior quality in comparison with the images obtained with a conventional unit.

From a biomechanical standpoint, McGill et al. (11) compared the position of the muscles in the trunk in a standing posture with their position in a supine posture. They found that the flexor moment arm of the anterior abdominal wall increases about 30% in the standing posture, whereas the moment arm of the erector spinae group increases between 3% and 12%. Thus, both the position of the muscles and their activity differ dramatically between standing and supine postures. Thevenon and Delcambre (18) noted that muscles participate not only in movement itself but also in controlling movement and in maintaining spinal stability and that the action of muscles also depends on the effect of gravity.

The MR phenomenon was first reported by Bloch (3) and Purcell et al. (14), but it was not until the early 1970s that Damadian (5) and Lauterbur (9) were able to use the technique to construct images. The technique was first used clinically in studies performed at University of Aberdeen (10), and Aberdeen contributed the basic mathematical theory (13). It became self-evident through the publications of Smith (6,17) that the importance of MRI lay in its excellent soft tissue contrast resolution, multiplanar imaging, lack of use of ionizing radiation in biomechanical studies, and the capacity to characterize pathologic tissue directly. It was obviously of great use in the axial skeleton. With further experience, it became clear that MR images of the spine must be interpreted in the context of the clinical findings. Wood et al. (20) examined the thoracic spine of asymptomatic persons to determine the prevalence of abnormal anatomic findings. Positive anatomic findings at one level or more were noted in 73% of asymptomatic persons. These included herniation of a disc in 37%, bulging of a disc in 53%, annular tear in 58%, deformation of the spinal cord in 29%, and Scheuermann endplate irregularities or kyphosis in 38%. Likewise, Jensen et al. (8) found that 36% of asymptomatic subjects had normal discs at all levels of the lumbar spine, 52% had a bulge at one level, 27% had a protrusion, and 1% had an extrusion. The most common abnormalities not involving the intervertebral discs were Schmorl nodes in 19%, annular defects in 14%, and facet arthropathy in 8%. It was concluded that the discovery by MRI of bulges or protrusions in people with low back pain may frequently be coincidental. Because these findings may well be quite different in the supine position, it is of great interest to examine people while they are under the influence of the gravitational vector.

Traditionally, MRI of the lumbar spine has been performed with the patient supine. We have developed and are evaluating an MRI scanner that images patients in both erect and supine positions. Six volunteers, four with back pain and two without, have been examined while in an erect, weight-bearing position and while lying down. Significant differences in the appearance of the lumbar intervertebral discs have been observed between the two positions. Another patient, with a grade 2 spondylolisthesis, has been imaged in the neutral, flexed, and extended positions while standing.

METHODS

A 0.6-T "stand-up" Indomitable MRI scanner (Fonar Corporation, Melville, NY, U.S.A.) has been used to examine six volunteers, four with back pain and two without, while in an erect, weight-bearing position and while lying down. Another patient, with a grade 2 spondylolisthesis, has been imaged in neutral, flexed, and extended positions while standing. A series of seven sagittal T2-weighted images were obtained in both the supine and erect, weight-bearing positions. In one case, axial T2-weighted images were obtained through the intervertebral discs in both the erect and supine positions. The dimensions of all five lumbar intervertebral discs were measured by two independent observers using the measurement software provided with the MRI scanner. A consensus opinion about the appearances of the nerve root canals and exit foramina in the patient with spondylolisthesis was reached after a discussion with four independent observers.

In a further study, we examined the shape of the spine in five men and five women without low back pain. We palpated the posterior superior iliac spine and drew a line at L5, as one would with the modified Schober test. Plaster of paris was then placed over the spinous processes and the external shape of the spine obtained in both the standing and supine postures. The cast impressions were cut in the midsagittal plane for further analysis, which consisted of drawing tangents at S2, L4, and T12 according to the method of Burton (4).

RESULTS

When the dimensions of the 30 intervertebral discs in the erect and supine images were compared, the following observations were made. Twenty-one discs with normally hydrated nuclei in the absence of annular bulge or prolapse were classified as normal; in nine discs, loss of signal from the nuclei was associated with annular bulge or prolapse.

A reduction in vertical height of between 10% and 15% (mean, 12.6%) was observed in the 21 normal discs when the volunteers were imaged in the erect position. In this group, the anteroposterior diameter of the discs increased less than 5% in the erect position. The discs with degenerate nuclei and annular prolapse (four at the L4–5 level, four at the L5–S1 level, and one at the L3–4 level) showed a decrease in vertical height posteriorly of more than 20% and an increase in height anteriorly of more than 15%. The anteroposterior diameter increased in each of these discs by more than 10%. Observation of the patient with a grade 2 spondylolisthesis showed that this was a stable spondylolisthesis, but the degree of protrusion of the disc annulus at the L4–5 level differed significantly between flexion, the neutral position, and extension. The disc protruded more prominently on the left and less on the right between full extension and flexion.

The mean loss of disc volume, when loss of disc height and the mean increase in diameter in the vertical position were taken into account, was calculated to be 20%.

Use of the replica method to determine the lumbosacral angle demonstrated a mean angle of 38.6 degrees during standing and 25.3 degrees during lying down.

DISCUSSION

We believe that these observations, made with a scanner specifically designed by us to image in both the erect and supine positions, support the belief that imaging of the lumbar spine in patients with back or leg symptoms is most logically performed with the patient in the erect position. They show a significant difference in appearance between images obtained in the two positions in addition to the potential for imaging the lumbar spine in cases of suspected lumbar instability. Figures 9.1 through 9.4 demonstrate the potential of the technique in some clinical case studies.

It is clear that many anatomic changes occur between the erect and supine positions. The vertical height of the normal discs was reduced in the erect position. The reduction was accompanied by an increase in the anteroposterior diameter of the discs. The discs with identifiable pathology showed greater differences. The overall shape of the lumbar

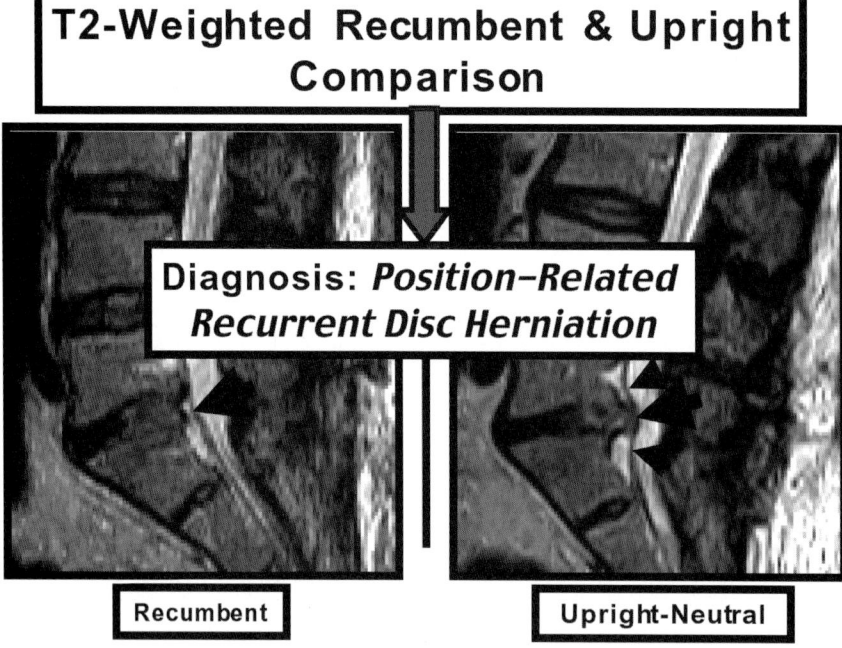

FIG. 9.1. T2-weighted recumbent and upright comparison. The diagnosis was position-related recurrent disc herniation. (Courtesy of M. Rose, M.D.)

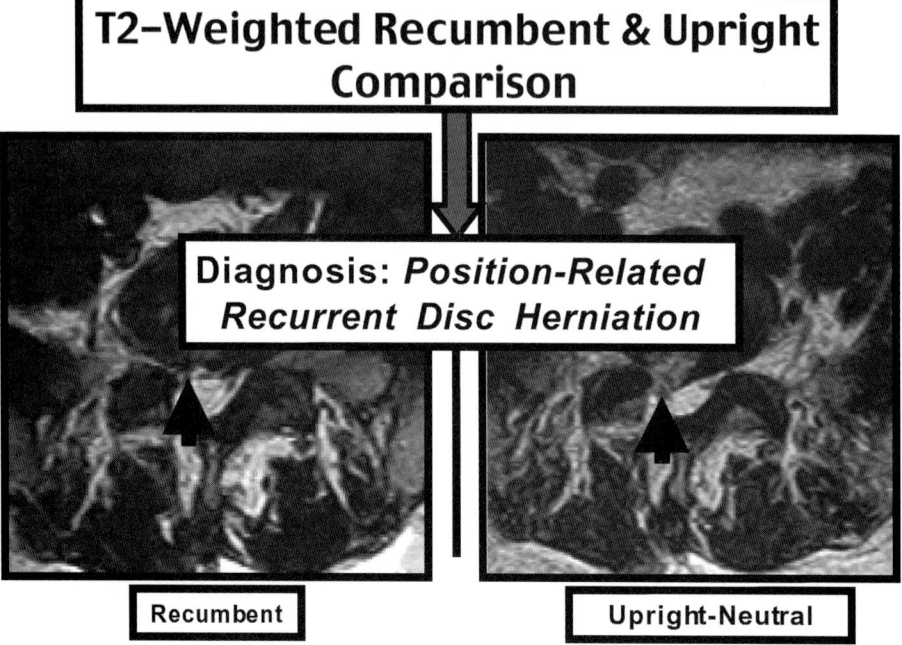

FIG. 9.2. T2-weighted recumbent and upright comparison (axial). The diagnosis was position-related recurrent disc herniation. (Courtesy of M. Rose, M.D.)

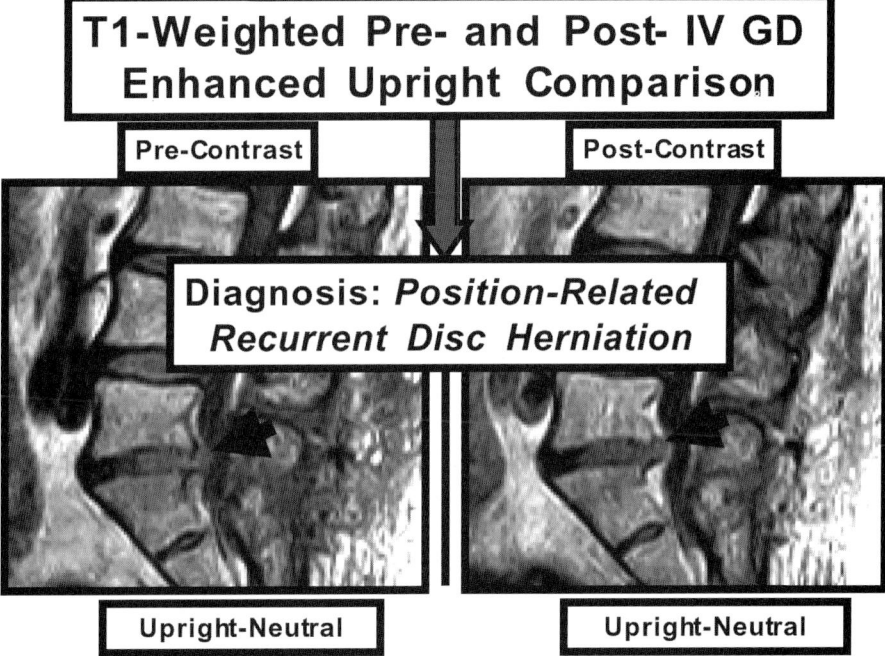

FIG. 9.3. T1-weighted upright comparison before and after intravenous (*IV*) gadolinium (*GD*) enhancement. The diagnosis was position-related recurrent disc herniation. (Courtesy of M. Rose, M.D.)

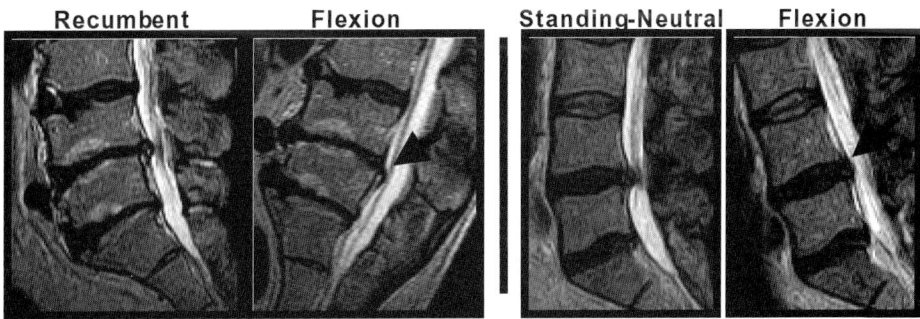

FIG. 9.4. Clinical case studies showing dynamic fluctuations in recurrent disc herniations. Patient No. 1: The recumbent image **(far left)** shows a posterior disc herniation at L4–5. In the upright-flexion image **(center left)**, the posterior disc herniation at L4–5 becomes less prominent *(arrow)*. At the same time, new anterior disc protrusions are noted at L3–4, L4–5, and L5–S1. Patient No. 2: The standing-neutral image **(center right)** shows a posterior disc herniation at L4–5. In the upright-flexion image **(far right)**, the posterior disc herniation at L4–5 becomes less prominent *(arrow)*. *Note:* These studies show that focal disc herniations may fluctuate. Fluctuation can be of significance in that some surgeons operate with patients in specific positions that may minimize posterior disc herniations at the time of surgery.

spine is different in the standing position. Significant lordosis is lost in the supine position, and the muscle lever arms change. In addition, the standing posture causes a rapid loss of hydration. Mechanical loading is dramatically different. In the standing posture, the dorsal muscles are active, and the gravitational vector is parallel to the midsagittal axis.

Nachemson (12) proposed that in a young disc, with a fluid nucleus pulposus, compressive stresses are resisted by the hydrostatic pressure in the nucleus pulposus, whereas high hoop stresses are present in the annulus fibrosus. In degenerate discs, the measured swelling pressures decrease with the severity of degeneration and approach zero. The finite element model of Shirazi-Adl et al. (16) demonstrated that the endplates in degenerate discs are subjected to less pressure in the center and that loads are distributed around the periphery. The axial stress is compressive, and the circumferential stress is close to zero. Horst and Brinckmann (7) showed that the annulus fibrosus in a mature disc resists compressive stresses perpendicular to the endplates. Thus, the degenerate disc behaves like a thick-walled cylinder rather than a pressurized vessel. This fundamental behavior is absent in the supine posture and leads to misleading MRI findings. The disc is an osmotic system for the exchange of ions and fluid. The macromolecules in the disc interior have such a high hydroscopic capacity that they can take up fluid even when under pressure. Osmotic fluid flow takes place until the osmotic pressure and loading pressure are in equilibrium. The system behaves in a fundamentally different mode in the supine posture. Both disc height and overall body height decrease with applied loads. Under prolonged loading, the disc continues to lose height after an initial deformation that immediately follows application of the load. The height and area of the disc vary within the disc itself, between levels, between people, between genders, with aging, and during the day. The body height changes after different stress environments, including vibration, gravity inversion, space flight, traction, and increased loading. Alterations in spinal height depend on body forces, externally applied forces, and disc properties.

Adams et al. (1) subjected cadaveric lumbar spines to periods of vertical creep loading to show a disc height change similar to the physiologic change. As a result, discs bulge more and become stiffer in compression and more flexible in bending. Disc tissue becomes more elastic as its water content falls. The neural arch and associated ligaments resist an increasing proportion of the compressive and bending stresses acting on the spine.

REFERENCES

1. Adams MA, Dolan P, Hutton WC, et al. Diurnal changes in spinal mechanics and their clinical significance. *J Bone Joint Surg Br* 1990;72:266–270.
2. Beattie PF, Brooks WM, Rothstein JM, et al. Effect of lordosis on the position of the nucleus pulposus in supine subjects. A study using magnetic resonance imaging. *Spine* 1994;19:2096–2102.
3. Bloch F. Nuclear induction. *Phys Rev* 1940;70:460–475.
4. Burton AK. Regional lumbar sagittal mobility; measurement by flexicurves. *Clin Biomech* 1986;1:20–26.
5. Damadian R. Tumor detection by nuclear magnetic resonance. *Science* 1971;171:1151–1153.
6. Harvey SB, Smith FW, Hukins DW. Measurement of lumbar spine flexion-extension using a low-field open-magnet magnetic resonance scanner. *Invest Radiol* 1998;33:439–443.
7. Horst M, Brinckmann P. Measurement of the distribution of axial stress on the end-plate of the vertebral body. *Spine* 1981;6:217–232.
8. Jensen MC, Brant-Zawadzki MN, Obuchowski N, et al. MRI of the lumbar spine in people without low back pain. *N Engl J Med* 1994;331:69–73.
9. Lauterbur PC. Image formation by induced local interactions: examples employing nuclear magnetic resonance. *Nature* 1973;242:190–191.
10. Mallard JR. A brief personal account of the Aberdeen story—with particular reference to SPECT and MRI. *J Med Eng Technol* 1993;17:176–179; discussion 197–198.

11. McGill SM, Juker D, Axler C. Correcting trunk muscle geometry obtained from MRI and CT scans of supine postures for use in standing postures. *J Biomech* 1996;29:643–646.
12. Nachemson AL. Lumbar intradiscal pressure. *Acta Orthop Scand Suppl* 1960;43:1–104.
13. Norris DG, Hutchison JM. Concomitant magnetic field gradients and their effects on imaging at low magnetic field strengths. *Magn Reson Imaging* 1990;8:33–37.
14. Purcell EM, Torrey HC, Pound RV. Resonance absorption by nuclear magnetic moments in solids. *Phys Rev* 1946;69:37–38.
15. Putz RL, Muller-Gerbl M. The vertebral column—a phylogenetic failure? A theory explaining the function and vulnerability of the human spine. *Clin Anat* 1996;9:205–212.
16. Shirazi-Adl SA, Shrivastava SC, Ahmed AM. Stress analysis of the lumbar disc body unit in compression: a three-dimensional non-linear finite element study. *Spine* 1984;9:120–126.
17. Smith F. The Williams S. Moore Award. *J Magn Reson Imaging* 1993;3:311.
18. Thevenon A, Delcambre B. Movements of the lumbar spine. A biomechanical study. *Rev Rhum Mal Osteoartic* 1988;55:367–373.
19. Weishaupt D, Schmid MR, Zanetti M, et al. Positional MR imaging of the lumbar spine: does it demonstrate nerve root compromise not visible at conventional MR imaging? *Radiology* 2000;215:247–253.
20. Wood KB, Garvey TA, Gundry C, et al. Magnetic resonance imaging of the thoracic spine. Evaluation of asymptomatic individuals. *J Bone Joint Surg Am* 1995;77:1631–1638.
21. Zamani AA, Moriarty T, Hsu L, et al. Functional MRI of the lumbar spine in erect position in a superconducting open-configuration MR system: preliminary results. *J Magn Reson Imaging* 1998;8:1329–1333.

10
Lumbar Discography

Asif Saifuddin

Department of Radiology, Royal National Orthopaedic Hospital, NHS Trust, Middlesex, United Kingdom

Discography is a technique in which contrast medium is injected into an intervertebral disc. It may be performed at the cervical, thoracic, or lumbar level, although lumbar discography is by far the most frequently performed. Lumbar discography has been used for more than 50 years to investigate disc degeneration, disc herniation, and low back pain (LBP). The requirement for discography to demonstrate disc degeneration and herniation decreased after the introduction of computed tomography (CT) and particularly magnetic resonance imaging (MRI). However, with the continued failure of MRI as a technique for accurately identifying the source of symptoms in patients with mechanical LBP thought to be if disc origin (discogenic LBP), discography continues to be an important investigation in patients with chronic LBP (2,25,74).

PATHOPHYSIOLOGY OF DEGENERATIVE DISC DISEASE

The normal and pathologic anatomy of the lumbar intervertebral disc and the pathophysiology of degenerative disc disease have been extensively reviewed (2,25,74), and they are considered here only briefly. Whereas disc prolapse and disc bulge are clearly evident on axial imaging studies, such as CT and MRI, the pathologic process associated with discogenic LBP, termed *internal disc disruption* (18), is not seen on CT and may be evident in only a minority of cases on MRI, appearing as a high-intensity zone (HIZ) (4). Internal disc disruption refers to changes within the nucleus, such as fragmentation and displacement, and annular pathology, such as fissures, which may be of partial or full thickness. Such abnormalities are most clearly demonstrated by CT discography (25), and positive findings on discography are considered a requirement for the diagnosis of discogenic back pain (66).

The production of pain as a result of disc injection appears to have two major components, chemical and mechanical (2,25). It is known that pain-receptive nerve endings are found in the inner third of the degenerate disc annulus (17) and that the degenerate nucleus pulposus contains a variety of pain-provoking chemical agents (56). The chemical stimulation of nerve endings within radial annular tears is considered to be a major source of discogenic LBP. Injecting such "chemically sensitive" discs typically causes pain at low volumes and pressures (2). Disc injection is also associated with changes in the pattern of loading of the posterolateral annulus and nucleus (45) and with mechanical deformation of the posterior annulus (52). This may result in stretching of the outer annular nerve fibers, a further possible mechanism of pain.

The vertebral endplate is a further potential source of pain, being very sensitive to the mechanical stimulation of a misplaced discography needle. Discography is reported to cause endplate deflection *in vitro* (26) and to increase intervertebral disc height, as assessed by *in vivo* MRI studies (61). Endplate deflection may result in changes in intraosseous pressure (26), and such changes have been suggested as a cause of false-positive results of discography obtained during the injection of a normal disc adjacent to a degenerate painful disc. Finally, the direct intraosseous extension of injected contrast medium through defects in the cartilaginous endplate has been reported in 14 of 692 disc injections and resulted in concordant pain at 13 levels (29).

Discography is undoubtedly associated with the production of pain radiating to the lower limbs (48,60). The injection of cadaveric intervertebral discs has demonstrated leakage of injected contrast medium through a ruptured annulus in 14% of discs and contact between injected contrast medium and adjacent nerve roots in 27% of leaking discs (41). The direct chemical irritation of nerve roots has been proposed as a further cause of pain at discography. However, several studies have clearly documented that the incidence of the radiation of pain to the buttocks, groins, and lower limbs after injection is the same in patients with full-thickness annular ruptures as in those with only partial-thickness annular ruptures (48,60). This finding indicates that direct involvement of the nerve root is not a requirement for referral of pain. Such pain may be mediated through chemical changes in the dorsal root ganglion, which have been demonstrated following injection into canine intervertebral discs (78). The complex nature of pain reproduction at discography is further illustrated by the lack of a relationship between the side of annular disruption of a concordantly painful disc and the side of the patient's low back symptoms (70).

INDICATIONS

Despite the accuracy of MRI in the diagnosis of disc degeneration, associated features such as the HIZ and reactive endplate (Modic) changes, although relatively specific, are not sufficiently sensitive to identify symptomatic disc levels (11,31,37,53,59,63,65,71,79). Therefore, the major indication for lumbar discography is to identify symptomatic discs in patients with chronic LBP who may be candidates for lumbar spinal fusion (16,20,47,64,67). Discography may also be used to investigate discs adjacent to a spondylolisthesis and determine whether additional levels should be included in the fusion (3), and it is valuable in identifying the cause of LBP in adults with painful scoliosis (23).

Discography is a prerequisite for various percutaneous disc therapies, including chemonucleolysis (40), percutaneous discectomy (15), the administration of intradiscal steroids (69), and more recently intradiscal electrothermal therapy (54).

Postoperatively, discography has been used to investigate persistent LBP following discectomy (27), lumbar pseudarthrosis (32), and posterolateral fusion (3). CT discography is also reported to be more accurate in the differentiation of recurrent disc prolapse and epidural scar (6).

TECHNIQUE AND FINDINGS

MRI is a prerequisite for discography (2,25,57,74). Depending on the practice of the individual surgeon, the presence of more than one or two degenerate discs may render the patient unsuitable for fusion, and therefore discography is not justified.

After the technique and risks have been fully explained and consent has been obtained, the patient is placed on the x-ray table. Discography can be performed with the patient either prone or in the decubitus position. When the patient is placed in the decubitus position, a pillow should be inserted into the small of the back to straighten the spine and open the disc spaces on the side of the injection. Reitman et al. (52) noted that the behavior of the posterior annulus varies during disc injection with the spinal position, and based on their experimental studies of fresh spine specimens, they suggested that the patient's position during discography should be standardized.

Mild intravenous sedation may be administered, but only to a level at which the discographer can still communicate clearly with the patient. The need for routine antibiotic cover is somewhat controversial. Discitis following discography results from the introduction of skin bacteria into the disc via a contaminated needle tip. Osti et al. (50) suggested that antibiotics should be administered routinely, either intravenously 30 minutes before the procedure or into the disc at the time of disc injection. However, Guyer and Ohnmeiss (25), in a position statement of the North American Spine Society, concluded that routine antibiotic cover is unnecessary because the reported incidence of discitis is very low.

Following skin cleansing, local anesthetic is infiltrated into the skin and subcutaneous tissues to the level of the facet joint. A posterolateral approach is now the standard technique (43), and the entry point for each disc is approximately 10 cm from the midline. It is important to screen each disc level individually and ensure that the disc space is imaged tangentially, so that the needle entry point is correct. Therefore, it is advantageous to have a fluoroscopic system that can be angled along the length of the x-ray table. A dual-needle technique is recommended for two reasons. First, the ability to curve the inner needle facilitates injection of the L5–S1 disc (36). Second, because the inner needle does not touch the skin, the incidence of discitis should be reduced (21). Various needle combinations have been reported. The outer needle is inserted into the outer annulus via a route that lies lateral to the facet joint and medial to the exiting nerve root. Correct needle placement can be identified on lateral screening if the needle tip hits the annulus at the posterior disc margin. Slight further pressure on the needle lodges it into the outer annulus. Insertion into a degenerate disc can be painful. The inner needle is then placed through the outer needle such that its tip lies centrally within the nucleus; it should be remembered that the nucleus lies slightly posterior within the disc. The importance of correct needle placement has been emphasized by Urasaki et al. (75), who assessed the effect of needle tip placement on discograms obtained in the same patient at an interval of 2 weeks as a precursor to intradiscal steroid therapy. They found that if the placement of the needle was different in the two investigations, the appearance of the injected disc often differed significantly. Such differences were less likely if the needle tip placement was consistent between the two discograms. However, they did not relate needle tip position to patient response during the injection, so the relevance of these findings is unclear. A 2- to 3-mL syringe is used to inject contrast medium into the disc via connection tubing. This allows sufficient pressure to be achieved. With correct needle placement in the nucleus, contrast should flow freely away from the needle tip. If the contrast forms an oval or elongated pool with smooth margins, the injection is probably annular (Fig. 10.1). Contrast medium is injected until the nucleus is filled, and if the annulus is intact, a firm endpoint to the injection is reached. A normal disc typically accommodates 1.5 to 2.0 mL of contrast medium (Fig. 10.2). With a degenerate disc, various situations arise. Contrast medium may fill a radial annular tear, which may be of either partial or full thickness

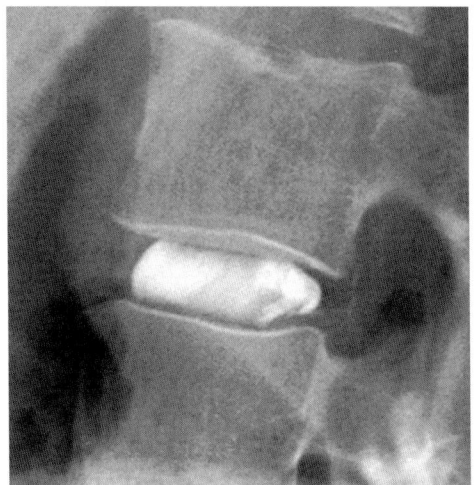 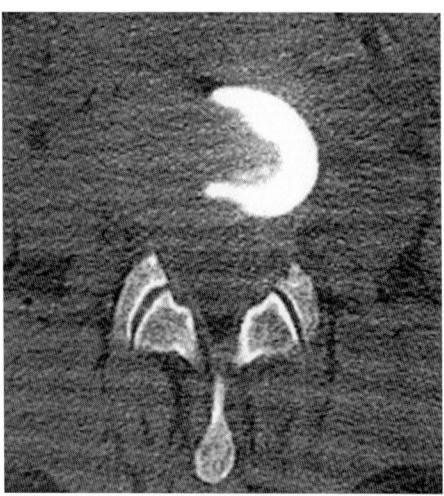

FIG. 10.1. Annular injection. **A:** Discographic appearance of an annular injection at L3–4. **B:** Computed tomography demonstrates contrast in the left side of the annulus.

(Fig. 10.3). In the latter situation, free spill of contrast medium into the epidural space may be seen. Rarely, contrast medium fills an adjacent nerve root sheath (Fig. 10.4) or the epidural venous plexus. Filling of an annular tear may be associated with the development of back pain, at which stage the injection is discontinued. Alternatively, with advanced disc degeneration and generalized annular disruption, several milliliters of contrast medium can be injected with little pressure.

The various discographic appearances of the nucleus were classified by Adams et al. (1). The normal nucleus may have either a "cotton wool" appearance (type 1) or a "hamburger" appearance caused by the intranuclear cleft (type 2) (Fig. 10.2). In the presence

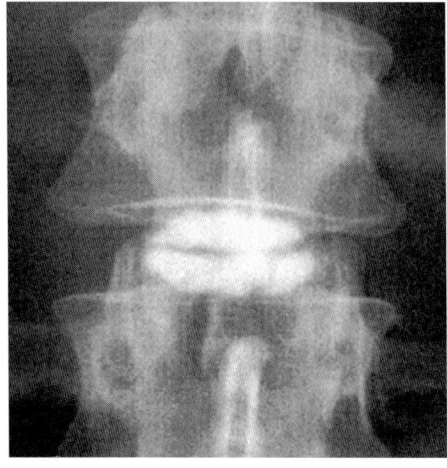 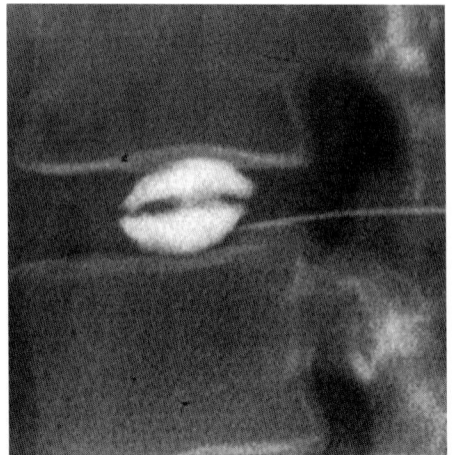

FIG. 10.2. Normal findings on discography at the L2–3 level. **A:** Anteroposterior image. **B:** Lateral image. Classic "hamburger" sign.

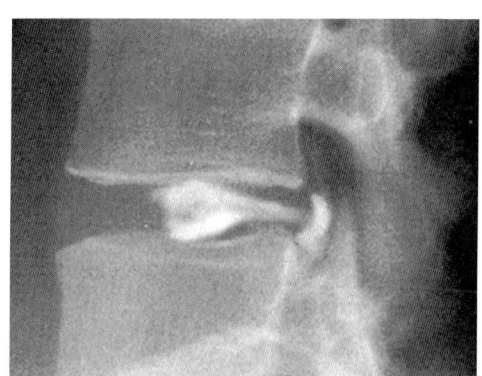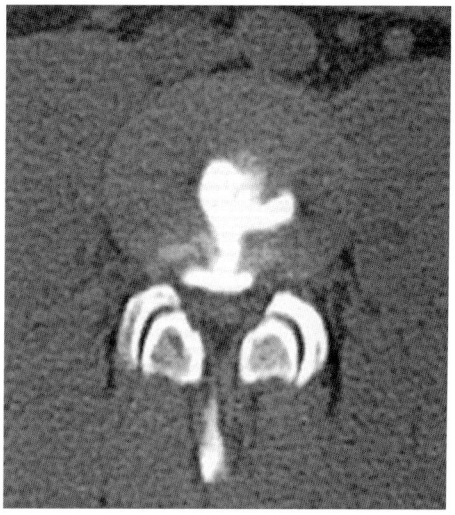

FIG. 10.3. Abnormal findings on computed tomographic (CT) discography at the L3–4 level. **A:** Lateral discogram shows incomplete filling of the nucleus with a full-thickness posterior annular rupture. **B:** CT discogram shows central posterior annular rupture.

of inner annular tears, the disc nucleus has an irregular outline (type 3). When radial tears extend into the outer annulus, the disc is described as being either fissured (type 4) or ruptured (type 5) (Fig. 10.3A). Lateral and anteroposterior images of the injected disc are obtained. The demonstration of an annular tear is important because this is the most common abnormal discographic finding associated with pain reproduction (46). However, annular pathology is optimally demonstrated by the addition of CT (CT discography) (5,44) (Fig. 10.3B). Using this technique, Sachs et al. (58) devised a system for record-

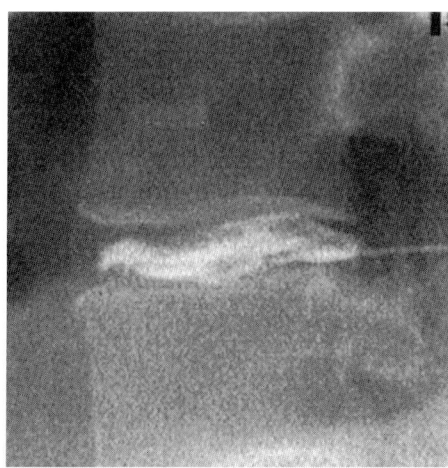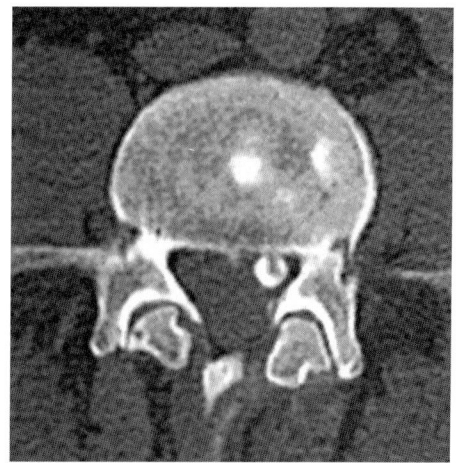

FIG. 10.4. Nerve root sheath filling following L3–4 discography. **A:** Lateral discogram showing advanced nuclear degeneration and posterior annular rupture. **B:** Computed tomographic discogram at the level of the L4 pedicle showing contrast medium in the left L4 nerve root sheath.

ing discographic findings, termed the *Dallas discogram description*, that considered five different categories of information: disc degeneration, annular disruption, provoked pain response, volume injected, and miscellaneous information.

Gadolinium has been used as an intradiscal contrast medium. T1-weighted postdiscography MRI, so-called MR discography, is as accurate as CT discography for demonstrating normal discs, disc degeneration, annular rupture, disc herniation, and contrast leak (30).

Although CT provides detailed images of the injected disc in the axial plane, it is associated with increases in cost, time, and dose of radiation delivered to the patient. It has also been suggested that the additional information obtained from CT discography is minimal (3) because the most important part of the study is the assessment of the patient's response to the disc injection. In some respects, this can be the most difficult aspect of discography.

The injection of a disc that appears normal on MRI should ideally be associated with no pain or at most a feeling of pressure. Such a response acts as an "internal control" for the assessment of the pain response at other disc levels. If the disc injection results in pain, the patient should be questioned about the nature, site, and severity of the pain and its relationship to daily symptoms. The latter can be recorded as dissimilar, similar, or an exact reproduction (58). Radiation into the buttocks, groins, or lower limbs should be recorded.

Various techniques have been reported that attempt to increase the specificity of the recorded pain response. Observation of the patient's facial expression at the time of the injection is particularly useful. Actual video recording of the patient's response has been suggested (2). Not uncommonly, severe pain reproduction corresponds to the filling of a radial annular tear.

Pain drawings have been used to identify patients likely to report pain during the injection of normal discs (49). Patients' pain drawings completed before CT discography were classified as either normal or abnormal. It was found that patients with abnormal pain drawings (indicating a nonanatomic pain pattern) were significantly more likely to report concordant pain reproduction during the injection of nondisrupted discs. The overall accuracy of pain drawings in identifying patients with false-positive pain reports was 78.0%.

Pressure recording at the time of disc injection has been used to identify chemically sensitive discs (positive result at a low injection pressure) and differentiate these from mechanically sensitive discs (positive result at a high injection pressure) (2). Such differentiation may have practical implications regarding the choice of surgical management. It has been suggested that patients with chemically sensitive discs do better with discectomy and interbody fusion, as opposed to an inter-transverse fusion (19).

COMPLICATIONS

A number of short- and long-term complications of lumbar discography have been reported. Complications developing during the procedure include nausea (2%), convulsions (4%), back pain (6%), and hypotension (10%); on the following day, severe headache (10%) and worsening back pain (81%) may occur. Headache may be related to a loss of cerebrospinal fluid resulting from inadvertent root sleeve puncture during needle placement (73).

The most common and serious long-term complication is discitis, with a reported occurrence in 0 to 4.92% of patients and in 0 to 2.99% of injected discs (25). The use of

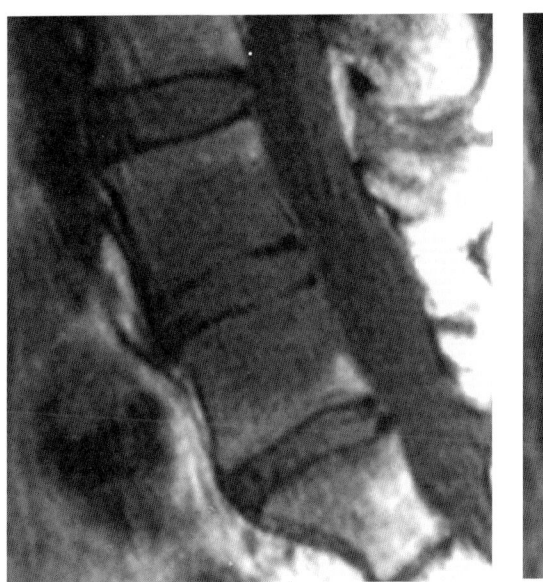 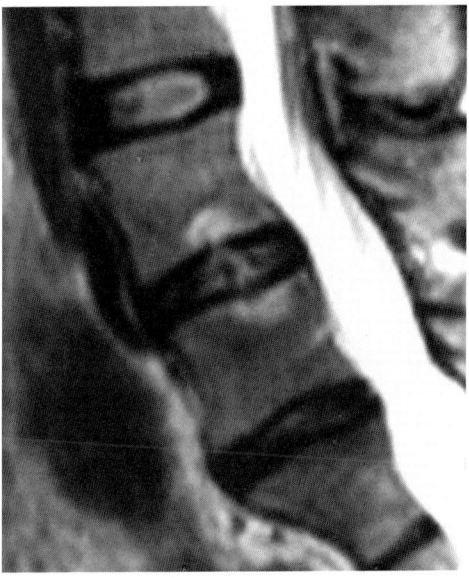

FIG. 10.5. Postdiscography discitis at L4–5. **A:** Sagittal T1-weighted magnetic resonance (MR) image showing extensive subchondral marrow edema in the L4 and L5 vertebral bodies. **B:** Sagittal T2-weighted MR image showing hyperintensity in the L4–5 disc with adjacent marrow edema.

prophylactic antibiotics and a double-needle technique can reduce this risk (50). Discitis manifests as a marked worsening of LBP with an associated raised erythrocyte sedimentation rate at a mean of 20 days after the procedure. The clinical diagnosis is confirmed by MRI, which shows typical features of a hyperintense disc on T2-weighted images and adjacent edematous vertebral marrow (24) (Fig. 10.5). Uncomplicated lumbar discography does not cause endplate changes identifiable by MRI (62). Lumbar discitis typically settles with conservative measures at 8 to 11 weeks (24).

Rarely reported complications include epidural abscess (34), retroperitoneal hemorrhage, and penetration of the dura (43).

Although studies are limited, discography does not appear to cause long-term damage to normal discs (33). However, back pain has been reported up to 1 year following discography in patients without low back symptoms but with significant emotional and chronic pain syndromes unrelated to the lumbar spine. Conversely, subjects with normal psychologic profiles do not report significant long-term back pain following discography (9).

VALIDITY

The validity of discography has been questioned because of the high proportion of false-positive results reported by some authors. The study by Holt (28), in which discography performed in asymptomatic prisoners had a false-positive rate of 37%, is commonly quoted, but these results have since been discredited by Simmons et al. (68). In a carefully controlled study, Walsh et al. (77) performed discography in seven symptomatic and 10 asymptomatic persons. Although 17% of the discs in 50% of the asymptomatic cases showed some abnormality on discography, none resulted in significant back pain. In this small group, therefore, the specificity of discography was considered to be 100%.

Many studies have reported the relationship between pain production at discography and the psychologic status of the patient. Block et al. (7) performed discography in a series of patients who had been assessed with the Minnesota Multiphasic Personality Inventory. They found that patients with significantly elevated scores for hypochondriasis, hysteria, and depression were more likely to report pain reproduction during injection of nondisrupted discs. They concluded that the pain reported at discography is not only a function of abnormal disc anatomy but also related to personality. Carragee et al. (14) performed several studies assessing the outcome of disc injection in asymptomatic persons and patients with various problems unrelated to the lower back. In a study of discography in 26 patients with no history of LBP, 10 were normal, 10 had chronic neck and arm pain, and six had a primary somatization disorder; significant positive pain responses and pain-related behavior were found in 10% of the pain-free group, 40% of the chronic cervical pain group, and 83% of the somatization disorder group (12). Similarly, when symptomatic and asymptomatic patients who had previously undergone discectomy were compared, discography was commonly found to produce pain on injection of previously operated discs in the asymptomatic group (10). Finally, discography was performed in a group of patients with no history of LBP who had undergone posterior iliac crest bone graft harvesting for nonthoracolumbar spinal procedures 2 to 4 months previously. A significant number of disc injections resulted in pain that was considered to be either similar to or exactly the same as pain experienced at the iliac crest bone graft harvest sites. The authors questioned the ability of patients to discriminate between pain of spinal and nonspinal origin following disc injection (13).

It is clear from these studies that assessment of the pain response can be very difficult, and the results underscore the need for extremely careful patient selection and discography technique. If these criteria are not met, discography may act as a tool for inappropriate surgery, as suggested by Bogduk and Modic (8).

OUTCOME STUDIES OF THE MANAGEMENT OF DISCOGRAM-POSITIVE LOW BACK PAIN

Management options for discogram-positive LBP include conservative treatment, minimally invasive therapies, and surgery.

Smith et al. (72) reported the outcome of nonoperative treatment in 25 patients with single-level, discogram-positive LBP, assessed at a minimum of 3 years and a mean of 4.9 years after discography. They found that 68% of the patients improved, 8% stayed the same, and 24% worsened. An older age at onset and a shorter duration of LBP were favorable indicators. Conversely, the presence of a psychiatric disorder was associated with a poor outcome. They concluded that conservative treatment was comparable with or better than surgical treatment for this condition.

Previously reported minimally invasive treatments that have used discography for the diagnosis include chemonucleolysis and percutaneous discectomy. However, current interest is focused on intradiscal electrothermal therapy, alternatively termed *intradiscal thermal annuloplasty* (35). Karasek and Bogduk (35) reported improvement in 53% of 35 patients at 12-months after intradiscal thermal annuloplasty. Saal and Saal (55) reported the 1- and 2-year outcomes of a cohort of 58 patients with chronic discogenic LBP who were treated with intradiscal electrothermal therapy following unsuccessful conservative treatment. They identified significant improvements in pain scores, functional outcome, and quality of life at 1 year, which had improved further by the time of the 2-year assessment.

Many studies have reported the outcome of surgery for discogenic LBP. Parker et al. (51) reviewed the literature published between 1980 and 1994 pertaining to spinal fusion for the condition they termed *idiopathic degenerative disc disease*; in the majority of cases, discography was used in the preoperative diagnosis. A satisfactory to good outcome was recorded in 35% to 92% of patients. The difficulty of comparing the multitude of studies relates to differences in patient characteristics, surgical techniques, and outcome measures. Isolated posterolateral fusion appears to be associated with the least optimal outcome (51,76). Conversely, combined posterolateral and interbody fusion, so-called 360-degree fusion, appears to give the best results (38,39,76).

Studies assessing the relevance of discography to surgical outcome are distinctly lacking. Colhoun et al. (16) reported a favorable clinical outcome in 89% of 137 patients who had pain reproduction at discography, versus only 52% of 25 patients who had abnormal disc images but no pain reproduction. This raises the question as to the reason for the improvement in the latter group. It has also been noted that despite solid fusion confirmed by "second look" exploration, not all patients are necessarily pain-free, indicating that a positive discography result is not the only factor in predicting surgical outcome (39). Gill and Blumenthal (22) compared the outcome of patients with a positive result of discography and normal or abnormal MRI findings at the L5–S1 level. Patients with an abnormal lumbosacral disc on both discography and MRI appeared to do better than those in whom the MRI appearance was normal and discography showed a contained annular tear. They suggested that discography should be performed only when MRI findings are abnormal. More recently, Madan et al. (42) compared the long-term outcome of spinal fusion in two groups of patients; the first group had been investigated without discography (group A) and the second with discography (group B). The characteristics of the two groups did not differ significantly. At the time of final follow-up, satisfactory outcomes were recorded in 75.6% of the group A patients and 81.2% of the group B patients. The authors concluded that screening provocative discography did not improve the surgical outcome after circumferential fusion for discogenic LBP.

CONCLUSIONS

Controversy surrounds all aspects of lumbar discography. This may, in part, be related to a lack of standardization of the technique. If discography is to be used in the preoperative assessment of LBP, particular care should be given to appropriate patient selection and assessment of the patient's response. Otherwise, the occurrence of false-positive results will continue to result in inappropriate surgery.

REFERENCES

1. Adams MA, Dolan P, Hutton WC. The stages of disc degeneration as revealed by discograms. *J Bone Joint Surg Br* 1986;68:36–41.
2. Anderson SR, Flanagan B. Discography. *Curr Rev Pain* 2000;4:345–352.
3. Antti-Poika I, Soini J, Tallroth K, et al. Clinical relevance of discography combined with CT scanning. A study of 100 patients. *J Bone Joint Surg Br* 1990;72:480–485.
4. Aprill C, Bogduk N. High-intensity zone: a diagnostic sign of painful lumbar disc on magnetic resonance imaging. *Br J Radiol* 1992;65:361–369.
5. Bernard TN Jr. Lumbar discography followed by computed tomography. Refining the diagnosis of low-back pain. *Spine* 1990;15:690–707.
6. Bernard TN Jr. Using computed tomography/discography and enhanced magnetic resonance imaging to distinguish between scar tissue and recurrent lumbar disc herniation. *Spine* 1994;19:2826–2832.
7. Block AR, Vanharanta H, Ohnmeiss DD, et al. Discographic pain report. Influence of psychological factors. *Spine* 1996;21:334–338.
8. Bogduk N, Modic MT. Lumbar discography. *Spine* 1996;21:402–404.
9. Carragee EJ, Chen Y, Tanner CM, et al. Can discography cause long-term back symptoms in previously asymptomatic subjects? *Spine* 2000;25:1803–1808.
10. Carragee EJ, Chen Y, Tanner CM, et al. Provocative discography in patients after limited lumbar discectomy: a controlled, randomized study of pain response in symptomatic and asymptomatic subjects. *Spine* 2000;25:3065–3071.

11. Carragee EJ, Paragioudakis SJ, Khurana S. 2000 Volvo Award in Clinical Studies. Lumbar high-intensity zone and discography in subjects without low back problems. *Spine* 2000;25:2987–2992.
12. Carragee EJ, Tanner CM, Khurana S, et al. The rates of false-positive lumbar discography in select patients without low back symptoms. *Spine* 2000;25:1373–1380.
13. Carragee EJ, Tanner CM, Yang B, et al. False-positive findings on lumbar discography. Reliability of subjective concordance assessment during provocative disc injection. *Spine* 1999;24:2542–2547.
14. Carragee EJ. Is lumbar discography a determinant of discogenic low back pain: provocative discography reconsidered. *Curr Rev Pain* 2000;4:301–308.
15. Castro WH, Jerosch J, Schilgen M, et al. Automated percutaneous nucleotomy: restricted indications based on CT scan appearance. *Neurosurg Clin N Am* 1996;7:43–47.
16. Colhoun E, McCall IW, Williams L, et al. Provocation discography as a guide to planning operations on the spine. *J Bone Joint Surg Br* 1988;70:267–271.
17. Coppes MH, Marani E, Thomeer RT, et al. Innervation of "painful" lumbar discs. *Spine* 1997;22:2342–2349.
18. Crock HV. Internal disc disruption. A challenge to disc prolapse fifty years on. *Spine* 1986;11:650–653.
19. Derby R, Howard MW, Grant JM, et al. The ability of pressure-controlled discography to predict surgical and nonsurgical outcomes. *Spine* 1999;24:364–371.
20. Fluke MM. The treatment of lumbar spine pain syndromes diagnosed by discography: lumbar arthrodesis. *Spine* 1995;20:501–504.
21. Fraser RD, Osti OL, Vernon-Roberts B. Discitis after discography. *J Bone Joint Surg Br* 1987;69:26–35.
22. Gill K, Blumenthal SL. Functional results after anterior lumbar fusion at L5-S1 in patients with normal and abnormal MRI scans. *Spine* 1992;17:940–942.
23. Grubb SA, Lipscomb HJ. Diagnostic findings in painful adult scoliosis. *Spine* 1992;17:518–527.
24. Guyer RD, Collier R, Stith WJ, et al. Discitis after discography. *Spine* 1988;13:1352–1354.
25. Guyer RD, Ohnmeiss DD. Lumbar discography. Position statement from the North American Spine Society Diagnostic and Therapeutic Committee. *Spine* 1995;20:2048–2059.
26. Heggeness MH, Doherty BJ. Discography causes end plate deflection. *Spine* 1993;18:1050–1053.
27. Heggeness MH, Watters WC 3rd, Gray PM Jr. Discography of lumbar discs after surgical treatment for disc herniation. *Spine* 1997;22:1606–1609.
28. Holt EP Jr. The question of lumbar discography. *J Bone Joint Surg Am* 1968;50:720–726.
29. Hsu KY, Zucherman JF, Derby R, et al. Painful lumbar end-plate disruptions: a significant discographic finding. *Spine* 1988;3:76–78.
30. Huang TS, Zucherman JF, Hsu KY, et al. Gadopentetate dimeglumine as an intradiscal contrast agent. *Spine* 2002;27:839–843.
31. Ito M, Incorvaia KM, Yu SF, et al. Predictive signs of discogenic lumbar pain on magnetic resonance imaging with discography correlation. *Spine* 1998;23:1252–1258.
32. Johnson RG, Macnab I. Localization of symptomatic lumbar pseudarthroses by use of discography. *Clin Orthop* 1985:164–170.
33. Johnson RG. Does discography injure normal discs? An analysis of repeat discograms. *Spine* 1989;14:424–426.
34. Junila J, Niinimaki T, Tervonen O. Epidural abscess after lumbar discography. A case report. *Spine* 1997;22:2191–2193.
35. Karasek M, Bogduk N. Twelve-month follow-up of a controlled trial of intradiscal thermal anuloplasty for back pain due to internal disc disruption. *Spine* 2000;25:2601–2607.
36. Kumar N, Agorastides ID. The curved needle technique for accessing the L5/S1 disc space. *Br J Radiol* 2000;73:655–657.
37. Lam KS, Carlin D, Mulholland RC. Lumbar disc high-intensity zone: the value and significance of provocative discography in the determination of the discogenic pain source. *Eur Spine J* 2000;9:36–41.
38. Lee CK, Vessa P, Lee JK. Chronic disabling low back pain syndrome caused by internal disc derangements. The results of disc excision and posterior lumbar interbody fusion. *Spine* 1995;20:356–361.
39. Leufven C, Nordwall A. Management of chronic disabling low back pain with 360 degrees fusion. Results from pain provocation test and concurrent posterior lumbar interbody fusion, posterolateral fusion, and pedicle screw instrumentation in patients with chronic disabling low back pain. *Spine* 1999;24:2042–2045.
40. Louwaege A, Goubau J, Deldycke H, et al. Efficiency of discography followed by chemonucleolysis in the treatment of sciatica. *J Belge Radiol* 1996;79:68–71.
41. MacMillan J, Schaffer JL, Kambin P. Routes and incidence of communication of lumbar discs with surrounding neural structures. *Spine* 1991;16:167–171.
42. Madan S, Gundanna M, Harley JM, et al. Does provocative discography screening of discogenic back pain improve surgical outcome? *J Spinal Disord Tech* 2002;15:245–251.
43. McCulloch JA, Waddell G. Lateral lumbar discography. *Br J Radiol* 1978;51:498–502.
44. McCutcheon ME, Thompson WC 3rd. CT scanning of lumbar discography. A useful diagnostic adjunct. *Spine* 1986;11:257–259.
45. McNally DS, Shackleford IM, Goodship AE, et al. In vivo stress measurement can predict pain on discography. *Spine* 1996;21:2580–2587.
46. Moneta GB, Videman T, Kaivanto K, et al. Reported pain during lumbar discography as a function of anular ruptures and disc degeneration. A re-analysis of 833 discograms. *Spine* 1994;19:1968–1974.

47. Murtagh FR, Arrington JA. Computer tomographically guided discography as a determinant of normal disc level before fusion. *Spine* 1992;17:826–830.
48. Ohnmeiss DD, Vanharanta H, Ekholm J. Degree of disc disruption and lower extremity pain. *Spine* 1997;22: 1600–1605.
49. Ohnmeiss DD, Vanharanta H, Guyer RD. The association between pain drawings and computed tomographic/discographic pain responses. *Spine* 1995;20:729–733.
50. Osti OL, Fraser RD, Vernon-Roberts B. Discitis after discography. The role of prophylactic antibiotics. *J Bone Joint Surg Br* 1990;72:271–274.
51. Parker LM, Murrell SE, Boden SD, et al. The outcome of posterolateral fusion in highly selected patients with discogenic low back pain. *Spine* 1996 15;21:1909–1916.
52. Reitman CA, Hipp JA, Kirking BC, et al. Posterior annular strains during discography. *J Spinal Disord* 2001;14: 347–352.
53. Ricketson R, Simmons JW, Hauser BO. The prolapsed intervertebral disc. The high-intensity zone with discography correlation. *Spine* 1996;21:2758–2762.
54. Saal JA, Saal JS. Intradiscal electrothermal treatment for chronic discogenic low back pain: a prospective outcome study with minimum 1-year follow-up. *Spine* 2000;25:2622–2627.
55. Saal JA, Saal JS. Intradiscal electrothermal treatment for chronic discogenic low back pain: prospective outcome study with a minimum 2-year follow-up. *Spine* 2002;27:966–973.
56. Saal JS. The role of inflammation in lumbar pain. *Spine* 1995;20:1821–1827.
57. Sachs BL, Spivey MA, Vanharanta H, et al. Techniques for lumbar discography and computed tomography/discography in clinical practice. *Orthop Rev* 1990;19:775–778.
58. Sachs BL, Vanharanta H, Spivey MA, et al. Dallas discogram description. A new classification of CT/discography in low-back disorders. *Spine* 1987;12:287–294.
59. Saifuddin A, Braithwaite I, White J, et al. The value of lumbar spine magnetic resonance imaging in the demonstration of anular tears. *Spine* 1998;23:453–457.
60. Saifuddin A, Emanuel R, White J, et al. An analysis of radiating pain at lumbar discography. *Eur Spine J* 1998;7: 358–362.
61. Saifuddin A, Remedios D, White J, et al. *Changes in intervertebral disc height during lumbar discography.* Presented at Worldspine I, Berlin, August 2000.
62. Saifuddin A, Renton P, Taylor BA. Effects on the vertebral end-plate of uncomplicated lumbar discography: an MRI study. *Eur Spine J* 1998;7:36–39.
63. Sandhu HS, Sanchez-Caso LP, Parvataneni HK, et al. Association between findings of provocative discography and vertebral endplate signal changes as seen on MRI. *J Spinal Disord* 2000;13:438–443.
64. Schechter NA, France MP, Lee CK. Painful internal disc derangements of the lumbosacral spine: discographic diagnosis and treatment by posterior lumbar interbody fusion. *Orthopedics* 1991;14.447 451.
65. Schellhas KP, Pollei SR, Gundry CR, et al. Lumbar disc high-intensity zone. Correlation of magnetic resonance imaging and discography. *Spine* 1996;21:79–86.
66. Schwarzer AC, Aprill CN, Derby R, et al. The prevalence and clinical features of internal disc disruption in patients with chronic low back pain. *Spine* 1995;20:1878–1883.
67. Simmons EH, Segil CM. An evaluation of discography in the localization of symptomatic levels in discogenic disease of the spine. *Clin Orthop* 1975;108:57–69.
68. Simmons JW, Aprill CN, Dwyer AP, et al. A reassessment of Holt's data on: "The question of lumbar discography." *Clin Orthop* 1988;237:120–124.
69. Simmons JW, McMillin JN, Emery SF, et al. Intradiscal steroids. A prospective double-blind clinical trial. *Spine* 1992;17:S172–S175.
70. Slipman CW, Patel RK, Zhang L, et al. Side of symptomatic annular tear and site of low back pain: is there a correlation? *Spine* 2001;26:165–169.
71. Smith BM, Hurwitz EL, Solsberg D, et al. Interobserver reliability of detecting lumbar intervertebral disc high-intensity zone on magnetic resonance imaging and association of high-intensity zone with pain and anular disruption. *Spine* 1998;23:2074–2080.
72. Smith SE, Darden BV, Rhyne AL, et al. Outcome of unoperated discogram-positive low back pain. *Spine* 1995;20:1997–2000.
73. Tallroth K, Soini J, Antti-Poika I, et al. Premedication and short-term complications in iohexol discography. *Ann Chir Gynaecol* 1991;80:49–53.
74. Tehranzadeh J. Discography 2000. *Radiol Clin North Am* 1998;36:463–495.
75. Urasaki T, Muro T, Ito S, et al. Consistency of lumbar discograms of the same disc obtained twice at a 2-week interval: influence of needle tip position. *J Orthop Sci* 1998;3:243–251.
76. Vamvanij V, Fredrickson BE, Thorpe JM, et al. Surgical treatment of internal disc disruption: an outcome study of four fusion techniques. *J Spinal Disord* 1998;11:375–382.
77. Walsh TR, Weinstein JN, Spratt KF, et al. Lumbar discography in normal subjects. A controlled, prospective study. *J Bone Joint Surg Am* 1990;72:1081–1088.
78. Weinstein J, Claverie W, Gibson S. The pain of discography. *Spine* 1988;13:1344–1348.
79. Weishaupt D, Zanetti M, Hodler J, et al. Painful lumbar disk derangement: relevance of endplate abnormalities at MR imaging. *Radiology* 2001;218:420–427.

11

Disc Degeneration and Low Back Pain

*†Michel Benoist and ‡Philippe Boulu

*University of Paris VII, Paris, France; Departments of †Rheumatology and ‡Neurology, Hôpital Beaujon, Clichy, France

Low back pain (LBP) is the scourge of modern society. In rheumatology clinics, it is a predominant cause of consultation. At the individual level, the exact source of pain is difficult to identify and often remains unknown. It is generally admitted that degenerative changes of the disc are responsible for most cases of low back and radicular painful episodes, and the classic concept is that loss of integrity of the disc is followed by the development of LBP. However, many sources of nociception are found in other structures of the motion segment, including facets, ligaments, and muscles. Yet it is generally recognized that degenerative changes in the facets and ligaments follow degeneration of the intervertebral disc (23).

The purpose of this chapter is to discuss the relationship between disc degeneration and low back and radicular pain. We attempt to answer the following questions:

1. Can the biochemical and biomechanical changes implicated in or resulting from disc degeneration lead to nociception and pain production?
2. Can LBP symptoms be correlated with signs of degeneration seen on imaging studies?
3. Is it possible to recognize the degenerated disc(s) responsible for LBP or radicular pain?

DISC DEGENERATION AND NOCICEPTION

The generation of LPB or radicular pain requires three key factors: (a) nociceptors in the tissue in which the nociceptive message is produced, (b) the liberation in tissue of pain-producing substances capable of lowering the response threshold of the nociceptors, and (c) biomechanical alterations that physically stimulate the nociceptors.

Schematically, persons whose pain can be attributed to disc degeneration comprise two categories: those with acute, subacute, or chronic pure LBP and those with a radiculopathy. We discuss, in turn, how the process of degeneration can be implicated in nociception in these two groups of patients. In the case of radicular pain caused by a herniated disc, the nerve root is the nociceptive receptor responsible for transmitting the pain message. In the case of pure LBP, the nerve fibers located in the degenerated disc and relevant to pain sensation comprise a receptor unit.

Disc Degeneration and Radicular Pain

A direct link between degenerative changes in the disc and radicular pain was established many years ago when Mixter and Barr demonstrated that compression of a nerve root by a disc herniation, the ultimate complication of disc degeneration, could cause sciatica. Disc degeneration always precedes disc herniation (29).

Mechanical deformation of the nerve root has long been thought to be the primary source of radicular pain. However, some clinical observations have progressively cast doubt on this theory. For example, in some conservatively treated patients, pain disappears despite persistence of a disc herniation on imaging studies. In contrast, some patients with no evidence of a disc herniation or stenosis have a severe radiculopathy. These observations, in addition to the occasional spontaneous resorption of a disc herniation, led to experimental studies that explored the biologic activity of the prolapsed degenerated disc (3).

Clinical studies have shown that touching a healthy nerve root under local anesthesia is not painful. In contrast, touching a nerve root compressed by a disc herniation reproduces the usual radicular pain. This observation indicates that some kind of sensitization by the disc tissue is necessary to induce radicular pain (22). Thus, two questions can be asked: What are the biologic mechanisms involved in sensitization of the nerve root by the degenerated disc tissue, and how is this phenomenon linked to disc degeneration?

A new avenue of research was opened in 1993 by a report indicating that nucleus pulposus implanted without compression on the nerve roots of pigs induces both a significant reduction in conduction velocity and nerve fiber degeneration (28). In subsequent studies, it was shown that the axonal changes, including myelin injury, increased vascular permeability, and intravascular coagulation, in addition to the functional changes induced in the nerve roots by the application of nucleus pulposus could be eliminated if the cells were killed by freezing. These experiments demonstrated that the biologic effect of nucleus pulposus is related to the cell population (25). These studies in pigs also implicated a chondrocyte-like product in nerve root dysfunction and altered structure, but the production of pain was not clearly demonstrated.

In two experimental studies (20,27), pain behavior in rats was observed to assess whether nucleus pulposus could also cause pain sensation. Both studies examined the response thresholds to thermal and mechanical stimuli after the application of nucleus pulposus to nerve roots. In both studies, behavioral consequences characterized by allodynia were noted. In the study by Olmarker and Myers (27), pain behavior was present only if a slight mechanical deformation was associated with the application of nucleus pulposus. It has been rightly argued that the notochordal cells of the animals used in the experiments suggesting that disc cells can produce neurotoxic factors (pigs, rats, mice) are different from the chondrocyte-like cells in the human nucleus (35). However, other studies, in which control normal human disc specimens and herniated disc tissue from patients undergoing surgery were used, have shown that the cells of the intervertebral discs are biologically active.

In studies performed by Kang et al. (18,19), herniated lumbar discs in culture media spontaneously produced increased amounts of nitric oxide, prostaglandin E_2 (PGE_2), interleukin-6 (IL-6), and matrix metalloproteinases (MMPs) in comparison with normal control discs. In a further study by the same authors, stimulation with IL-1β dramatically increased the production of nitric oxide, IL-6, and PGE_2 in normal, nondegenerate discs. Production was also increased in degenerate discs, but to a lesser degree.

Takahashi et al. (33) detected inflammatory cytokines, including IL-1α, IL-1β, IL-6, tumor necrosis factor-α (TNF-α), and granulocyte–macrophage colony–stimulating factor, at sites of lumbar disc herniation in homogenates of degenerate disc tissue obtained from patients undergoing surgery for disc herniation. Cells producing cytokines were also detected with immunohistologic staining. In tissues from patients with protrusion-type herniations, most of the cells were chondrocytes. In the samples from patients with extruded or sequestrated fragments, the cells in the granulation tissue surrounding the herniation and in the disc tissue were macrophages, fibroblasts, and endothelial cells. Moreover, the production of PGE_2, also detected in the culture, was dramatically increased by the addition of IL-1α and decreased by betamethasone. Proinflammatory cytokines can contribute to pain indirectly by increasing the production of PGE_2 by cells. PGE_2 plays an important role in pain production by directly stimulating nerve fibers or by enhancing sensitivity to other pain-producing substances such as bradykinin (33).

The biologic effects of degenerate disc tissue have been attributed to the cytokines present in granulation tissue and in the herniation. Neurotoxic properties have been demonstrated in various cytokines, such as IL-1α, interferon-γ, and TNF-α (32). Another study (26) has shown that TNF-α is the key substance in inducing the inflammatory neuropathy associated with the application of disc tissue. The topical application of TNF-α to the nerve roots of rats induces histologic changes, including endoneural edema, demyelination, and wallerian degeneration of the axons. The same study has shown that in addition to neuropathologic changes, behavior deficits similar to those observed after the application of nucleus pulposus develop after mechanical and thermal stimulation (17). More recently, Aoki et al. (1) have shown that unlike other cytokines, TNF-α locally applied to cauda equina of pigs induces a reduction in nerve conduction velocity even more pronounced than that induced with nucleus pulposus. It had previously been shown that the epidural application of substances could result in direct transport to axons by the route between the epidural space and intraneural capillaries (6). It has been suggested that TNF α liberated at the site of the nerve root barrier reaches the axons in this way. A subsequent cascade of neuropathic changes includes the activation of Schwann cells and the recruitment of additional macrophages, which inside the endoneurium further stimulate the production of TNF-α with ensuing inflammatory neuropathy (36). Because TNF-α alone can cause allodynia and morphologic changes that mimic human radiculopathy, it has been suggested that anti-TNF drugs be given to patients with sciatica (1). In a pilot study, 10 patients with acute sciatica and discal herniation were treated with infliximab. Treatment was highly effective and caused no adverse reactions (21).

What is the biologic link between LBP and radicular pain and disc degeneration? Numerous factors influence degeneration of the disc, including genetic factors, aging, excessive loading, and nutrition (35). The role of MMPs in matrix degradation has been emphasized (15,30). MMPs can be produced by endogenous cells and also by cells of the invading vessels. They are able to degrade proteoglycans and collagen and play an important role in disc degeneration. In a study in which immunohistochemistry methods were used (38), all four MMPs (collagenase, gelatinase, stromelysin, membrane-type MMP) were expressed in disc tissue obtained at surgery. Surgical specimens were obtained from patients of different ages (age range, 11 to 68 years). This study was able to demonstrate greater MMP expression with advancing age. MMP expression was also correlated with the formation of tears and clefts. Interestingly, the production of these enzymes depends on a number of cytokines, such as IL1-α, IL-1β, and TNF-α (15). Thus, proinflammatory cytokines are directly involved in the process of matrix degradation and also, especially TNF-α, the pathophysiology of acute sciatica. The cytokine network is the biologic link between disc degeneration and radicular pain (Fig. 11.1).

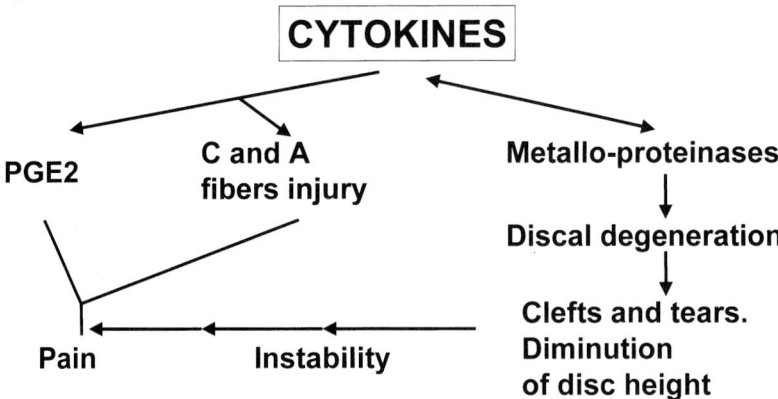

FIG. 11.1. Cytokines responsible for the production of pain also up-regulate the production of proteinases. *PGE2*, prostaglandin E$_2$.

Disc Degeneration and Discogenic Low Back Pain

In patients with radicular pain, the relationship between pain and disc degeneration is clearly established. Both depend on a failure of cellular activity that leads to the production of pain-producing substances and matrix-degrading proteolytic enzymes. However, the etiologic conditions and mechanisms associated with pure LBP are less well documented. As previously mentioned, several structures of the motion segment can be implicated in the generation of pain. For example, nociceptors have been described in facet joints, ligaments, and muscles. However, the intervertebral disc is generally considered the primary source of pure LBP. The term *discogenic low back pain*, generally used to designate nonspecific LBP, reflects the focus of the medical community on intervertebral disc pathology. The question that can be asked is: Can a degenerate disc be a source of nociception causing LBP?

If a tissue is to be a source of nociception, nerve fibers relevant to the sensation of pain must be present. Nociceptors of painful stimuli include the free nerve endings of small myelinated A-δ nerve fibers, high-threshold nociceptors responding to firm mechanical pressure, and the free endings of polymodal nociceptive unmyelinated nerve fibers responding to various activating stimuli, including mechanical, chemical, heat, and ischemic stimuli.

Studies have shown the presence of nociceptive nerve fibers in the annulus and also in the inner nucleus of the intervertebral disc. Roberts et al. (31) used immunohistochemistry to investigate samples of human intervertebral discs from patients undergoing anterior fusion for LBP or scoliosis. Mechanoreceptors were found in 50% of the discs from patients with LBP and 15% of the discs from patients with scoliosis. Coppes et al. (8) used neurofilament and substance P immunocytochemistry to investigate the anterior segment of 10 degenerate discs from patients undergoing anterior fusion for chronic LBP and two control discs. Nerve fibers of different diameters were found in the outer region of the disc. Eight of 10 degenerate discs contained nerve fibers invading to a level deeper than the outer third of the disc. The presence of innervation expressing substance P in the inner part of the annulus and in the nucleus has been demonstrated in the study by Freemont et al. (13). In this study, 43 discs were obtained from 35 patients undergoing anterior surgery for chronic LBP. Preoperative discography assessed the anatomic pain level by reproducing the original pain. Thirty symptomatic levels and 16 nonsymptomatic levels were defined by discography. In eight patients, samples were taken from both painful and nonpainful levels. In addition, 34 control samples were obtained from cadavers without a history of LBP. Analysis of the samples included a standard histologic examination and immunohistochemistry studies for protein gene product 9.5, general nerve marker, substance P, and growth-associated protein, expressed during axonogenesis. Innervation of the inner third of the annulus was detected in 57% of the painful levels and 25% of the nonpainful levels, and never in the control discs. Innervation of the nucleus was found in 30% of the painful levels and 6% of the nonpainful levels. Most of the nerve fibers identified by immunochemistry accompanied blood vessels; this topographic relation, already reported in other studies (8,31), suggests a role for vascular regulation of these nerves. However, another set of neural elements independent of vessels, expressing substance P and with a morphology of nociceptive nerve terminals, have been found in the nucleus of 30% of painful discs and never in control or nonpainful discs (13). Taken together, these observations indicate the presence of nociceptors in degenerate discs and particularly in painful degenerate discs. This important finding strongly suggests a role for nerve terminals in the pathogenesis of LBP.

An innervated disc can be a source of nociception. The nerve terminals can be sensitized in three different ways. Figure 11.2 presents a hypothetical and rough sketch of the biologic events leading to the sensitization of nerve terminals and the generation of LBP. First, neuropeptides, such as substance P and calcitonin gene–related peptide, expressed by nerve fibers can have a vasodilator effect, including an increase in the local microcirculation and extravasation of plasma. Neurogenic inflammation releases inflammatory

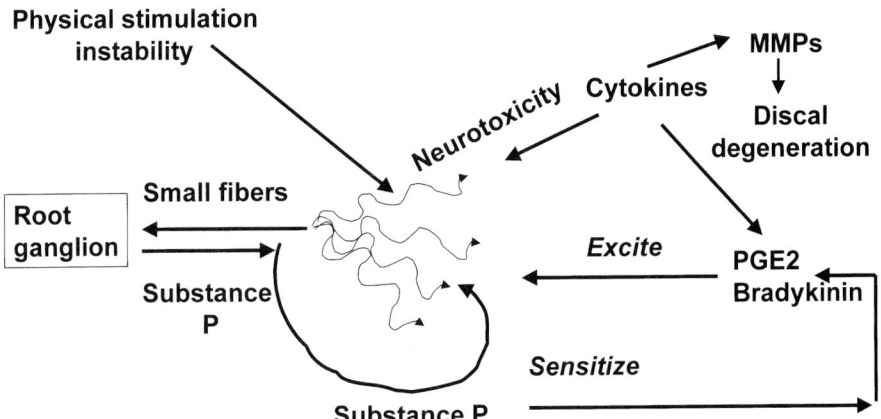

FIG. 11.2. Hypothetical sketch of peripheral sensitization of nerve terminals found in denervated painful discs. Substance P released from the nerve endings directly excites the nociceptors and induces neurogenic inflammation. Cytokines have a neurotoxic effect and enhance the production of chemical substances that excite the nociceptors. Mechanical stimuli, even micromovements of the motion segment, may excite the sensitized nerve endings. *MMPs,* matrix metalloproteinases; *PGE2,* prostaglandin E_2.

substances (histamine, serotonin, bradykinin), which in turn excite and sensitize the sensory nerve terminals (9,31).

Second, proinflammatory mediators, including PGE_2 and cytokines (IL-6, IL-7, and IL-8) have been found at high levels in tissue cultures of patients undergoing lumbar interbody fusion for "discogenic low back pain" (5). IL-1 and TNF-α have been detected in homogenates of contained subligamentous disc herniations inside the intervertebral space (33). These cytokines are potent stimulators of prostaglandins, which in turn sensitize the afferent pain fibers. The neurotoxic effect of TNF-α has already been discussed.

Third, disc degeneration can contribute to the production of nonspecific LBP through mechanical mechanisms. Tears and clefts of the disc and a diminution of disc height, which are the macroscopic hallmarks of disc degeneration, lead to mechanical instability of the motion segment. Even micromovements may cause pain when sensitized nerve terminals are stimulated (5).

DIAGNOSIS OF DISCOGENIC LOW BACK PAIN

Basic and clinical science has clearly established that disc degeneration is a potential source of nociception capable of generating LBP and radicular pain. From a clinical point of view, the question that can be asked is: Can LBP symptoms be correlated with specific clinical and imaging signs?

In the case of radicular pain, clinical examination and modern imaging techniques can easily demonstrate a degenerate disc fragment compressing a nerve root. In the case of pure LBP, the etiologic role of the disc, although commonly recognized, is more difficult to establish because other structures of the motion segment can also be a source of nociception. However, disabling low back illness not responding to medical treatment may require surgical management, such as various types of fusion or implants. At that point, if surgical treatment is considered, it is imperative to recognize with accuracy the disc(s) responsible for the pain because the aim of the surgical procedure is to eliminate the source of nociception. In cases of knee or hip osteoarthritis, specific clinical signs or symptoms can indicate precisely the generator of pain. Unfortunately, this is not possible in the face of nonspecific LBP.

Can low back symptoms be correlated with radiographic changes consistent with disc degeneration? In other words, in a patient presenting with a subacute or chronic LBP, can disc degeneration demonstrated on plain radiographs be considered the source of pain? Numerous studies have compared radiographs from patients with LBP and those of asymptomatic persons (14,34). The conclusion of these studies has been that plain radiographs are of little value in detecting the exact cause of nonspecific LBP. It is well-known that radiographs of asymptomatic persons may reveal major degenerative changes of the disc.

Magnetic resonance imaging (MRI) noninvasively provides precise information about the status of the disc. Moreover, the diagnosis of disc degeneration by MRI makes it possible to correlate morphologic findings with LBP. Can MRI recognize precisely the painful lesions of the disc(s)? A few studies have attempted to answer this question. In the first study, by Boden et al. (4), disc degeneration on MRI was not necessarily correlated with pain because MRI disclosed disc degeneration in more 30% of 67 asymptomatic subjects. Vertebral endplate changes described by Modic et al. (24) and the high-intensity zone (HIZ) described by Aprill and Bogduk (2) have been considered specific markers of painful discs. Such findings are controversial because HIZs and Modic changes of the endplate are also found in asymptomatic subjects (12). The temporal relationship between the incidence of LBP and the appearance of disc degeneration on MRI has been in examined a 5-year longitudinal study of asymptomatic persons (12). MRI was performed in 41 asymptomatic subjects at baseline and at 5-year follow-up. MRI changes rated included disc degeneration, bone marrow changes of the endplates, and HIZs. Of the 41 subjects, 17 (41%) with deterioration of disc degeneration reported LBP more frequently, experienced longer episodes of LBP, and required more medical consultations than did the subjects without progression of disc degeneration. However, probably because of the small size of the sample, the difference did not reach statistical significance. Bone marrow changes and HIZs were not associated with pain variables. These studies emphasize the difficulty of identifying the source of LBP by MRI abnormalities.

For this reason, the diagnosis of LBP related to disc degeneration includes a morphologic abnormality of the disc on MRI associated with concordant pain at discography, which is used as the gold standard to designate a painful disc. However, the value of provocative discography to identify painful degenerate discs is controversial. Holt (16) was the first to show that asymptomatic persons may have abnormal findings on discograms coupled with a positive pain response at discography. In a later study (37), no positive test result was obtained in 10 asymptomatic volunteers without any history of LBP. A positive test result included an abnormal discogram, noted in 17% of the discs injected, and an associated pain reaction, noted in none of the 10 asymptomatic subjects. Therefore, the false-positive rate was zero and the specificity was 100%. The limitations of this study were the small size of the sample and the young age of the paid volunteers (24 years), which was well below the average age of the symptomatic patients (44 years) examined in the same study. Therefore, the results cannot be applied to the general population of persons with LBP.

More recently, Carragee et al. (7) studied a group of asymptomatic patients with a mean age of 43 years. Of these, 10 were pain-free, 10 had chronic neck and arm pain but no LBP, and six had primary somatization without low back symptoms. A positive pain response and pain-related behavior were observed at discography in 10% of the pain-free group, 40% of the chronic cervical pain group, and 83% of the somatization group. This study demonstrates that persons with psychologic factors are likely to have higher pain scores than normal persons. In patients with chronic LBP, psychosocial factors frequently reduce the ability to analyze concordance of pain. In addition, chronic pain may sensitize and activate the central nervous system and thereby increase the responsiveness to a normally innocuous stimulus. As suggested by Deyo (11), the subjectivity of the test for both patients and investigators creates a real problem in accurately identifying the disc(s) responsible for nociception. It has also been suggested that one way to determine the value of a positive result of discography would be to compare the outcome of fusion with a positive result of preoperative discography. Such studies have been performed and indicate a low predictive value and specificity of the test (11).

What can be concluded?

First, accurate recognition of the painful disc(s) is mandatory only in the limited group of LBP patients for whom conservative therapy has failed and for whom a surgical option is being considered. Second, MRI accurately reflects the morphologic structure of the disc(s) and the degree and extent of degeneration, but it cannot precisely predict the symptomatic disc, especially in cases with degeneration at multiple levels. However, if an abnormality is seen on MRI at a single level, the source of the pain is identified.

118 CLINICAL PRESENTATION

Third, reproduction of the patient's pain by discography is the gold standard for identifying the generator of pain. However, as emphasized by Carragee et al. (7), the test is subjective and should be performed by competent investigators on psychologically sound patients.

Fourth, in the preoperative management of patients with discogenic LBP, MRI and discography are complementary and should both be performed, with discography restricted to the discs that appear abnormal on MRI.

CONCLUSIONS

At the beginning of this chapter, we questioned whether a degenerate disc could be a source of nociception and whether the disc(s) responsible for pain could be identified. The following conclusions can be drawn.

First, a degenerate disc is biologically active and can be a source of nociception. Disc degeneration depends on a failure of cellular activity that leads to the production of degradative enzymes and proinflammatory neurotoxic mediators causing pain. The cytokine network is the link between disc degeneration and pain. Increasing knowledge about the molecular mechanisms of tissue degradation and pain-generating factors may make it possible to develop new therapeutic strategies, such as pain therapy targeting the nociceptive cytokine or gene therapy to restore matrix production.

Second, even though the source of nociception has been identified (e.g., by discography), it must be remembered that pain is a complex phenomenon involving not only peripheral nociception but also the central nervous system, including the spinal cord and brain (Fig. 11.3). When massive signals reach spinal nociceptive neurons, the central nervous system may become sensitized. The release of large amounts of glutamate and substance P cause a permanent hyperexcitability of the neurons despite the diminution or

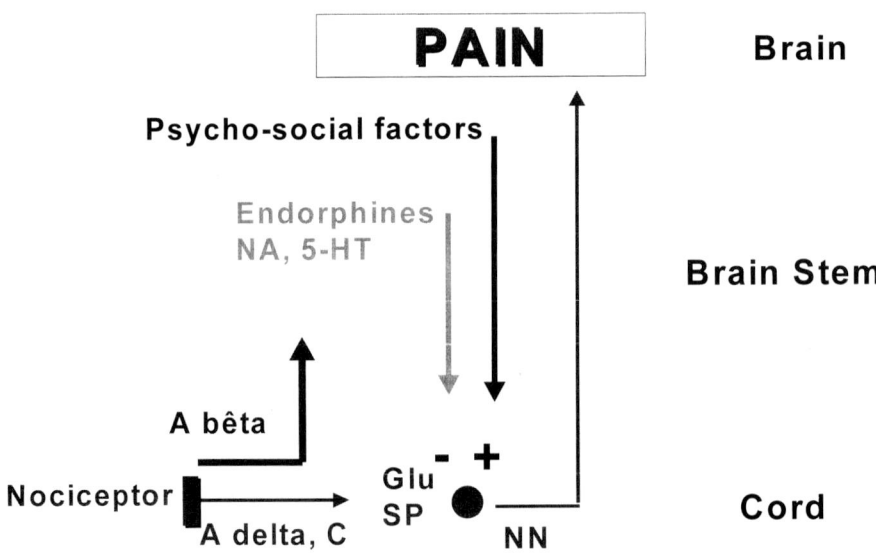

FIG. 11.3. Pain is a complex phenomenon involving not only peripheral nociception but also the central nervous system, including the spinal cord and brain, as shown.

even disappearance of the initial nociceptive message. When the treatment of chronic LBP is undertaken, peripheral and central parameters must be carefully analyzed, especially if fusion is being considered. Sensitization of the central nervous system can in itself be responsible for chronic LBP (10).

REFERENCES

1. Aoki Y, Rydevik B, Kikuchi S, et al. Local application of disc-related cytokines on spinal nerve roots. *Spine* 2002;27:1614–1618.
2. Aprill C, Bogduk N. High intensity zone. A diagnostic sign of painful lumbar disc on magnetic resonance imaging. *Br J Radiol* 1992;65:361–369.
3. Benoist M. The natural history of lumbar disc herniation and radiculopathy. *Joint Bone Spine* 2002;69:155–160.
4. Boden SD, Davis DO, Dina T, et al. Abnormal magnetic resonance scans of the lumbar spine in asymptomatic subjects: a prospective investigation. *J Bone Joint Surg Am* 1990;72:403–408.
5. Burke JG, Watson RW, McCormack D, et al. Intervertebral discs which cause low back pain secrete high levels of proinflammatory mediators. *J Bone Joint Surg Br* 2002;84:192–202.
6. Byrod G, Olmarker K, Konno S, et al. A rapid transport route between the epidural space and the endoneural capillaries of the nerve roots. *Spine* 1995;20:138–143.
7. Carragee EJ, Tanner CM, Khurana S, et al. The rates of false positive lumbar discography in select patients without low back symptoms. *Spine* 2000;25:1373–1381.
8. Coppes MA, Marani E, Thomeer RT, et al. Innervation of "painful" lumbar discs. *Spine* 1997;22:3242–3248.
9. Cuello AC, Matthews MK. In: Wall PD, Melzack R, eds. *Textbook of pain*. New York: Churchill Livingstone, 1985:65–79.
10. Deleo JA, Winkelstein BA. Physiology of chronic spinal pain syndromes. *Spine* 2002;27:2526–2537
11. Deyo RA. Reproducibility and accuracy of lumbar spine imaging studies. In: Wiesel SW, Weinstein JN, Kerkowitz H, et al., eds. *The lumbar spine*, 2nd ed, vol 1. Philadelphia: WB Saunders, 1996:434–446.
12. Effering A, Sommer N, Birkhofer D, et al. Young Investigator Award 2001. Risk factors for lumbar disc degeneration. A 5-year prospective MRI study in asymptomatic individuals. *Spine* 2002;27:125–134.
13. Freemont AJ, Peacock TE, Goupille P, et al. Nerve ingrowth into diseased intervertebral disc in chronic back pain. *Lancet* 1997;350:178–181.
14. Frymoyer JW, Newberg A, Pope M, et al. Spine radiographs in patients with low back pain. An epidemiological study in men. *J Bone Joint Surg Am* 1984;66.1048–1055.
15. Grange L, Gaudin F, Troeme C, et al. Dégénérescence discale et hernie discale. Rôle des métalloprotéases et cytokines. *Rev Rhum* 2001;68:613–619.
16. Holt AP. The question of lumbar discography. *J Bone Joint Surg Am* 1968;50:720–725.
17. Igarashi T, Kikuchi S, Shubayev V, et al. 2000 Volvo Award winner in basic science studies: Endogenous tumor necrosis factor alpha mimics nucleus pulposus–induced neuropathology: molecular, histologic and behavioral comparisons in rats. *Spine* 2000;25:2975–2980.
18. Kang JD, Georgescu H, McIntyre L, et al. Herniated lumbar intervertebral discs spontaneously produce matrix metalloproteinases, nitric oxide, interleukin 6, and prostaglandin E_2. *Spine* 1996;21:271–277.
19. Kang JD, Stefanovic-Racic M, McIntyre LA, et al. Toward a biochemical understanding of human intervertebral disc degeneration. Contributions of nitric oxide, interleukins, prostaglandin E_2, and matrix metalloproteinases. *Spine* 1997;22:1065–1073.
20. Kawakami M, Tamaki T, Weinstein JN, et al. Pathomechanism of pain-related behavior produced by allografts of intervertebral disc in the rat. *Spine* 1996;21:2101–2107.
21. Korhonen T, Karppinen Y, Malmivaara, et al. *Treatment of sciatic pain with infliximab, a monoclonal humanised chimaeric antibody against TNF-alpha*. Presented at the 29th annual meeting of the International Society for the Study of the Lumbar Spine, Cleveland, OH, 2002(abst).
22. Kuslich SD, Ulstrom CL, Michael CY. The tissue origin of low back pain and sciatica: a report of pain response to tissue stimulation during operations on the lumbar spine using local anesthesia. *Orthop Clin North Am* 1991;22:181–187.
23. Lorenz M, Patwardhan AG. The three joint complex. In: Wiesel SW, Weinstein JN, Kerkowitz H, et al., eds. *The lumbar spine*, 2nd ed, vol 1. Philadelphia: WB Saunders, 1996:52–57.
24. Modic MT, Steinberg PM, Ross JS, et al. Degenerative disc disease: assessment of changes in vertebral body bone marrow with MR imaging. *Radiology* 1988;166:193–199.
25. Olmarker K, Brisby H, Yabuki S, et al. The effects of normal, frozen, and hyaluronidase-digested nucleus pulposus on nerve root structure and function. *Spine* 1997;24:471–475.
26. Olmarker K, Larsson K. Tumor necrosis factor alpha and nucleus pulposus–induced nerve root injury. *Spine* 1998;23:2538–2544.
27. Olmarker K, Myers RR. Pathogenesis of sciatic pain: role of herniated nucleus pulposus and deformation of spinal nerve root and dorsal root ganglion. *Pain* 1998;78:99–105.
28. Olmarker K, Rydevik B, Nordborg C. Autologous nucleus pulposus induces neurophysiologic and histologic changes in porcine cauda equina nerve roots. *Spine* 1993;18:1425–1432.

29. Rannou F, Poiraudeau S, Corvol M, et al. Contraintes mécaniques et disque intervertébral lombaire. *Rev Rhum* 2000;67[Suppl 4]:219–224.
30. Roberts S, Caterson B, Menage J, et al. Matrix metalloproteinases and aggrecanase: their role in disorders of the human intervertebral disc. *Spine* 2000;25:3005–3013.
31. Roberts S, Eisenstein SM, Menage Y, et al. Mechanoreceptors in intervertebral discs. Morphology, distribution and neuropeptides. *Spine* 1995;20:2645–2651.
32. Sorkin LS, Xiao WH, Wagner R, et al. Tumor necrosis factor-alpha induces ectopic activity in nociceptive primary afferent fibers. *Neuroscience* 1997;81:255–262.
33. Takahashi H., Suguro T, Okazima Y, et al. Inflammatory cytokines in the herniated disc of the lumbar spine. *Spine* 1996;21:218–224.
34. Torgeson W, Dotter W. Comparative roentgenographic study of asymptomatic and symptomatic lumbar spine. *J Bone Joint Surg Am* 1976;58:850–853.
35. Urban JPG. Degeneration of the lumbar spinal unit: biochemical aspects. In: Deburge A, Benoist M, Morvan G, et al., eds. *Monographie des journées de l'Hôpital Beaujon*. Montpellier: Sauramps Medical, 1999:25–38.
36. Wagner R, Myers RR. Schwann cells produce tumor necrosis factor alpha: expression in injured and noninjured nerves. *Neuroscience* 1996;73:625–629.
37. Walsh TR, Weinstein JN, Sprott RF, et al. Lumbar discography in normal subjects. *J Bone Joint Surg Am* 1990;72:1081–1086.
38. Weiler C, Nerlich AG, Zipperer Y, et al. Expression of major matrix metalloproteinases is associated with intervertebral disc degradation and resorption. *Eur Spine J* 2002;11:308–320.

12
Disc Degeneration in Children and Adolescents

*†Federico Balagué and ‡§Jean Dudler

*Department of Rheumatology, Physical Medicine, an Rehabilitation, Cantonal Hospital, Fribourg, Switzerland; †Department of Orthopedic Surgery, New York University School of Medicine, New York, New York; ‡Department of Rheumatology, Physical Medicine, and Rehabilitation, University of Lausanne; and §Service of Rheumatology, Physical Medicine, and Rehabilitation, Centre Hospitalier Universitaire, Vaudois, Lausanne, Switzerland

At first glance, the concepts of degeneration and youthfulness may seem antinomic, except in some very uncommon conditions presenting with premature aging. Classically, physiologic events, such as growth, maturation, and aging, have been distinguished from degeneration, which is by nature pathologic (5). Perhaps this distinction cannot be straightforwardly applied to intervertebral discs. According to Boos et al. (12), if the degree of disc degeneration is related to age, substantial individual differences can be observed in the sense that young persons exhibit the disc of elderly persons and vice versa. Overall, the most recent studies on this topic indicate that aging and degeneration cannot be differentiated (5,12).

Apart from the difficulties of distinguishing between normal aging and disease, this topic is further complicated by the absence of any satisfactory animal models, humans being the only obligate bipedal vertebrate (23). Furthermore, the different studies focusing on disc degeneration in young persons have unfortunately used different definitions and methodologies, so that comparisons are made difficult.

With these limitations in mind, we have reviewed the literature (Medline) and summarized the data, separating general population studies from data on specific spinal disorders, either congenital or acquired.

GENERAL POPULATION STUDIES

Studies of disc degeneration in the general population can be schematically separated into autopsy and imaging studies. If by definition autopsy studies miss the clinical and prospective dimensions, most imaging studies unfortunately also fail to establish a causal correlation between findings and symptoms.

Autopsy Studies

If macroscopic disc degeneration can be observed in adolescents and rarely in children, no studies have demonstrated such lesions in infants. Twomey and Taylor (60) reported on 204 cadavers, including subjects ages 0 to 19 years at the time of death. The quality of the lumbar discs was assessed visually in 37 specimens according to a four-point scale described by Rolander (46a). All the discs of the subjects up to 1 1/2 years of age (n = 6) were normal (grade 0). Most of the children and young adolescents (age range, 1.5 to 12 years; n = 18) had normal discs (13 of 18); however, five subjects had nucleus pulposus more fibrous than normally expected, even though it was still clearly distinct from the annulus. Finally, in the subjects ages 13 to 19 years (n = 23), not a single disc obtained a perfect score of 0. One L4–5 disc was graded 2 (i.e., less distinct boundary between nucleus and annulus, color yellowish brown, and isolated fissure), and one L5–S1 disc was frankly degenerate. Miller et al. (35), using a similar four-point scoring system on 600 autopsy specimens including those from 10 children (0 to 9 years) and 43 teenagers (10 to 19 years), also demonstrated perfectly normal discs in all children (both genders) and teenage girls. However, 7 of 19 boys in their second decade were given a grade of 2, regarded as disc degeneration.

More recent studies do not rely solely on visual macroscopic grading but also include histologic and immunohistochemical analyses. Nerlich et al. (37) reported on 229 lumbar motion segments obtained from 47 persons whose ages ranged from fetal to 86 years. No macroscopic evidence of disc degeneration was found in the fetal and juvenile specimens. The histologic findings were also normal in the fetal (25 to 33 weeks of gestation) and infantile (1 day to 28 months of age) discs. The earliest histologic signs of disc alteration, with focal nuclear chondrocyte proliferation and beginning granular changes with slight abnormalities of the extracellular matrix, appeared between the ages of 8 and 13 years. Positive staining for N-carboxymethyl-lysine on immunohistochemical analyses as an indicator of oxidative stress was reported in the nucleus pulposus of juveniles as young as 13 years and in the endplate chondrocytes of 2-year-old specimens.

In another immunohistochemical study, Weiler et al. (66) analyzed cadaveric and surgical specimens. Fetal and infantile discs were included among the autopsy specimens; the age of the youngest surgical patient was 11 years. Again, fetal and infantile discs showed almost no histologic signs of degenerative lesions, and discs from adolescents between 10 and 15 years of age demonstrated only slight focal chondrocyte proliferation and minimal granular changes. However, significant degenerative alterations (e.g., extensive formation of clefts and tears, focal chondrocyte proliferation, significant granular matrix degeneration, focal minor mucoid degeneration) were noted in subjects ages 16 to 30 years. These lesions were located mostly in the nucleus pulposus. The same authors also looked for matrix metalloproteinases (MMPs) expression. Fetal, infantile, and young adolescent tissues showed almost no staining for MMP-1, -2, -3, and -9. However, the tissues of adolescents older than 15 years exhibited significant expression of MMP-1, -2, and -3. Moreover, phagocytic cells (CD68$^+$) were observed only after the age of 15 years. The authors stated that their study supports the notion that disc degeneration starts in childhood and early adolescence. In agreement with this notion, Gruber and Hanley (25) demonstrated apoptotic nuclei, which can probably be regarded as the earliest sign of degeneration and aging, in half of the discs in eight specimens from 0 to 4.7 years of age, even though they were grade 1 on the Thompson scale.

In a study aimed at distinguishing patterns of disc matrix turnover during growth, maturation, aging, and degeneration, Antoniou et al. (5) reported on 121 intervertebral discs from 25 cadaveric lumbar spine specimens. Macroscopically, the specimens were normal in the subjects ages 0 to 15 years (Thompson grade 1); in the subjects 15 to 25 years of age, 50% of the discs were grade 1, 40% grade 2, and 10% grade 3. Unfortunately, the data for older adolescents were pooled with those for young adults, so it was impossible to date the appearance of disc degeneration. The water content of the nucleus was 90% in infants, and this proportion dropped to just above 80% in the 15- to 25-year-old age group; the water content in elderly subjects or clearly degenerated discs was significantly lower. The glycosaminoglycan content in the nucleus pulposus was also higher in the young. Type II collagen was reported to account for all collagen in the nucleus pulposus in subjects younger than 5 years. The proportion of denatured type II collagen increased with age; it was lowest in the 0- to 2-year-old age group and did not differ significantly between the regions of the disc; the percentage increased significantly in all regions except the posterior annulus in the subjects 2 to 15 years of age. The levels of 846 epitope of aggrecan and the propeptide of collagen II were highest in the nucleus of neonates and those ages 2 to 5 years. The levels dropped markedly in those 5 to15 years old and continued to decrease afterward. The level of propeptide of collagen I was also highest in the neonates and lowest in the 5- to 15-year-old group. However, unlike the level of propeptide of collagen II, it increased again thereafter, leading the authors to identify three phases (growth, aging and maturation, and degeneration) based on the profile of collagen synthesis and degradation.

The extensive and very impressive study of Boos et al. (12) best summarizes our current knowledge of disc degeneration. They analyzed the characteristics of cadaveric spines and surgical specimens ranging in age from fetal to 88 years; included among other material were nine fetal discs, 13 discs from newborns ages 0 to 1 month, 17 discs from children ages 2 months to 2 years, five discs from children ages 3 to10 years, eight discs from adolescents ages 11 to 16 years, and eight discs from subjects 17 to 20 years old. The macroscopic aspect (according to the Thompson scale) and multiple histologic variables concerning both intervertebral discs and endplates were described. The main finding was that the diminution of blood supply in the endplates, which induces tissue breakdown beginning in the nucleus pulposus, starts in the second decade of life. The obliteration of blood vessels in the endplates gradually increases between 1 month and 16 years and is paralleled by different structural modifications. These first reach a peak in the group 11 to 16 years of age, in whom disc alterations begin to increase. In another cadaveric study that included material from eight fetuses 24 to 41 weeks of gestational age and two children, one age 10 months and one age 6 years, in whom no degenerative changes were present, specimens showed numerous and dilated blood vessels (46).

Finally, Boos et al. (12) also developed an original histologic classification system, and decision tree analysis was used to evaluate the ability of histologic findings to predict age and macroscopic disc degeneration. It appears that disc histologic markers are more accurate than endplate markers in predicting both age and macroscopic degeneration. However, the nature and the harvest site of the histologic markers are important, and histology patterns are not always consistent with conventional assessments of the disc.

Imaging Studies

If osteophytes and diminished intervertebral space height are classic signs of disc disease on standard radiographs, magnetic resonance imaging (MRI) would be nowadays considered the gold standard to define disc degeneration. However, it probably would be better regarded as the best available surrogate marker in the absence of a well-demonstrated correlation with clinical and pathologic variables.

Shao et al. (53) reported measurements performed on plain lateral views of the lumbar spine. None of 87 men and 86 women ages 20 to 29 years had osteophytes. Unexpectedly, the intervertebral space height appeared to increase with age in parallel with increasing concavity of the endplates.

In a cross-sectional study of 32 children (mean age, 8 years) referred for lumbar MRI and 49 controls of the same age with no spinal symptoms, Salo et al. (49) reported normal MRI findings in 56% of patients and 78% of controls. Overall, some alterations of the discs were noted 13% of the patients and 22% of the controls that involved 3.1% and 4.5% of the examined discs, respectively. Alterations in signals were interpreted as definite signs of disc degeneration by the authors, who stated that no disc degeneration was found in subjects younger than 10 years. In another cross-sectional study, which compared persons with chronic (symptoms for longer than 12 weeks) low back pain (LBP) and age-matched asymptomatic controls, Paajanen et al. (40) retrospectively analyzed the MR images of 20 subjects ages 10 to 14 years (10 from each group) and 140 subjects ages 15 to 19 years (70 from each group). The difference between the percentages of MR images with one or more degenerate lumbar discs was statistically significant in the 15- to 19-year-olds ($P = 0.014$); however, alterations were also seen in one asymptomatic child and 18 control adolescents. In another MRI study of 35 gymnasts (mean age, 12 ± 2.6 years; mean practice time, 12 ± 5.5 h/wk) and 10 asymptomatic subjects (mean age, 12 ± 2.5 years), three gymnasts and one control had signs of disc degeneration, but no clear correlation was found with LBP or low back trauma (58).

Other areas of the spine have also been studied. Goh et al. (24) published a retrospective MRI study of the vertebral bodies and discs of the thoracic spine in different age groups. The youngest subgroups, ages 1 to 20 years, included 15 girls (mean age, 12.3 ± 5 years) and 11 boys (mean age, 10.2 ± 5.2 years). Four regions of the disc (nucleus, annulus, endplates, and disc margins) were graded 1 to 3 according to a modified Thompson scale for normal to severe degenerative changes independently in three segments of the thoracic spine: T1–T4, T5–T8, and T9–T12. Finally, both genders were analyzed separately. The boys had almost no disc abnormalities in the thoracic spine, whereas a small minority of the girls (fewer than 20%) had moderate changes limited to the nucleus pulposus of the mid and lower thoracic segments. MRI of the cervical discs of 497 asymptomatic volunteers, including 39 male and 37 female subjects ages 10 to 19 years, was performed by Matsumoto et al. (34). Fewer than 5% of the evaluated discs in this age group showed degenerative changes, posterior protrusion, or narrowing.

Sequential studies of a cohort by a Finnish group provide some insights into the value of lumbar MRI in adolescents. In an initial study in which a 0.02-T MRI system was used, Tertti et al. (59) compared the findings in 39 patients ages 15 years reporting continuous or recurrent LBP or sciatica with those in asymptomatic controls matched for age, gender, and school class. Roughly 12% of the examined discs showed incipient or total degeneration, but no significant difference was found between the symptomatic and asymptomatic subjects. Both disc protrusion and Scheuermann-type changes were associated with MRI disc degeneration, but only in the LBP group. Disc protrusions were also significantly more common in the LBP group (8 vs. 1), but not Scheuermann-type changes. The same cohort was reexamined 3 years later with another imager (0.1 T). The participation rate at follow-up was 79%, and overall disc degeneration increased, particularly among the subjects with LBP. It should also be highlighted that a few discs with mild degeneration or even protrusions at baseline were classified as normal at follow-up (19). Finally, when the same cohort was surveyed at the age of 23 years, it appeared that disc degeneration at the age of 15 years on initial imaging was a significant predictor of recurrent LBP (48).

SPINAL DISORDERS

Specific spinal disorders range from common to rare congenital conditions, and we have attempted to collect information on disc degeneration in such conditions.

Disc Herniation

The topic of disc herniation in children and teenagers has been reviewed extensively (7,50).

A study of 15 adolescents who underwent a surgical procedure for disc herniation reported degenerative signs after histologic analysis of all the disc material (31). However, it is unknown whether these degenerative changes were limited to the single herniated disc or part of a more general disorder. Other studies partially answer this question. Luukkonen et al. (32) followed 12 subjects operated on for a lumbar disc herniation at 15 years of age or younger for up to 6.2 years (range, 3.5 to 9.1 years). The follow-up MRI showed disc degeneration at unoperated levels in 67% of the patients, but without clear correlation between imaging and clinical symptoms. Similarly, Poussa et al. (43) reported multilevel disc degeneration in all cases with 10 years of follow-up, even those with favorable clinical results. Another approach to the concept of a more general disorder was taken by Matsui et al. (33). In an interesting case control study, they demonstrated an increased prevalence of high-grade disc degeneration among the first-degree relatives of patients ages 15 to 60 years operated on for disc herniation, suggesting some genetic background. However, another article highlighted the difficulties of analyzing genetic influences in disc herniation (3).

Scoliosis

The role of disc degeneration in scoliosis is unknown. Some radiologic studies have addressed the quality of the discs in addition to the risk for degenerative changes in unfused levels after surgery. Numerous studies have also evaluated biochemical markers in surgical specimens, but it appears that they have often been used as control specimens for studies of disc degeneration, rather than to specifically address the question of degeneration in scoliosis.

Wedging and morphologic modifications are obvious in scoliosis. In a retrospective review of radiographs from 27 patients with idiopathic scoliosis and 17 patients with scoliosis associated with cerebral palsy performed by Stokes and Aronsson (54), vertebral wedging was more prominent than disc wedging at the thoracic level, whereas the opposite was found in the lumbar and thoracolumbar regions. No significant difference between the two groups of patients with scoliosis was observed. The correlation of disc wedging with degeneration is unknown. Takahashi et al. (57) reported a group of 30 patients operated on at the average age of 17 years; only two patients had degenerative signs with disc narrowing or osteophytes at 5 to 9 years of follow-up (average, 6.2 years). However, Danielsson et al. (14,15), in an impressive controlled follow-up MRI study of persons who had been surgically treated for idiopathic scoliosis as adolescents 25 years earlier, found significantly more degenerative changes that in matched controls at the level of the lowest unfused disc. Another MRI study with 3 years follow-up that included 14 surgically treated scoliotic subjects ages 16 to 66 years also reported a 23% incidence of disc degeneration below the fusion, which was furthermore correlated with pain (9).

With the limitations previously stated kept in mind, different studies have shown biochemical or histologic modification in scoliotic discs, often between the concave and the convex sides. Duance et al. (17), analyzing 29 discs from eight scoliotic patients ages 10 to 23 years, showed a difference in reducible cross-linking between sides, indicating more rapid turnover and extensive tissue remodeling on the convex side. However, turnover was elevated on both sides in comparison with normal discs. Another study, of 29 discs in seven patients ages 13 to 27 years, found significantly decreased concentrations of sulfated glycosaminoglycans, collagen, MMP-2, and MMP-9 in the annulus on the concave side (13). Transport of nitrous oxide (62), expression of collagen type X (1), and modifications in cellularity (61), oxygen concentration (10,42), cell viability (10), lactate concentration (10), and glucose concentration (10) have also been analyzed in scoliotic discs.

In summary, multiple biochemical events have been described in these patients, interpreted by Antoniou et al. (4) as ineffective matrix turnover in comparison with that in normal discs. Another review article suggested that genetic factors may play an important role in the premature degradation of intervertebral scoliotic discs (11).

Finally, and despite all these clues, the relationship between scoliosis, disc degeneration, and LBP is far from strong. Ramirez et al. (44) retrospectively studied 2,442 patients with idiopathic scoliosis and found no association between pain and magnitude or type of curve, spinal alignment, or discrepancy in limb length, among other variables explored. In their cohort of 426 adolescents, Joncas et al. (28) found no correlation between back pain and severity of scoliosis, whereas Weinstein (67), in his review of the topic, stated that the incidence of back pain in patients with scoliosis is comparable with that in the general population.

Spondylolisthesis

MRI (0.04 T), discography, and plain x-rays were used, but not in all cases, in a cross-sectional study of 27 patients (mean age, 14.4 years) with isthmic L5 spondylolisthesis. Standard radiographs correlated poorly with the other two techniques. Disc degeneration below the slipped vertebra was the rule, and a high frequency of degenerative changes was also found in the disc above the slipped vertebra (51). However, another MRI study, which compared 40 patients with 40 age- and sex-matched controls, found no difference between patients and controls in the disc above the level of spondylolisthesis, and rare cases of disc degeneration below the slipped vertebra in young patients, even though patients older than 25 years showed significantly more disc degeneration than controls at that level (56).

Finally, Seitsalo et al. (52), using standard radiographs, reported 82 conservatively treated and 145 surgically treated patients (age at diagnosis, 13.8 years) followed for an average of 15.4 years. Disc degeneration correlated significantly with lack of mobility below the slipped vertebra. The incidence of disc degeneration above the spondylolisthetic vertebra was 26% in the conservatively treated group and 31% in the fusion group (difference not significant), and the presence of degenerative changes was significantly associated with a more severe slip, but not with LBP.

Scheuermann Disease

Based on a study of 12 cases (mean age, 16 years), Swischuk et al. (55) suggested that Scheuermann disease, Schmorl nodes, limbus vertebra, and ordinary disc degeneration can be grouped together as different forms of the same disorder.

An MRI study of 146 intervertebral spaces in 21 patients with Scheuermann disease (mean age, 13 ± 2.6 years) and those of 34 volunteers with no history of LBP demonstrated increased abnormalities in the patients with Scheuermann disease (55% of discs) in comparison with the healthy controls (10%). However, disc degeneration was significantly associated with some radiologic signs, including narrowed discs (25 of 26), Schmorl nodes (37 of 41), and marginal sclerosis (50 of 66), whereas 16 of 54 spaces free of such radiologic signs showed MRI signs of disc degeneration (39). A cadaveric study comparing radiographic and pathologic findings in an elderly population demonstrated an association between Schmorl nodes and moderate but not advanced degenerative changes (41). Therefore, it is difficult to guess the long-term effect of such lesions on the intervertebral discs.

Finally, acute Schmorl nodes have been described in two articles that shed some light on a possible relationship with disc degeneration (20,65).

Fractures

Kerttula et al. (29,30), in a report on 17 patients who had sustained vertebral fractures (age 11.8 years at the time of injury and 15.5 years at follow-up), found significantly more frequent disc degeneration in the patients than in 20 asymptomatic controls (57% vs. 7%). These modifications were significantly associated with endplate damage, as well as with an age older than 15 years at follow-up.

Another study looked prospectively at the effect on intervertebral discs of two types of surgical orthopedic treatment for vertebral fractures. Only discs adjacent to the fracture showed signs of degeneration on MRI at follow-up (mean follow-up between implant removal and MRI, 301 days), and no difference was seen between treatments (Harrington rods vs. transpedicular fixation). None of the uninjured discs demonstrated any significant signal decrease on T2-weighted images (64). However, only two patients in this study were younger than 20 years of age.

Transitional Vertebra

In an extensive study, Hsieh et al. (27) demonstrated a significantly smaller L5–S1 disc height in patients with transitional vertebra. This was even more marked when the transverse processes of L5 were fused to the sacrum. The findings were unrelated to age or sex. The case of a teenage girl with a reduced height of the last two lumbar intervertebral spaces but with perfectly normal disc signal intensity on MRI has been reported (8). Therefore, the possibility of morphologic anomalies located on discs that do not harbor any degenerative pathology should be kept in mind. An MRI study of 21 patients (age range, 20 to 27 years) with segmental lumbar spine anomalies (transitional or rudimentary discs) demonstrated normal signal intensity of the discs but a lack of the intranuclear cleft (16).

Down Syndrome

According to the cross-sectional radiographic study of Van Dyke and Gahagan (63), indirect evidence is found of disc degeneration with C1–2 instability, even in children, and other degenerative signs in adults. In a letter, Fidone (22) reported an increased prevalence of radiographic degenerative signs with age. (The youngest patient was 21 years old.)

Calcification

Calcifications in the nucleus pulposus of the thoracic vertebrae were reported in an 11-month-old girl with mucolipidosis II, or I-cell disease (36). Wong et al. (68) reported four cases of cervical disc calcification in children ages 6 to 10 years followed for 2 to 16 years in whom permanent deformities of the adjacent vertebral bodies, possibly associated with early degenerative signs, were observed. Finally, Dussault and Kaye (18) reported 28 patients with disc calcifications associated with spine fusions secondary to various congenital or acquired disorders. Even though the population characteristics were not described in detail, some were children or young adults. Calcifications were interpreted as signs of degeneration, but no patient had symptoms related to the calcifications.

Diastrophic Dysplasia

Diastrophic dysplasia is a rare autosomal-recessive inherited skeletal dysplasia. The most typical findings are short-limbed short stature, spinal deformities, multiple joint contracture, and early degeneration of joints (45). Remes et al. (45) reported 88 patients, including 10 children ages 0 to 10 years and 14 patients ages 11 to 20 years. None of these young patients reported LBP, even though the discs were abnormal in all. The number of bulging and prolapsed discs was very low in the thoracic spine (2% bulge and no prolapse during the first decade, 7% bulge and 1% prolapse in the 11- to 20-year-olds) but was much higher between T12 and S1 (77% bulge and no prolapse during the first decade, 46% bulge and 7% prolapse in the 11- to 20-year-olds).

Klippel–Feil Syndrome

Allsopp et al. (2) reported the case of a 5-year-old girl with a cervical disc herniation. At surgery, the defect was found in the posterior part of the annulus, suggesting a disc malformation rather than early degeneration from mechanical stress caused by the fused segments. In adult patients whose disease was diagnosed during childhood (average age at diagnosis, 9 years; age at follow-up, 35 years), 100% of patients had degenerative changes of the discs on MRI. Moreover, 16 of the 22 patients had disc protrusions, and four had osteophytes (26).

Spina Bifida Occulta

No specific information is available for children with this congenital malformation. However, Avrahami et al. (6), reporting the computed tomographic findings in 1,200 patients (50% women) ages 18 to 72 years, found that the prevalence of the malformation was higher in younger patients and decreased with age. Furthermore, spina bifida occulta of S1 was significantly associated with posterior disc herniation. However, by design, all patients had LBP with or without sciatica and a clinical diagnosis of disc herniation.

Others

Ruffing (47) reported 480 patients with thalidomide-induced embryopathy. Most of the subjects were 12 to 15 years of age, and the study focused on spinal lesions evaluated with standard radiographs. Only 28.1% of the patients had normal radiographic findings.

Among the various spinal lesions, narrowing of the intervertebral space was found at one to seven levels per subject. The prevalence of such lesions was not reported in the article; however, they were the third most frequent pathology in this sample.

Nerlich et al. (38) described the histologic and biochemical alterations found in a 9-year-old girl who died of abdominal and vascular lesions associated with Ehlers–Danlos syndrome type IV. Among the various tissue samples, the authors included an intervertebral disc in which a decreased amount of collagen type III and an enhanced perifibrillar deposition of proteoglycans in comparison with normal tissue could be demonstrated. Moreover, some findings suggest that other collagen types may also be affected by the defective deposition of collagen type III in this condition.

Finally, Farrior et al. (21) reviewed the etiology of progressive vertebral fusion after describing an intriguing case of progressive fusion of the intervertebral spaces that started in a child at about 4 years of age and continued for several years without any underlying disease being identified.

CONCLUSIONS

Based on the macroscopic analysis of autopsy material, disc degeneration starts at the middle of the second decade of life. More recent and extensive microscopic studies suggest that the process begin even earlier, in childhood. Degeneration appears to be linked to physiologic modifications of the vascularization of the disc, so that the distinction between physiologic aging and degeneration is difficult. MRI studies have confirmed an unexpectedly high prevalence of disc degeneration among teenagers. However, the correlation between the imaging findings and symptoms is far from perfect.

Morphologic or physiologic changes of the intervertebral discs have also been reported in several spinal disorders, either congenital or acquired. Again, correlation with symptoms is controversial in the reviewed literature, and the role of disc degeneration in such disorders is far from clearly understood.

REFERENCES

1. Aigner T, Greskötter K, Fairbank J, et al. Variation with age in the pattern of type X collagen expression in normal and scoliotic human intervertebral discs. *Calcif Tissue Int* 1998;63:263–268.
2. Allsopp G, Griffiths S, Sgouros S. Cervical disc prolapse in childhood associated with Klippel-Feil syndrome. *Childs Nerv Syst* 2001;17:69–70.
3. Annunen S, Paassilta P, Lohiniva J, et al. An allele of COL9A2 associated with intervertebral disc disease. *Science* 1999;285:409–412.
4. Antoniou J, Arlet V, Goswami T, et al. Elevated synthetic activity in the convex side of scoliotic intervertebral discs and endplates compared with normal tissues. *Spine* 2001;26:E198–E206.
5. Antoniou J, Steffen T, Nelson F, et al. The lumbar human intervertebral disc. Evidence for changes in the biosynthesis and denaturation of the extracellular matrix with growth, maturation, ageing, and degeneration. *J Clin Invest* 1996;98:996–1003.
6. Avrahami E, Frishman E, Fridman Z, et al. Spina bifida occulta of S1 is not an innocent finding. *Spine* 1994;19:12–15.
7. Balagué F, Kaelin A. Intervertebral disc herniation in children. In: Gunzburg R, Szpalski M, eds. *Lumbar disc herniation*. Philadelphia: Lippincott Williams & Wilkins, 2002:50–61.
8. Balagué F, Sadry F. Narrowed intervertebral disks in a teenager: should these be considered pathologic? *J Clin Rheumatol* 1995;1:253–255.
9. Balderston R, Albert T, McIntosh T, et al. Magnetic resonance imaging analysis of lumbar disc changes below scoliosis fusions. *Spine* 1998;23:54–58.
10. Bibby S, Fairbank J, Urban M, et al. Cell viability in scoliotic discs in relation to disc deformity and nutrient levels. *Spine* 2002;27:2220–2228.
11. Bibby S, Jones D, Lee R, et al. Biochimie, biologie et physiologie du disque intervertbral. *Rev Rhum (Ed Fr)* 2001;68:903–907.

12. Boos N, Weissbach S, Rohrbach H, et al. 2002 Volvo Award in Basic Science Studies. Classification of age-related changes in lumbar intervertebral discs. *Spine* 2002;27:2631–2644.
13. Crean J, Roberts S, Jaffray D, et al. Matrix metalloproteinases in the human intervertebral disc: role in disc degeneration and scoliosis. *Spine* 1997;22:2877–2884.
14. Danielsson A, Cederlund C, Ekholm S, et al. The prevalence of disc aging and back pain after fusion extending into the lower lumbar spine. A matched MR study twenty-five years after surgery for adolescent idiopathic scoliosis. *Acta Radiol* 2001;42:187–197.
15. Danielsson A, Wiklund I, Pehrsson K, et al. Health-related quality of life in patients with adolescent idiopathic scoliosis: a matched follow-up at least 20 years after treatment with brace or surgery. *Eur Spine J* 2001; 10:278–288.
16. Desmond P, Buirski G. Magnetic resonance appearance of developmental disc anomalies in the lumbar spine. *Australas Radiol* 1993;37:26–29.
17. Duance V, Crean J, Sims T, et al. Changes in collagen cross-linking in degenerative disc disease and scoliosis. *Spine* 1998;23:2545–2551.
18. Dussault R, Kaye J. Intervertebral disk calcification associated with spine fusion. *Radiology* 1977;125:57–61.
19. Erkintalo M, Salminen J, Alanen A, et al. Development of degenerative changes in the lumbar intervertebral disk: results of a prospective MR imaging study in adolescents with and without low-back pain. *Radiology* 1995; 196:529–533.
20. Fahey V, Opeskin K, Silberstein M, et al. The pathogenesis of Schmorl's nodes in relation to acute trauma. An autopsy study. *Spine* 1998;23:2272–2275.
21. Farrior J, Weaver D, Kling T, et al. Progressive vertebral fusion of unknown etiology: a case report. *Am J Med Genet* 2002;112:221–227.
22. Fidone G. Degenerative cervical arthritis and Down's syndrome. *N Engl J Med* 1986;314:320.
23. Freemont A, Watkins A, Le Maitre C, et al. Current understanding of cellular and molecular events in intervertebral disc degeneration: implications for therapy. *J Pathol* 2002;196:374–379.
24. Goh S, Tan C, Price R, et al. Influence of age and gender on thoracic vertebral body shape and disc degeneration: an MR investigation of 169 cases. *J Anat* 2000;197:647–657.
25. Gruber H, Hanley E. Ultrastructure of the human intervertebral disc during aging and degeneration. *Spine* 2002;27:798–805.
26. Guille J, Miller A, Bowen J, et al. The natural history of Klippel-Feil syndrome: clinical, roentgenographic, and magnetic resonance imaging findings at adulthood. *J Pediatr Orthop* 1995;15:617–626.
27. Hsieh C, Vanderford J, Moreau S, et al. Lumbosacral transitional segments: classification, prevalence, and effect on disk height. *J Manipulative Physiol Ther* 2000;23:483–489.
28. Joncas J, Labelle H, Poitras B, et al. Douleur dorso-lombaire et scoliose idiopathique de l'adolescence. *Ann Chir* 1996;50:637–640.
29. Kerttula L, Kurunlahti M, Jauhiainen J, et al. Apparent diffusion coefficients and T2 relaxation time measurements to evaluate disc degeneration. *Acta Radiol* 2001;42:585–591.
30. Kerttula L, Serlo W, Tervonen O, et al. Post-traumatic findings of the spine after earlier vertebral fracture in young patients. *Spine* 2000;25:1104–1108.
31. Lee J, Ernestus R, Schrder R, et al. Histological study of lumbar intervertebral disc herniation in adolescents. *Acta Neurochir (Wien)* 2000;142:1107–1110.
32. Luukkonen M, Partanen K, Vapalahti M. Lumbar disc herniations in children: a long-term clinical and magnetic resonance imaging follow-up study. *Br J Neurosurg* 1997;11:280–285.
33. Matsui H, Kanamori M, Ishihara H, et al. Familial predisposition for lumbar degenerative disc disease. A case-control study. *Spine* 1998;23:1029–1034.
34. Matsumoto M, Fujimura Y, Suzuki N, et al. MRI of cervical intervertebral discs in asymptomatic subjects. *J Bone Joint Surg Br* 1998;80:19–24.
35. Miller J, Schmatz C, Schultz A. Lumbar disc degeneration: correlation with age, sex, and spine level in 600 autopsy specimens. *Spine* 1988;13:173–178.
36. Mogle P, Amitai Y, Rotenberg M, et al. Calcification of intervertebral disks in I-cell disease. *Eur J Pediatr* 1986;145:226–227.
37. Nerlich A, Schleicher E, Boos N. 1997 Volvo Award in Basic Science Studies. Immunohistologic markers for age-related changes of human intervertebral discs. *Spine* 1997;22:2781–2795.
38. Nerlich A, Stoess H, Lehmann H, et al. Pathomorphological and biochemical alterations in Ehlers-Danlos syndrome type IV. *Pathol Res Pract* 1994;190:697–706.
39. Paajanen H, Alanen A, Erkintalo M, et al. Disc degeneration in Scheuermann disease. *Skeletal Radiol* 1989;18: 523–526.
40. Paajanen H, Erkintalo M, Parkkola R, et al. Age-dependent correlation of low-back pain and lumbar disc degeneration. *Arch Orthop Trauma Surg* 1997;116:106–107.
41. Pfirrmann C, Resnick D. Schmorl nodes of the thoracic and lumbar spine: radiographic-pathologic study of prevalence, characterization, and correlation with degenerative changes of 1,650 spinal levels in 100 cadavers. *Radiology* 2001;219:368–374.
42. Poitras B, Mayo N, Goldberg M, et al. The Ste-Justine adolescent idiopathic scoliosis cohort study. Part IV: Surgical correction and back pain. *Spine* 1994;19:1582–1588.

43. Poussa M, Schlenzka D, Mäenpää S, et al. Disc herniation in the lumbar spine during growth: long-term results of operative treatment in 18 patients. *Eur Spine J* 1997;6:390–392.
44. Ramirez N, Johnston C, Browne R. The prevalence of back pain in children who have idiopathic scoliosis. *J Bone Joint Surg Am* 1997;79:364–368.
45. Remes V, Tervahartiala P, Poussa M, et al. Thoracic and lumbar spine in diastrophic dysplasia. *Spine* 2001; 26:187–195.
46. Repanti M, Korovessis P, Stamatakis M, et al. Evolution of disc degeneration in lumbar spine: a comparative histological study between herniated and postmortem retrieved specimens. *J Spinal Disord* 1998;11:41–45.
46a. Rolander SD. Motion of the lumber spine with special reference to the stabilizing effect of posterior fusion. An experimental study on autopsy specimens. *Acta Orthop Scand* 1966;90 (suppl):1–144.
47. Ruffing L. Die Wirbelsäule bei der Thalidomid-Embryopathie. *Fortschr Med* 1980;98:405–409.
48. Salminen J, Erkintalo M, Pentti J, et al. Recurrent low back pain and early disc degeneration in the young. *Spine* 1999;24:1316–1321.
49. Salo S, Paajanen H, Alanen A. Disc degeneration of pediatric patients in lumbar MRI. *Pediatr Radiol* 1995;25: 186–189.
50. Schlenzka D. Intervertebral disc herniation in adolescents. In: Gunzburg R, Szpalski M, eds. *Lumbar disc herniation*. Philadelphia: Lippincott Williams & Wilkins, 2002:62–64.
51. Schlenzka D, Poussa M, Seitsalo S, et al. Intervertebral disc changes in adolescents with isthmic spondylolisthesis. *J Spinal Disord* 1991;4:344–352.
52. Seitsalo S, Schlenzka D, Poussa M, et al. Disc degeneration in young patients with isthmic spondylolisthesis treated operatively or conservatively: a long-term follow-up. *Eur Spine J* 1997;6:393–397.
53. Shao Z, Rompe G, Schiltenwolf M. Radiographic changes in the lumbar intervertebral discs and the lumbar vertebrae with age. *Spine* 2002;27:263–268.
54. Stokes I, Aronsson D. Disc and vertebral wedging in patients with progressive scoliosis. *J Spinal Disord* 2001; 14:317–322.
55. Swischuk L, John S, Allbery S. Disk degenerative disease in childhood: Scheuermann's disease, Schmorl's nodes, and the limbus vertebra: MRI findings in 12 patients. *Pediatr Radiol* 1998;28:334–338.
56. Szypryt E, Twining P, Mulholland R, et al. The prevalence of disc degeneration associated with neural arch defects of the lumbar spine assessed by magnetic resonance imaging. *Spine* 1989;14:977–981.
57. Takahashi S, Delécrin J, Passuti N. Changes in the unfused lumbar spine in patients with idiopathic scoliosis. *Spine* 1997;22:517–524.
58. Tertti M, Paajanen H, Kujala U, et al. Disc degeneration in young gymnasts. A magnetic resonance imaging study. *Am J Sports Med* 1990;18:206—208.
59. Tertti M, Salminen J, Paajanen H, et al. Low-back pain and disk degeneration in children: a case-control MR imaging study. *Radiology* 1991;180:503–507.
60. Twomey L, Taylor J. Age changes in lumbar intervertebral discs. *Acta Orthop Scand* 1985;56:496–499.
61. Urban M, Fairbank J, Bibby S, et al. Intervertebral disc composition in neuromuscular scoliosis. *Spine* 2001;26:610–617.
62. Urban M, Fairbank J, Etherington P, et al. Electrochemical measurement of transport into scoliotic intervertebral discs in vivo using nitrous oxide as a tracer. *Spine* 2001;26:984–990.
63. Van Dyke D, Gahagan C. Down syndrome. Cervical spine abnormalities and problems. *Clin Pediatr* 1988;27: 415—418.
64. Vornanen M, Böstman O, Keto P, et al. The integrity of intervertebral disks after operative treatment of thoracolumbar fractures. *Clin Orthop* 1993;297:150–154.
65. Walters G, Coumas J, Akins C, et al. Magnetic resonance imaging of acute symptomatic Schmorl's node formation. *Pediatr Emerg Care* 1991;7:294–296.
66. Weiler C, Nerlich A, Zipperer J, et al. 2002 SSE Award Competition in Basic Science. Expression of major matrix metalloproteinases is associated with intervertebral disc degradation and resorption. *Eur Spine J* 2002; 11:308–320.
67. Weinstein S. Natural history. *Spine* 1999;24:2592–2600.
68. Wong C, Pereira B, Pho R. Cervical disc calcification in children. A long-term review. *Spine* 1992;17:139–144.

13

Gene Therapy Approach for the Treatment of Disc Degeneration

S. Tim Yoon

Department of Orthopedics, Emory University; and Department of Orthopedics, Atlanta VA Medical Center, Decatur, Georgia

Intervertebral disc degeneration is an extremely common phenomenon, with up to 90% of all persons older than 60 years of age having at least one degenerate intervertebral disc (6). The frequency of disc degeneration increases with age (39). The biologic changes of disc degeneration are associated with back pain and other spinal disorders, such as disc herniation, spondylolisthesis, facet arthropathy, and spinal stenosis. Currently, no method of reversing or even retarding disc degeneration is known. Many different strategies can be used for the biologic treatment of the disc. Delivery of a therapeutic gene into the disc is a relatively new strategy and, therefore, very little data on this topic have been published. Because the gene therapy approach may provide a long-lasting effect, it is one of the most promising strategies under investigation. This chapter discusses the biologic changes involved in disc degeneration, other approaches to the biologic treatment of disc degeneration, and the current state of research in the gene therapy–based approach to treat disc degeneration.

THE CLINICAL PROBLEM

Disc degeneration is a very common affliction and is a major cause of low back pain (LBP). A lifetime prevalence of LBP of up to 80% has been reported in Western society (13). The painful disc can be identified by a combination of imaging and clinical methods (36). Unfortunately, no biologic treatment for the degenerate disc is currently available (16). Patients with intractable LBP and lumbar disc degeneration at a single level sometimes undergo disc excision and spinal fusion with anterior interbody fusion (11). This procedure successfully relieves pain in only 70% to 80% of cases, even under the best of circumstances (11). In less favorable situations, as in cases of multiple-level disc degeneration, the success of fusion surgery drops substantially (25). A method of reversing or retarding disc degeneration could revolutionize spinal care by obviating the need for painful and destructive fusion surgery that has a variable success rate.

DISC COMPOSITION AND METABOLISM

The disc is composed primarily of water, proteoglycans (PGs), and collagens. Water constitutes 70% to 80% of the weight of the nucleus (5). The concentration of PGs and water is much higher in the nucleus than in the annulus (2,5). The nucleus functions as a shock absorber and provides resistance to compressive loads across the disc (40). The annulus encapsulates the nucleus with well-ordered sheets of collagen (32). It has excellent mechanical strength and provides most of the resistance to tensile loads across the disc (1,12,14). The disc matrix determines the mechanical property of the disc (40).

Aggrecan is the major PG in the intervertebral disc (34). It is characteristic of cartilaginous tissue, such as disc and articular cartilage. Aggrecan molecules are attached to hyaluronan to form aggregates with a very large molecular weight. The highly negatively charged sulfated glycosaminoglycan (sGAG) molecules in aggregated aggrecan attract water molecules into the disc, producing high hydrostatic pressures in the normal disc nucleus (12,17). Disc degeneration is characterized by a loss of aggrecan core protein, sGAG molecules, and water from the nucleus (2). The loss of PGs results in a decrease in nucleus hydrostatic pressure, which then increases loads on the annulus and facet joints (26) with resultant pathology.

Several different types of fibrillar and nonfibrillar collagens are found in the disc, with collagen types I and II comprising most of the disc collagens (10,32). Collagen type I is found primarily in the annulus fibrosus and much less in the nucleus pulposus (33). It is not specific for cartilage or disc. Collagen type II is found throughout the disc and is the major fibrillar collagen in the nucleus (33,34). It forms a fibrillar network that serves as a scaffold for the PGs (10,33). A decrease of collagen type II synthesis is another hallmark of disc degeneration (2).

The turnover of disc matrix components is thought to occur gradually during many years (4). Disc degeneration as measured by magnetic resonance imaging (MRI) evolves very slowly through many years (9). The best available data suggest that degradation of the disc matrix arises from small imbalances between synthesis and degradation that accumulate with time (3,30). As a result, the goal of a biologic strategy to prevent disc degeneration must strive for small changes in the balance between disc matrix synthesis and degradation that have cumulative effects with time, rather than massive shifts in matrix metabolism. Even a small increase in the rate of synthesis of disc matrix components can have a significant beneficial effect during the course of many years.

OTHER BIOLOGIC APPROACHES TO TREAT DISC DEGENERATION

Many treatment strategies have been tested in attempts to restore discs or retard disc degeneration, such as mechanical stabilization with a plate and screws across a sheep disc injured with a partial-thickness annulotomy (27). This injury model had previously been shown to lead to progressive degeneration. Interestingly, mechanical stabilization had no statistically significant effect on the progression of disc degeneration. Another approach has been to inject cells or transplant disc material into the disc (15,29). This strategy has yielded mixed results, and obtaining appropriate cells or donor disc tissue has been problematic.

A more recent strategy has been to deliver therapeutic molecules to disc cells directly as a protein. *in vitro* studies using this strategy have demonstrated the anabolic effects of certain cytokines. Preliminary *in vivo* data also suggest that this strategy may be successful (37). Takegami et al. (37) demonstrated that direct injection of bone morphogenetic protein-7 (BMP-7) can lead to an increase in disc height and disc sGAG in normal rabbit discs for up to 4 weeks. However, the direct protein injection method may have only transient effects because of diffusion and protein inactivation (35) and, therefore, it is not likely to be a viable approach for the treatment of a long-term process such as disc degeneration. To obtain longer-term effects, gene therapy strategies are being investigated.

GENE THERAPY

Therapeutic Gene

The gene therapy approach requires a careful choice of the therapeutic gene. Candidate genes can be grouped into structural and regulatory genes. Structural genes encode structural proteins that may be important in disc degeneration. Examples of such genes are aggrecan core protein or collagen type II genes. Gene therapy with a structural gene, however, theoretically requires that a fairly large number of disc cells be transduced with the therapeutic gene. Furthermore, because more than one structural protein is deficient or abnormal in disc degeneration, it may be necessary to transduce more than one structural gene. Because of these potential limitations, more work has been carried out with regulatory genes.

Regulatory genes encode anabolic molecules such as cytokines or transcriptional factors that can enhance disc matrix production, or molecules that can down-regulate the catabolic process of disc metabolism. Regulatory genes have two major advantages over structural genes. First, regulatory genes that lead to the secretion of cytokines may have a multiplier effect by inducing the secretion of the regulatory cytokine that can positively affect neighboring cells that do not carry the transduced gene. Secondly, regulatory genes may lead to the regulation of more than one structural protein and have a cascade effect. In theory, regulatory genes that control multiple other regulatory genes may be the most potent or physiologic of the candidate therapeutic genes.

Cytokines with known anabolic effects on disc cells can be classified as mitogens or morphogens. Insulin-like growth factor-1 (IGF-1), epithelial growth factor (EGF), fibroblast growth factor (FGF), and fetal calf serum are known to stimulate disc cell numbers in culture *in vitro* (39). EGF and fetal calf serum are both effective in stimulating PG production, especially in nucleus cells. Although mitogenic cytokines may be useful, it is unclear whether it is always desirable to increase cell mitosis in the disc. Mammalian cells can undergo a limited number of cell divisions before they become senescent and much less synthetic (21). Furthermore, because the nutrition of the disc is limited as a consequence of its avascularity, increasing cell density may be deleterious in certain situations (18).

Morphogens act primarily by promoting cell differentiation without having much mitogenic effect. BMP-2 and BMP-7 are morphogens that have been shown to increase the production of extracellular matrix per cell (28,38,42). These cytokines increase the chondrocyte phenotype of disc cells and increase the synthesis of aggrecan and type II collagen *in vitro*. No comparative tests have been carried out to establish differences in the way the many BMP family members affect disc cells. Transforming growth factor-β1 (TGF-β1) is another morphogen that has been shown to increase PG and collagen type II synthesis *in vitro* (28,39). However, it is not a BMP; rather, it is part of the larger TGF-β superfamily.

Extensive human clinical experience has been acquired with BMP-2 and BMP-7 in relation to bone formation (23,41). BMP-2 has been approved by the Food and Drug Administration for intervertebral fusion with titanium cages, and BMP-7 is undergoing pivotal studies in posterolateral lumbar spine fusion (23). No complications of the use of BMP-2 or BMP-7 have yet been reported in human clinical trials, and antibody responses have been low or nonexistent in most situations. This level of safety is not matched by any other cytokine in spine fusion. BMPs have not been tested intradiscally in humans, but they have been tested in normal animal discs *in vivo*, and no unwanted side effects have been noted. Intradiscal bone formation has not occurred, even after the injection of up to 100 μg of BMP-7 and 42 μg of BMP-2 (22,42). In a study of *ex vivo* gene therapy with BMP-7, disc height and sGAG content were increased in comparison with those in controls in a rabbit experiment. The ability to increase disc matrix synthesis is exciting because it may be possible to reverse or at least retard the biochemical hallmarks of disc degeneration (loss of PG, nucleus hydration, and collagen type II). However, BMPs have not been tested in animal models of normal disc degeneration because a good model of natural disc degeneration does not exist.

LIM mineralization protein-1 (LMP-1) is a relatively recently discovered gene that is known to induce multiple BMPs (BMP-2, -4, -6, and -7) when overexpressed in osteoblasts, fibroblasts, and leukocytes (7,20,24). The transduction of LMP-1 in very low doses of adenovirus leads to bone formation *in vitro* and *in vivo* (7,8). A likely reason why LMP-1 is so potent is that it induces heterodimeric forms of BMPs, which are known to be 20 times more effective than homodimer BMPs *in vitro* and up to 10 times more effective in forming cartilage and bone *in vivo* (19). LMP-1 is an intracellular regulator that is necessary for osteoblast differentiation (7). It is thought that LIM domain proteins are involved in protein–protein interactions and function as intracellular mediators of signal transduction (20). The transduction of LMP-1 by adenovirus has been shown to increase disc cell sGAG production threefold *in vitro* (31). Furthermore, LMP-1 has been shown to induce the up-regulation of multiple BMPs, including BMP-2 and BMP-7. Therefore, although LMP-1 itself encodes an intracellular protein, it increases the production and secretion of cytokines (BMPs) that can then have paracrine effect on neighboring cells.

Delivery Mechanism

The gene delivery mechanism can be either *ex vivo* or *in vivo*. With *ex vivo* gene therapy, cells are transduced with the therapeutic gene *in vitro*, then the transduced cells are transferred into the disc *in vivo*. Gene transduction can be performed *ex vivo* with a wide variety of nonviral methods. For instance, the gene gun method, in which a monolayer of cells is blasted with tiny gold particles coated with the DNA of interest, can be used only *ex vivo*. Other methods, such as lipofection and electroporation, also are available only *ex vivo*. Another advantage of *ex vivo* gene therapy is that cell transduction can often be verified before the cells are transferred into the disc. The major disadvantages of *ex vivo* gene therapy are obtaining cells and culturing them *ex vivo*. For an application that requires long-term gene expression, cells must survive for an extended period of time. This makes autograft cells a necessity. Because harvesting autograft disc cells is not reasonable in clinical practice, other tissues, such as cartilage from a non–weight-bearing surface of the knee or perhaps bone marrow stem cells, must be used. This involves a potentially invasive procedure and increases cost. Furthermore, culturing the cells *ex vivo* entails a significant risk for cell contamination or transformation before reintroduction into the patient. For these reasons, *ex vivo* therapy may be useful in proof-of-concept experiments but is not ideal for clinical use.

In vivo gene therapy is the approach that appears most promising in clinical practice. With this method, the choice of delivery mechanism is more limited. Virally mediated gene delivery has been the most popular method under investigation. Adenovirus can infect non-dividing cells from a wide variety of tissue types and is currently extensively used in research. However, adenovirus vectors induce the production of viral proteins, and these cause an immune reaction that suppresses expression of the therapeutic gene. Adeno-associated virus, which is much less immunogenic than adenovirus, allows longer-term gene expression. However, the initial level of transgene expression is usually lower with adeno-associated virus. Retrovirus vectors can lead to permanent integration of the therapeutic gene into the host chromosome. However, retrovirus can integrate only into mitotic cells, which limits its usefulness.

Marker gene experiments with adenovirus vector have demonstrated successful infection of cells in both nucleus and inner annulus with doses of 1 million viral particles per rabbit lumbar disc (28). Marker genes induced by adenoviral vector can be detected in the rabbit discs for up to 1 year after viral injection. Nishida et al. (28) demonstrated the feasibility of *in vivo* gene therapy with adenovirus-delivered TGF-β1. This approach led to an increase in TGF-β1 and PG synthesis from explanted disc cells cultured *in vitro*, but no *in vivo* effect on the discs was demonstrated.

CONCLUSIONS

Research in biologic methods of treating disc degeneration is still in its infancy. Of the many different strategies, gene therapy is one of the most promising. Many different candidate therapeutic genes are being evaluated *in vitro*. BMP-7, TGF-β1, and LMP-1 are being actively investigated in both *in vivo* and *ex vivo* methods of gene therapy. Current research is focused on demonstrating *in vivo* efficacy in animal models of disc degeneration. The next step will be primate and human trials.

REFERENCES

1. Acaroglu ER, Iatridis JC, Setton LA, et al. Degeneration and aging affect the tensile behavior of human lumbar anulus fibrosus. *Spine* 1995;20:2690–2701.
2. Antoniou J, Steffen T, Nelson F, et al. The human lumbar intervertebral disc: evidence for changes in the biosynthesis and denaturation of the extracellular matrix with growth, maturation, ageing, and degeneration. *J Clin Invest* 1996;98:996–1003.
3. Bayliss MT, Johnstone B, O'Brien JP. 1988 Volvo Award in Basic Science. Proteoglycan synthesis in the human intervertebral disc. Variation with age, region and pathology. *Spine* 1988;13:972–981.
4. Bayliss MT, Urban JP, Johnstone B, et al. In vitro method for measuring synthesis rates in the intervertebral disc. *J Orthop Res* 1986;4:10–17.
5. Bibby SR, Jones DA, Lee RB, et al. The pathophysiology of the intervertebral disc. *Joint Bone Spine* 2001;68:537–542.
6. Boden SD, Davis DO, Dina TS, et al. Abnormal magnetic-resonance scans of the lumbar spine in asymptomatic subjects. A prospective investigation. *J Bone Joint Surg Am* 1990;72:403–408.
7. Boden SD, Liu Y, Hair GA, et al. LMP-1, an LIM-domain protein, mediates BMP-6 effects on bone formation. *Endocrinology* 1998;139:5125–5134.
8. Boden SD, Titus L, Hair G, et al. Lumbar spine fusion by local gene therapy with a cDNA encoding a novel osteoinductive protein (LMP-1). *Spine* 1998;23:2486–2492.
9. Borenstein DG, O'Mara JW Jr, Boden SD, et al. The value of magnetic resonance imaging of the lumbar spine to predict low-back pain in asymptomatic subjects: a seven-year follow-up study. *J Bone Joint Surg Am* 2001;83:1306–1311.
10. Buckwalter JA. Aging and degeneration of the human intervertebral disc. *Spine* 1995;20:1307–1314.
11. Burkus JK, Gornet MF, Dickman CA, et al. Anterior lumbar interbody fusion using rhBMP-2 with tapered interbody cages. *J Spinal Disord Tech* 2002;15:337–349.
12. Ebara S, Iatridis JC, Setton LA, et al. Tensile properties of nondegenerate human lumbar anulus fibrosus. *Spine* 1996;21:452–461.
13. Frymoyer JW, Cats-Baril WL. An overview of the incidences and costs of low back pain. *Orthop Clin North Am* 1991;22:263–271.
14. Fujita Y, Duncan NA, Lotz JC. Radial tensile properties of the lumbar annulus fibrosus are site and degeneration dependent. *J Orthop Res* 1997;15:814–819.

15. Gruber HE, Johnson TL, Leslie K, et al. Autologous intervertebral disc cell implantation: a model using *Psammomys obesus*, the sand rat. *Spine* 2002;27:1626–1633.
16. Han SM, Lee SY, Cho MH, et al. Disc hydration measured by magnetic resonance imaging in relation to its compressive stiffness in rat models. *Proc Inst Mech Eng [H]* 2001;215:497–501.
17. Hayes AJ, Benjamin M, Ralphs JR. Extracellular matrix in the development of the intervertebral disc. *Matrix Biol* 2001;20:107–121.
18. Horner HA, Urban JP. 2001 Volvo Award in Basic Science Studies. Effect of nutrient supply on the viability of cells from the nucleus pulposus of the intervertebral disc. *Spine* 2001;26:2543–2549.
19. Israel DI, Nove J, Kerns KM, et al. Heterodimeric bone morphogenetic proteins show enhanced activity in vitro and in vivo. *Growth Factors* 1996;13:291–300.
20. Liu Y, Hair GA, Boden SD, et al. Overexpressed LIM mineralization proteins do not require LIM domains to induce bone. *J Bone Miner Res* 2002;17:406–414.
21. Martin JA, Buckwalter JA. Aging, articular cartilage chondrocyte senescence and osteoarthritis. *Biogerontology* 2002;3:257–264.
22. Masuda, K, An HS, Thonar E. *OP-1 stimulates proteoglycan synthesis in a C-ABC injured disc*. Presented to the International Society for the Study of the Lumbar Spine, Cleveland, 2002(abst).
23. McKay B, Sandhu HS. Use of recombinant human bone morphogenetic protein-2 in spinal fusion applications. *Spine* 2002;27:S66–S85.
24. Minamide A, Boden SD, Viggeswarapu M, et al. Mechanism of bone formation with gene transfer of the cDNA encoding for the intracellular protein LMP-1. *J Bone Joint Surg Am* 2003;85:1030–1039.
25. Moore KR, Pinto MR, Butler LM. Degenerative disc disease treated with combined anterior and posterior arthrodesis and posterior instrumentation. *Spine* 2002;27:1680–1686.
26. Moore RJ, Crotti TN, Osti OL, et al. Osteoarthrosis of the facet joints resulting from anular rim lesions in sheep lumbar discs. *Spine* 1999;24:519–525.
27. Moore RJ, Latham JM, Vernon-Roberts B, et al. Does plate fixation prevent disc degeneration after a lateral anulus tear? *Spine* 1994;19:2787–2790.
28. Nishida K, Kang JD, Gilbertson LG, et al. Modulation of the biologic activity of the rabbit intervertebral disc by gene therapy: an in vivo study of adenovirus-mediated transfer of the human transforming growth factor beta 1 encoding gene. *Spine* 1999;24:2419–2425.
29. Nomura T, Mochida J, Okuma M, et al. Nucleus pulposus allograft retards intervertebral disc degeneration. *Clin Orthop* 2001;94–101.
30. Ohshima H, Urban JP. The effect of lactate and pH on proteoglycan and protein synthesis rates in the intervertebral disc. *Spine* 1992;17:1079–1082.
31. Park J, Yoon ST, Kim K, et al. LMP-1 overexpression in intervertebral disc cells increases BMP-2 gene expression and up-regulates proteoglycan production. *Transactions of the Orthopaedic Research Society (2003)*.
32. Roberts S. Disc morphology in health and disease. *Biochem Soc Trans* 2001;30:864–869.
33. Roberts S, Menage J, Duance V, et al. 1991 Volvo Award in Basic Sciences. Collagen types around the cells of the intervertebral disc and cartilage end plate: an immunolocalization study. *Spine* 1991;16:1030–1038.
34. Roughley PJ, Alini M, Antoniou J. The role of proteoglycans in aging, degeneration and repair of the intervertebral disc. *Biochem Soc Trans* 2001;30:869–874.
35. Seeherman H, Wozney J, Li R. Bone morphogenetic protein delivery systems. *Spine* 2002;27:S16–S23.
36. Silveri CP, Simeone FA. Lumbar disc disease. In: An HS, ed. *Principles and techniques of spine surgery*. Baltimore: Williams & Wilkins, 1998:425–442.
37. Takegami K, Masuda K, An HS, et al. In vivo administration of osteogenic protein-1 increases proteoglycan content and disc height in rabbit intervertebral disc. *Transactions of the Orthopaedic Research Society* 25(0338), 2000(abst).
38. Takegami K, Thonar EJ, An HS, et al. Osteogenic protein-1 enhances matrix replenishment by intervertebral disc cells previously exposed to interleukin-1. *Spine* 2002;27:1318–1325.
39. Thompson JP, Oegema TR Jr, Bradford DS. Stimulation of mature canine intervertebral disc by growth factors. *Spine* 1991;16:253–260.
40. Urban JP, McMullin JF. Swelling pressure of the intervertebral disc: influence of proteoglycan and collagen contents. *Biorheology* 1985;22:145–157.
41. Vaccaro AR, Anderson DG, Toth CA. Recombinant human osteogenic protein-1 (bone morphogenetic protein-7) as an osteoinductive agent in spinal fusion. *Spine* 2002;27:S59–S65.
42. Yoon ST, Kim K, Li J, et al. The effect of bone morphogenetic protein-2 on rat intervertebral disc cells in vitro. *Spine* 2003.

14

Bone Graft Alternatives in Spinal Surgery

*Angelo M. Ciminiello, †David H. Kim, and ‡§Alexander R. Vaccaro

*Department of Orthopedic Surgery, University of Connecticut Health Center,
Farmington, Connecticut; †The Boston Spine Group, New England Baptist Hospital,
Boston, Massachusetts; ‡Reconstructive Spine Service, The Rothman Institute;
and §Department of Orthopedic Surgery, Thomas Jefferson University Hospital,
Philadelphia, Pennsylvania

A fundamental goal of spinal surgery is the maintenance or restoration of stability to the injured or diseased spine. Modern surgical techniques include the use of complex instrumentation systems to achieve early stability, but long-term stability requires the creation of a solid biologic fusion. The successful accomplishment of such a fusion depends not only on the rigid biomechanical environment provided by surgical instrumentation but also on the biologic environment provided by local tissue.

The use of autogenous bone graft can enhance the local biology, making it more favorable for the development of a healthy fusion. The outcome of such bone grafting depends on the successful achievement of three distinct biologic processes: osteoconduction, osteoinduction, and osteogenesis. *Osteoconduction* is defined as the apposition of growing bone to the three-dimensional surface of the graft structural scaffold. *Osteoinduction* is the cytokine-mediated recruitment and differentiation of various cell types essential for bone formation. *Osteogenesis* is the process of new bone formation occurring at a cellular level and implies the recruitment of osteoprogenitor stem cells.

PRINCIPLES OF BONE GRAFTING IN SPINAL FUSION

A robust spinal fusion depends on the successful interaction of multiple factors, both biologic and biomechanical. The local tissue environment of the placed graft is of critical importance. An adequate blood supply is essential and can be promoted through careful surgical technique. Exposure of the spine should be limited to the extent required for the visualization of landmarks and adequate decortication. Excessive muscle stripping reduces the vascularity of underlying bone, creates potential dead space for seroma and hematoma formation, and causes tissue necrosis that may contribute to delayed wound healing and infection. An intact blood supply to local tissue maintains the oxygen tension and nutrient levels necessary for cellular synthetic activity, promotes neovascularization, and allows cellular migration into the developing fusion mass. The risk for infection must be minimized because local infection drains available nutrients and disturbs the delicate balance of local cytokines responsible for the evolving fusion mass.

A systemic illness such as diabetes can also have an adverse impact on fusion rates, most likely by impairing vascular ingrowth. Cigarette smoking is another well-established risk factor for pseudarthrosis (5), most likely as a result of the effect of nicotine on the vascular supply. Malnutrition is associated with a general impairment of wound healing and may also have a specific effect on fusion rates.

The importance of local biomechanical factors depends on the nature and position of the bone graft. Because anterior interbody structural grafts are placed under local compressive forces, they must contribute immediate support and stability, and precise contouring and position may be the difference between successful fusion and pseudarthrosis. Posterior grafts, in contrast, are placed along the tension side of the spinal column, serve no immediate structural function, and are not as directly affected by local biomechanical factors. Nevertheless, even in the posterior position, mechanical instability with excessive strain may allow injury to fragile new blood vessels growing into the graft and result in a fibrous nonunion.

Osteogenic cells are an absolute requirement for successful fusion. The origin of such cells varies with different grafting strategies. A fresh autograft directly provides viable, although few, progenitor stem cells and mature osteoblasts. The extracellular matrix of the autograft and local wound hematoma are sources of osteoinductive factors, such as bone morphogenetic proteins (BMPs). These factors play a critical role in the formation and maturation of new bone and stimulate the recruitment of additional osteogenic cells. The hydroxyapatite and collagen of the autograft act as an osteoconductive lattice within the developing fusion mass for new blood vessels and migrating stem cells (50).

The osteoconductive properties of graft material depend in part on the similarity of various biomechanical properties between the implanted graft and native bone. Specifically, elastic modulus, pore size, and three-dimensional interconnectivity of host and donor tissue must be closely matched to allow migration of osteoblastic precursor cells and ingrowth of new bone (50).

AUTOLOGOUS BONE GRAFT

The gold standard for bone graft material in spinal surgery is autologous iliac crest graft. The term *autograft* (formerly *homograft*) refers to bone taken from one anatomic site and transplanted to another site in the same individual. A unique advantage of autograft is the presence of a viable population of osteoblasts and osteogenic precursor cells with predictable osteoconductive, osteoinductive, and osteogenic properties. Moreover, because the graft originates from the individual patient, autograft harvest is generally rapid and convenient.

The biomechanical properties of structural autograft have been well studied in the appendicular skeleton (9). The mineralized collagen matrix of an autograft provides an initial lattice with relatively less strength and stability than those of intact bone. As fusion proceeds, the voids between graft and host bone are bridged by new bone formation. Segmental stiffness increases as new bone is deposited onto the osteoconductive matrix of the autograft and then further remodeled. New bone formation and remodeling occur during a period of several months.

Autologous bone theoretically provides a favorable microenvironment for new bone formation by creeping substitution (9). Unfortunately, the full potential of autograft is most likely not realized in actual practice (19). The process of graft harvesting and transplantation is inherently damaging to the graft tissue. Cells that survive the initial harvest and transplantation initially depend on passive diffusion for oxygenation. Anoxic death probably occurs in significant numbers of cells before sufficient neovascularization can reestablish a blood supply into the developing fusion mass.

The principal disadvantage of autograft is morbidity associated with graft harvest. In anterior cervical discectomy procedures, complications are more commonly associated with the graft harvest site than with the primary surgical site. Reported donor site complication rates vary from 4% to 49% (19). Major complications associated with graft harvest include chronic pain, infection, prolonged wound drainage, hematoma formation, pelvic ring destabilization, enterocutaneous fistula, local and regional sensory loss, gait disturbance, and bowel herniation.

The morbidity associated with autograft has led to development of numerous alternatives, including allograft bone, demineralized bone matrix (DBM), recombinant bone growth factors (e.g., BMPs), and synthetic implants. These alternatives can be used in isolation or more effectively in combination with autologous bone marrow or as autograft extenders. It should be emphasized that no commercially available alternative to autograft effectively provides all three fundamental properties of autograft bone—namely, osteogenicity, osteoconductivity, and osteoinductivity. Nevertheless, the use of autograft alternatives has become established in modern spine surgery. In the setting of an insufficient supply of autograft, alternatives may be used as graft extenders.

Clinical studies suggest that acceptable fusion rates may be achieved in specific surgical procedures without autograft—for example, the use of structural allograft in single-level anterior cervical discectomy and fusions followed by plating. In these specific situations, the morbidity of autograft harvest can be avoided without compromising outcome (1,2,18,57).

BONE MARROW ASPIRATE

Bone marrow aspirate is a readily available alternative source of osteoprogenitor cells. The marrow cell population contains mesenchymal stem cells that can be induced by specific cytokines to differentiate along the osteoblast lineage. The percentage of stem cells has been shown to vary according to patient age, with elderly patients demonstrating significantly smaller numbers of inducible stem cells (28). In young patients, the ratio of stem cells to the total number of nucleated cells has been estimated to be 1:50,000. In elderly patients, the ratio decreases to 1:2,000,000. The concentration of stem cells and efficiency of osteogenesis can be increased through centrifugation of the marrow aspirate. Preliminary results of clinical studies have demonstrated good results in long-bone unions with the use of this technique of "medullary osteogenesis" (12).

The minimal morbidity associated with iliac crest bone marrow aspiration encourages its use as an adjunct to grafting procedures for spinal fusion. The osteogenic property of bone marrow aspirate can be augmented through the addition of bone extracts containing BMPs, which further enhance its potential usefulness. Currently, bone marrow aspirate is often added to various autograft alternatives to provide osteogenicity to the osteoinductive and osteoconductive properties of the graft material.

ALLOGRAFT BONE

Allograft bone is the most commonly used alternative to autograft in spinal fusion. An *allograft* is defined as an organ or tissue transferred from one member of a species to another member of the same species. The use of allograft has greatly increased as a result of improved methods of procurement, preparation, and storage. Infection remains the most commonly expressed concern among patients. Large follow-up studies suggest that the risk for HIV infection is less than 1 per 1 million uses of allograft sources (8). The risk for hepatitis B or C transmission may be slightly greater.

Allograft bone is available in different forms, including strips, cubes, wedges, shafts, and machined dowels. It is considered both osteoconductive and weakly osteoinductive, with the degree of osteoinductivity varying according to the method of preparation and sterilization. During processing, cells and debris are removed from allograft bone to minimize the risk for infection and reduce immunogenicity (19). As a result, allografts do not contain living cells and have no osteogenic potential.

The fate of allograft material partially depends on its anatomic location within the spine. The placement of allograft in the anterior column, where it is exposed to compressive forces, has resulted in higher rates of fusion (5). Excellent results have been reported for the use of allograft in adolescent patients undergoing instrumented spinal fusion for scoliosis (4). Dodd et al. (17). reviewed the results in 40 patients with idiopathic scoliosis in whom fusions were performed with either femoral head allograft or iliac crest autograft. Radiographic union was successfully achieved in all patients. Patients receiving allograft experienced less operative blood loss and postoperative pain and had a relatively low infection rate.

In comparison with isolated allograft placed in the anterior column, isolated allograft applied in a posterior or posterolateral position under neutral load is associated with fusion rates lower than those achieved with autograft bone. In this position, allograft is more extensively resorbed, incorporated more slowly, and possibly associated with a greater risk for infection than autologous bone graft (26,32,33).

DEMINERALIZED BONE MATRIX

DBM is a product of more extensive allograft bone processing. The mineral content of bone is removed through mild acid extraction to leave an organic product containing BMPs, collagen, and various noncollagenous proteins (28). Extensive processing makes DBM the least immunogenic of all currently available allograft bone products. Excellent results have been reported with the use of DBM in stable and well-supported skeletal defects in animal studies and in the treatment of giant cell tumors of bone in humans (40,41). In addition, Glowacki and Mulliken (23) reported that DBM and marrow composite grafts are comparable in efficacy to autogenous iliac crest bone grafts in certain clinical situations requiring arthrodesis.

DBM is commercially available in different preparations. One example is Grafton Allogenic Bone Matrix (Osteotech, Eatontown, NJ, U.S.A.). This product consists of DBM in a glycerol carrier and is available in three different forms (28). Grafton DBM Gel consists of particulate DBM, Grafton DBM Putty contains DBM in fiber form, and Grafton DBM Flex is a nonwoven sheet of DBM fibers. Grafton has proven osteoinductive properties in animal models, and preclinical studies yielded favorable results when Grafton was used alone or as an autograft extender.

Other commercially available preparations of DBM include Opteform (Regeneration Technologies, Alachua, FL, U.S.A.), Osteofil (Regeneration Technologies), and Dynagraft (GenSci Regeneration Sciences, Toronto, Ontario, Canada). Fewer data are currently available regarding the experimental or clinical use of these products.

CERAMICS

Synthetic ceramics are bone graft alternatives that have the advantages of potentially limitless availability and essentially no increased risk for infection. Ceramics alone are purely osteoconductive without being osteogenic or osteoinductive. The two-dimensional surface of these graft alternatives provides an osteoconductive scaffold for the adherence and migration of bone-forming cells. However, the three-dimensional microarchitecture of these materials is a more important determinant of the speed of incorporation and remodeling. The highly porous, lower-density constructs offer a greater surface area for nutrient supply, neovascularization, and bony ingrowth (4).

Three different types of ceramics are currently available: sintered, replamiform, and collagen mesh. Sintered ceramics are porous forms of hydroxyapatite. Although the porous structure allows ingrowth of new bone, the three-dimensional structure lacks the interconnectivity of trabecular bone. Replamiform ceramic is chemically processed sea coral with a microarchitecture much more closely resembling that of bone. Collagen mesh and injected molded ceramics are relatively newer forms that may, in combination with bone marrow aspirate or recombinant BMPs, form composite grafts with clinical efficacy equivalent to that of autograft.

The major synthetic ceramics with demonstrated clinical application for spinal fusion are the calcium phosphate biomaterials hydroxyapatite (HA) and tricalcium phosphate (TCP) (28). These compounds have been used alone or in combination and appear to elicit little immunologic reaction in surrounding tissue, presumably because their biochemical makeup resembles that of normal bone. At first, the new ceramic graft lacks compressive or tensile strength, but the substance of the implant eventually attains mechanical strength similar to that of cancellous bone following successful incorporation into the fusion mass (22).

Synthetic ceramics have already demonstrated effectiveness in spinal fusion performed for deformity and trauma. A large prospective randomized study of 341 adolescents undergoing posterior spinal fusion for idiopathic scoliosis compared autograft with synthetic porous ceramic blocks [macroporous biphasic calcium phosphate (Triosite); Zimmer, Warsaw, IN, U.S.A.] (47). Overall fusion rates were comparable between the group receiving the synthetic ceramic and the group receiving traditional autograft, but the rate of wound complications was significantly decreased in the group receiving ceramic.

In another prospective study, of 106 patients with degenerative scoliosis or spondylolisthesis undergoing posterior lumbar fusion, macroporous biphasic calcium phosphate granules were used in combination with corticocancellous allograft bone chips and bone marrow aspirate (10). In all but six patients, radiographic fusion was achieved, suggesting that macroporous biphasic calcium phosphate is also an adequate substitute to autograft in this patient population.

Pro Osteon (Interpore Cross International, Irvine, CA, U.S.A.) is a commercially available form of ceramic graft derived from coral and composed primarily of calcium carbonate. The production of Pro Osteon involves chemical processing to transform calcium carbonate into hydroxyapatite. Different pore sizes can be created to yield a three-dimensional lattice structure resembling that of either cortical or cancellous bone. The initial formulation of Pro Osteon demonstrated extremely slow resorption rates in clinical follow-up studies—complete resorption occurred only after 15 to 20 years. The newer version of Pro Osteon is purported to demonstrate much more rapid resorption rates.

A major disadvantage of coralline ceramic is its relatively poor mechanical properties. Coralline hydroxyapatite is quite brittle and provides little fracture resistance or tensile strength. Structural grafts must be shielded from loading until substantial bone ingrowth occurs (13). Nevertheless, several clinical studies have demonstrated the successful use of structural anterior column coralline implants when they were protected by load-sharing internal fixation. Thalgott et al. (54) used Pro Osteon 200 in combination with rigid anterior plating in 26 patients undergoing anterior cervical decompression and fusion.

The fusion rate with a minimum 2-year follow-up was 100%, and the mean decrease in pain was 76%. In a separate study of 20 patients undergoing anterior–posterior lumbar fusion, Pro Osteon 200 was used for anterior lumbar interbody fusion (55). With a minimum 37-month follow-up, fusion rates were 93.7%, and pain decreased by an average of 61.8%.

Additional disadvantages of ceramic bone graft substitutes include the absence of osteoinductive or osteogenic properties and their relatively high cost. A more specific disadvantage of using ceramic as a structural bone graft substitute is the minimal initial strength of the implant. The absence of biologic activity is being addressed through the creation of composite implants containing both ceramic material and recombinant BMPs. The high price tag of ceramic implants may be at least partially offset by a reduction in surgical time and the rate of complications associated with autologous bone-grafting techniques.

A study of 12 patients with severe idiopathic scoliosis undergoing long posterior instrumented fusion examined the efficacy of HA/TCP alone or as an extender to autograft (42). In this small study, successful radiographic fusion was achieved in all patients, and postoperative clinical examination at 15 months revealed no significant differences between the two groups.

Vitoss (Orthovita, Malvern, PA, U.S.A.) is a commercially available ceramic bone graft alternative marketed as a highly porous β-TCP bone void filler. The implant material contains 90% interconnected void space designed to mimic the trabecular structure of cancellous bone (19). The microarchitecture contains a broad range of pore sizes, from 1 to 1,000 μm. The smallest pore sizes are purported to induce the capillary wicking of phagocytes for implant resorption in addition to bone-forming cells, nutrients, and cytokines for bone formation (4) (Fig. 14.1). The larger pore sizes are intended to encourage neovascularization and structural bone ingrowth. *In vivo* studies have shown that smaller particles demonstrate improved osteoconductive performance (19). Furthermore, a greater relative surface area theoretically results in higher resorption rates than are possible with denser forms of β-TCP. With normal cellular activity, nanometer-sized crys-

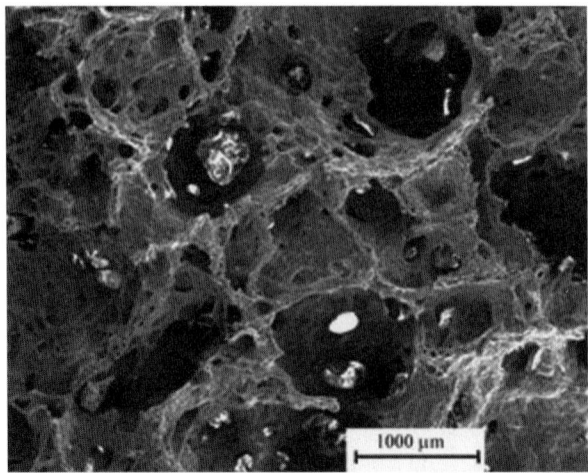

FIG. 14.1. Unimplanted Vitoss scaffold showing porous structure. (From *http://www.orthovita.com/products/vitoss.remodeling.html*, with permission.)

tallines are small enough for the body to digest (19), a property that is imperative for rapid resorption during bone remodeling.

The interconnected microporosity of Vitoss makes it an excellent candidate for use with bone marrow aspirate or recombinant BMPs in a composite implant. A Vitoss scaffold possesses favorable wicking and hydrophilic properties that encourage the retention of both seeded marrow cells and growth factors. The variable microarchitecture may also allow a greater penetration of bone-forming cells and phagocytes and enhance the diffusion of cytokines and nutrients from adjacent bone (4).

In a prospective study, 50 patients undergoing lumbar spinal fusion received Vitoss as an autograft extender (34). All patients underwent decompressive laminectomy with bilateral posterolateral intertransverse fusion in which Vitoss was used in combination with local or local and iliac crest autograft. Both noninstrumented and instrumented posterior fusions were performed, and some patients also underwent posterior lumbar interbody fusion with cages and autograft. Of the 32 patients examined at the 5- to 7-month follow-up, 100% demonstrated progressive radiographic bone graft consolidation. In seven (14%) of the 32 patients, the use of iliac crest bone graft was avoided entirely, and an average of 30% less autograft was required in those who required iliac crest autograft.

When combined with bone marrow aspirate or venous blood, Vitoss may be particularly well suited for use as a composite graft. In a small study, seven patients underwent anterior or posterior lumbar interbody fusion at a total of 12 levels with femoral ring allograft and Vitoss/venous blood without autograft (29). At both 3- and 6-month follow-up, 100% radiographic fusion was noted with no evidence of allograft subsidence, extrusion, fracture, or resorption (Figs. 14.2, 14.3).

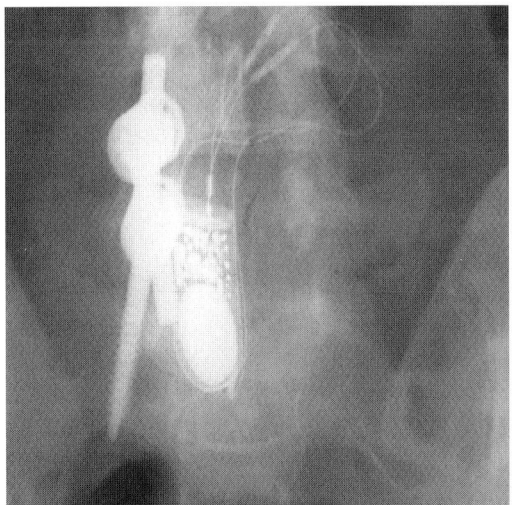
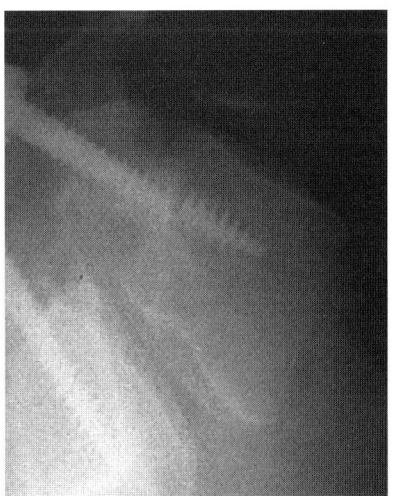

FIG. 14.2. A: Preoperative x-ray films showing an anteroposterior view of the unilateral pedicle screw fixation and placement of a direct current bone growth stimulator. **B:** Lateral view of the fatigue-fractured pedicle screw with no evidence of posterolateral bone. (From Linovitz RJ, Peppers TA. The use of an advanced formulation of beta-tricalcium phosphate as a bone extender in interbody lumbar fusion. *Orthopedics* 2002;25(5 Suppl):S585–S589, with permission.)

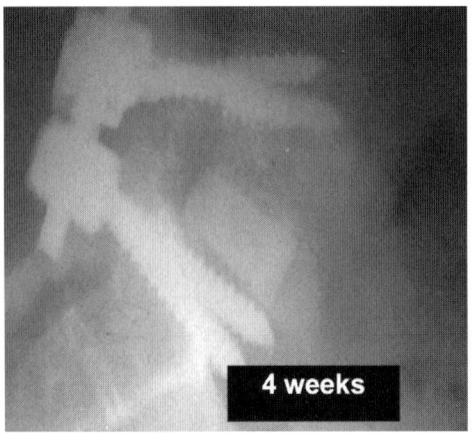 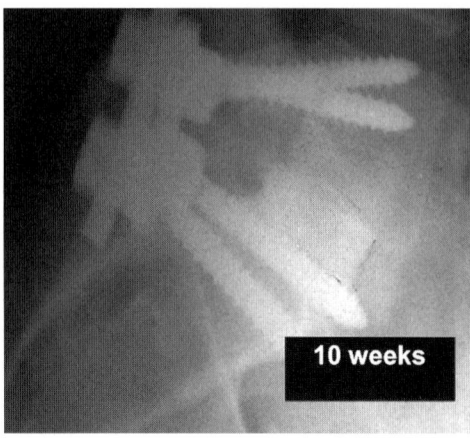

FIG. 14.3. Postoperative x-ray films following removal of instrumentation and anterior lumbar interbody fusion with a femoral ring allograft and a mixture of Vitoss and venous blood. Rapid incorporation of the interbody constructions is shown at 4 weeks **(A)** and 10 weeks **(B)**. The sentinel sign is present in both views. (From Linovitz RJ, Peppers TA. The use of an advanced formulation of beta-tricalcium phosphate as a bone extender in interbody lumbar fusion. *Orthopedics* 2002;25(5 Suppl):S585–S589, with permission.)

Injectable Ceramic Cements

A class of ceramic that combines the qualities of a cement with those of a bone void filler is injectable calcium phosphate (Norian SRS; Synthes-Stratec, Oberdorf, Switzerland). Norian cement contains α-TCP, calcium carbonate, and monocalcium phosphate monohydrate in a solution of sodium phosphate. The resulting ceramic is a pastelike material that can be injected by syringe into a bone defect or fracture site. *In vivo*, Norian hardens into a material that has an initial compressive strength comparable with that of cancellous bone. Within a few weeks after introduction, vascular channels invade the implant, osteoclastic activity appears, and new bone formation occurs in direct contact with the ceramic. Eventually, the implant undergoes remodeling and is ultimately replaced by host bone with minimal foreign body reaction (14).

Norian SRS has shown promising results in the treatment of distal radial fractures and vertebral compression fractures and in the reinforcement of pedicle screw fixation. It has been suggested that this material could be used prophylactically to improve the compressive strength of osteoporotic vertebral bodies even before fracture occurs (27). In a model of vertebral burst fracture, Norian SRS has been shown to enhance the strength of pedicle screw fixation (27), and it might eliminate the need for supplemental anterior reconstruction in these fractures. A potential concern regarding the liquid injectable cement is extraosseous extrusion.

COMPOSITE GRAFTS

Collagen is the most abundant protein in extracellular bone matrix and is conducive to mineral deposition, vascular ingrowth, and growth factor binding, providing both a physical and a chemical milieu favorable to bone regeneration (4). Collagraft (Zimmer, Warsaw, IN, U.S.A.) is a composite of collagen gel and granules of a biphasic ceramic consisting of 60% HA and 40% TCP. It is designed to mimic the composition of natural bone.

When mixed with a patient's own marrow, Collagraft provides both osteoconductive and osteogenic potential (3,15).

In a study of the treatment of long-bone fractures, Collagraft and autologous marrow were compared with iliac crest autograft. No significant differences were found in radiographic healing rates or functional outcomes; in addition, the use of Collagraft shortened the operative time and avoided the morbidity associated with harvesting iliac crest autograft (11).

BONE MORPHOGENETIC PROTEINS

BMPs are members of the transforming growth factor-β (TGF-β) superfamily and consist of at least 15 structurally related osteoinductive growth factors. These proteins were first identified in 1976 as the active osteoinductive fraction of DBM and were characterized by molecular cloning in 1988 (30). Like other members of the TGF-β superfamily, BMPs are multifunctional cytokines that subserve several critical functions. These include skeletal morphogenesis and development, angiogenesis, and tissue homeostasis. They promote the differentiation of mesenchymal stem cells into osteochondrogenic cells and regulate the proliferation, matrix synthesis, and apoptosis of osteoblasts, osteoclasts, and vascular endothelial cells.

The property of BMPs that has generated the most interest is the ability to stimulate new bone formation. A number of BMPs demonstrate the capacity to trigger a cascade of cellular events resembling ectopic endochondral ossification. The sequencing and cloning of specific BMPs has made it possible to produce an essentially unlimited supply of these proteins by means of recombinant gene technology. Recombinant human bone morphogenetic protein-2 (rhBMP-2; Wyeth Genetics Institute, Cambridge, MA, U.S.A.) and rhBMP-7 (Creative Biomolecules, Hopkinton, MA, U.S.A.) are the first two such products to undergo extensive testing (30).

Numerous applications of BMPs in orthopedic and spinal surgery are being investigated in clinical trials. In a small prospective study, 14 patients with lumbar degenerative disk disease underwent interbody fusion with threaded fusion cages filled with either an rhBMP-2/collagen sponge or autograft (7). At the 2-year follow-up, fusion had occurred in all 11 of the patients who received rhBMP-2, compared with two of the three patients who received autograft (Fig. 14.4). Oswestry Disability Index scores demonstrated more rapid postoperative improvement in the patients receiving rhBMP-2 than in those receiving autograft. Patients in the rhBMP-2 group also had shorter hospital stays, possibly because of the absence of pain at an autograft harvest site.

The use of an rhBMP-2/biphasic ceramic block composite has been compared with autograft in patients undergoing posterolateral lumbar fusion (49). Seven patients underwent unilateral implantation of the BMP/ceramic composite, whereas the contralateral side received autograft. Short-term results have revealed no significant difference in terms of radiographic appearance between the two sides. Bilateral implantation of rhBMP-2/ceramic, which eliminates the need for autograft altogether, is being examined in the second phase of this study.

In one study, 45 patients undergoing anterior cervical discectomy and fusion with autograft were examined (49). Various concentrations of rhBMP-2 were combined with a collagen sponge construct to repair the defect in the iliac crest resulting from graft procurement. Results have not yet been published.

RhBMP-7, also known as *recombinant human osteogenic protein-1 (rhOP-1)*, has been extensively studied in animal models of spinal fusion. In both rabbit and canine

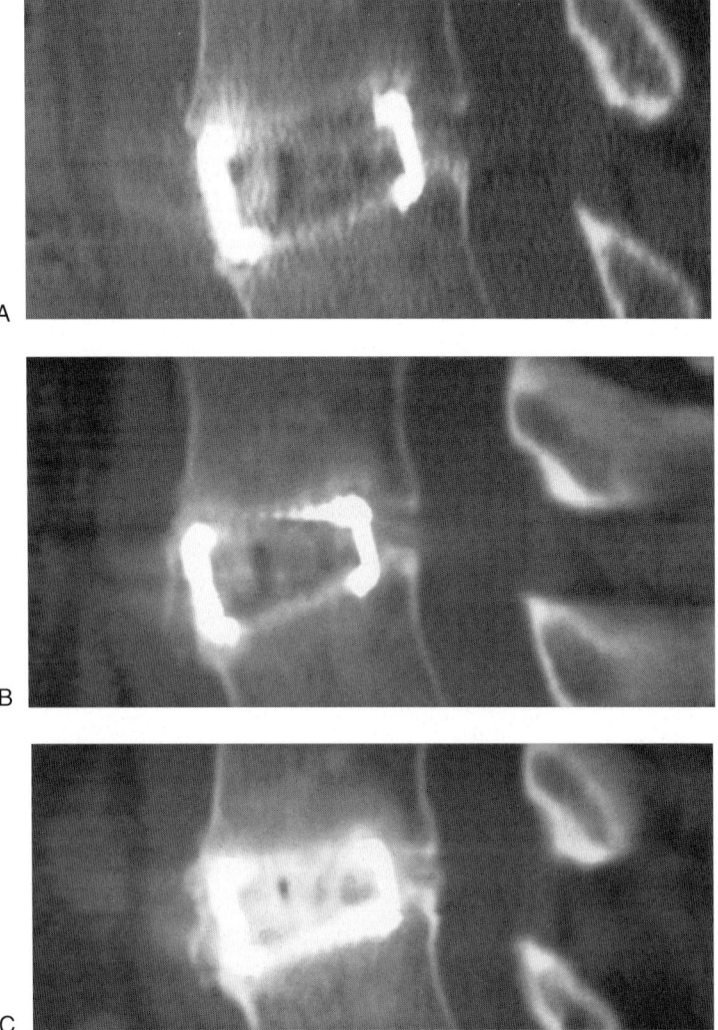

FIG. 14.4. Sagittal re-formations of a computed tomographic scan from a patient who underwent anterior lumbar interbody arthrodesis with a titanium-threaded fusion device filled with recombinant human bone morphogenetic protein-2 (rhBMP-2)/absorbable collagen sponge instead of autogenous bone graft. **A:** At 3 months after surgery, bone formation throughout the cage, in addition to partial anterior bridging in front of the cage, is seen. **B:** At 6 months after surgery, bone growth throughout the center of the cage and a complete bridge anterior to the cage are seen. **C:** At 1 year after surgery, more dense bone filling the entire cage, persistence of the anterior bridge of bone, and formation of a bridge of bone posterior to the cage are seen. (From Boden SD, Zdeblick TA, Sandhu HS, et al. The use of rhBMP-2 in interbody fusion cages. *Spine* 2000;25:376–381, with permission.)

models of posterolateral spinal fusion, the use of rhOP-1 has been associated with more reliable fusion rates and the histologic appearance of more mature lamellar bone than the use of autograft (16). In rabbits exposed to systemic nicotine, a well-known inhibitor of spinal fusion, the use of rhOP-1 was associated with a 100% fusion rate, whereas the fusion rate was only 25% with the use of autograft (43). The use of rhOP-1 may therefore be particularly appropriate in patients such as smokers, who are at high risk for pseudarthrosis.

The biomechanical properties of recombinant BMP-induced spinal fusion have been studied in a sheep model (31). Three groups of sheep underwent posterolateral spinal fusion with transpedicular instrumentation and were implanted with autograft iliac crest bone, deproteinized bovine hydroxyapatite, or rhOP-1 in a collagen matrix. Biomechanically, the resulting fusion was most rigid in the animals given both autograft and rhOP-1 (Figs. 14.5, 14.6). The use of deproteinized hydroxyapatite was associated with the formation of a dense pseudarthrosis and no evidence of continuous bony fusion. The bone density of the rhOP-1–induced fusions was 40% greater than the density of the fusions in the autograft group.

Considerable research is being directed toward identifying the optimal carrier for recombinant BMP delivery. Numerous carriers appear to be compatible with the osteoinductive activity of rhBMPs; however, at this time, only collagen-based carriers are being used in clinical trials (56). An absorbable collagen sponge produced from reconstituted bovine tendon and a collagen matrix derived from demineralized/guanidine-extracted bovine bone have been used successfully in the delivery of rhBMP-2 and rhBMP-7, respectively. An important advantage of collagen as a carrier material is that it is an endogenous protein that is readily metabolized by the body following implantation (56). A disadvantage is that collagen in its native form lacks significant biomechanical rigidity and therefore does not make a good structural graft. Further modification, such as the addition of hydroxyapatite, may provide useful biomechanical properties (38,52,53).

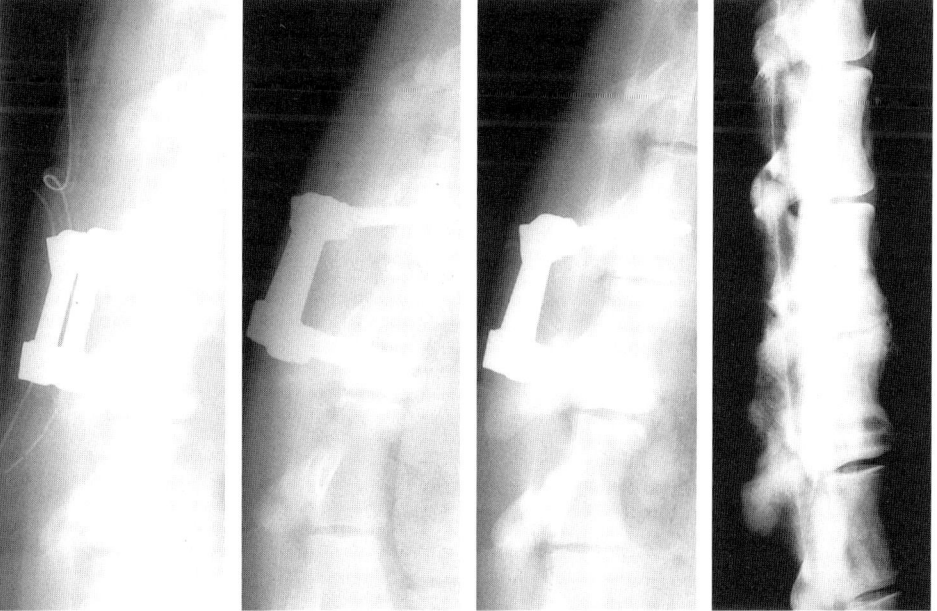

FIG. 14.5. Serial lateral radiographs of a sheep that underwent fusion with recombinant human osteogenic protein-1 (rhOP-1) show the fusion site at 2, 4, and 6 months after surgery. Complete fusion can already be seen at 4 months. [From Magin MN, Delling G. Improved lumbar vertebral interbody fusion using rhOP-1: a comparison of autogenously bone graft, bovine hydroxylapatite (Bio-Oss), and BMP-7 (rhOP-1) in sheep. *Spine* 2001;26: 469–478, with permission.]

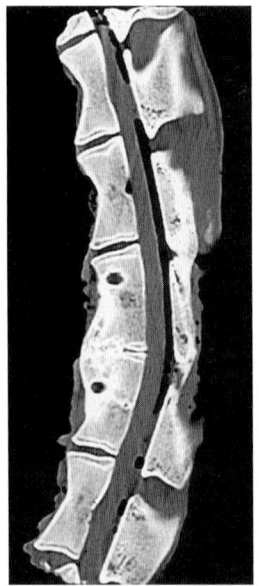 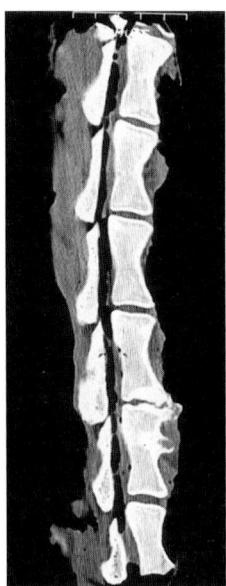 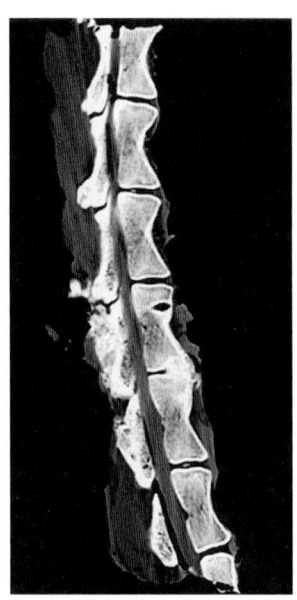

FIG. 14.6. A: A computed tomographic (CT) longitudinal image from a lumbar spinal segment after 6 months. In addition to the nonfused segments, very good bony fusion is clearly visible at L4–5, where autograft was used. The holes remaining in the adjacent vertebral bodies after removal of the internal fixator can be discerned. **B:** Another CT longitudinal image showing a pseudoarthrosis at L4–5. In this case, fusion was performed with bovine hydroxyapatite. **C:** A CT longitudinal image from a recombinant human osteogenic protein-1 fusion site showing homogenous bone formation. [From Magin MN, Delling G. Improved lumbar vertebral interbody fusion using rhOP-1: a comparison of autogenous bone graft, bovine hydroxyapatite (Bio-Oss), and BMP-7 (rhOP-1) in sheep. *Spine* 2001;26:469–478, with permission.]

Another study is examining the use of rhOP-1 in patients with degenerative disc disease (51). All patients underwent decompressive laminectomy and noninstrumented posterolateral lumbar fusion with the implantation of iliac crest autograft on one side and rhOP-1 in a collagen and carboxymethylcellulose carrier on the other side. Preliminary evaluation with flexion–extension radiography and computed tomography at the 6-month follow-up revealed equal or greater bone formation on the rhOP-1 side than on the autograft side.

An investigational device exemption study approved by the Food and Drug Administration evaluated the safety and efficacy of rhBMP-7 in treating patients with single-level degenerative spondylolisthesis and spinal stenosis (45). All patients were treated with a noninstrumented fusion in which iliac crest autograft was combined with rhOP-1 in a collagen and carboxymethylcellulose carrier. Radiographic evidence of fusion was determined by the observation of bony bridging on plain x-ray films and vertebral body stability on flexion–extension films. Clinical success was determined by a 20% improvement in the Oswestry score relative to the preoperative score. Preliminary results from 12 patients revealed a 55% radiographic success rate in the autograft plus rhOP-1 group after 12 months, with 92% of patients demonstrating new bone formation in the intertransverse region (44). These results are similar to those obtained with the use of autologous bone grafting alone in the setting of degenerative spondylolisthesis, as reported in the literature (20). No systemic toxicity or ectopic bone formation was associated with the use of rhOP-1. A clinical study of patients undergoing posterolateral fusion randomized to either iliac crest autograft or rhOP-1 in a collagen and carboxymethylcellulose carrier has been approved by the Food and Drug Administration and is ongoing.

Biodegradable Polymers As Bone Morphogenetic Protein Carriers

Two categories of polymeric membranes being investigated for use in bone grafting procedures are polytetrafluoroethylene and the biodegradable poly α-hydroxy acids polylactic acid (PLA) and polyglycolic acid (PGA) (4). In periodontal studies, the addition of bovine-derived BMP to both polytetrafluoroethylene and biodegradable membranes did not increase the healing rate of critically sized defects in rat mandibles, but rhBMP-2 did accelerate healing when used with PLA/PGA membranes (58). Poly [D,L-(lactide-glycide)] (PLGA) is a porous, biodegradable copolymer that has been evaluated in a canine spinal fusion model as a potential carrier for rhBMP-2 (37). The rhBMP-2/PLGA composite was compared with both autograft bone and PLGA alone; no differences were identified in terms of fusion rates or biomechanical properties between the rhBMP-2/PLGA composite and autograft bone groups. However, both of these treatments were superior to PLGA alone.

Although biodegradable polymers have little osteoconductive potential and have been associated with adverse foreign body reactions, their versatility in terms of various degradation rates and three-dimensional structure make them attractive as potential growth factor delivery vehicles (21). Biodegradable polymers, most notably PLA and PGA, are already in clinical use as absorbable suture or fixation materials, and early studies have shown promising results in terms of their use as potential growth factor carriers. A downside is that these polymers, compared with collagen sponge, appear to be less osteoconductive (25,35). A copolymer of PLA and polyethylene glycol (PLA–PEG) has been developed in which the plasticity, stiffness, and biodegradability of the polymer can be controlled by altering the ratio of PLA to PEG (36,48). In preliminary studies, this material has demonstrated good osteoinductivity and osteoconductivity when combined with BMPs.

GROWTH FACTOR ENHANCEMENTS

Another new strategy being pursued by multiple commercial ventures is growth factor enhancement. This technique is based on the concept that during an injury, white blood cells and platelets collect at the site of insult to secure a clot and deliver growth factors. A commercially available service, Autogenous Growth Factors (AGF; Interpore Cross, Irvine, CA, U.S.A.), collects and processes the platelet and leukocyte-rich buffy coat at the time of surgery, combines it with bone-grafting materials to decrease bone graft migration, and creates a constraining gel that fixes the bone graft in place (24). Such a product allows the surgeon to use only native tissue during grafting and at the same time expedites the natural healing process.

GENE THERAPY

As our understanding of the human genome and its role in disease has evolved, it has become imperative that this wealth of new information be used in the search for new treatments of various diseases. Although the original practice of limiting research to congenital and lethal diseases continues, researchers are now turning toward the treatment of nonlethal conditions. Applying this strategy to spine surgery, scientists are studying gene therapy and its role in spinal fusion.

The use of gene therapy to accomplish spinal fusion may have significant advantages over the local introduction of recombinant BMPs. In terms of both timing and concentration of growth factors, modified genetic material may be more physiologically useful than osteoconductive matrix. In degenerative disc disease, researchers have found that the progressive loss of proteoglycan in the nucleus pulposus leads to dehydration of the disc and subsequent degeneration of its load-bearing ability (46). Thus far, several genes directly applicable to spinal fusion have been successfully transferred. The successful transferral of one such gene, TGF-β1, into the nucleus pulposus of rabbit intervertebral discs has resulted in a doubling of proteoglycan synthesis (39). Additional research is investigating the potential benefits of transferring bone marrow cells with complementary DNA for the osteoinductive proteins LIM mineralization protein-1 (LMP-1) and BMP-2 as an adjunctive treatment for enhancing spinal fusion (6).

CONCLUSIONS

Failed spinal fusion accounts for a considerable number of unsatisfactory clinical outcomes of adult spine surgery. Although careful surgical technique supplemented with generous amounts of autograft bone has previously provided the most reliable means of achieving a rapid and robust fusion mass, results have nevertheless remained unpredictable, and the morbidity associated with graft harvest has often overshadowed the positive clinical results of the primary operation. Numerous alternatives to autograft bone have been developed, including allograft, DBM, and ceramics, none of which possess all three crucial properties of autograft—namely, osteoconductivity, osteoinductivity, and osteogenicity.

Recently developed composite grafts incorporating recombinant BMPs may provide fusion-enhancing capacity that matches or even exceeds the performance of autograft; however, their high initial cost will probably prohibit the extensive use of composite grafts in general spinal procedures. Moreover, the clinical safety and effectiveness of the newer graft alternatives remain to be demonstrated in large clinical trials. With advances in gene therapy and the availability of recombinant osteoinductive proteins, a new era of biotechnology in spine surgery is upon us, with the promise of more effective treatment for patients requiring spinal fusion.

REFERENCES

1. Arrington ED, Smith WJ, Chambers HG, et al. Complications of iliac crest bone graft harvesting. *Clin Orthop* 1996;329:300–309.
2. Banwart JA, Asher MA, Hassanein RS. Iliac crest bone graft harvest donor site morbidity. A statistical evaluation. *Spine* 1995;20:1055–1060.
3. Begley CT, Doherty MJ, Hankey DP, et al. The culture of human osteoblasts upon bone graft substitutes. *Bone* 1993;14:661–666.
4. Betz R. Limitations of autograft and allograft: new synthetic solutions. *Orthopedics* 2002;25(5 Suppl): S561–S570.
5. Boden SD, Schimandle JH. Biology of lumbar spine fusion and bone graft materials. In: International Society for Study of the Lumbar Spine Editorial Committee, eds. *The lumbar spine*, 2nd ed. Philadelphia: WB Saunders, 1996:1284–1306.
6. Boden SD, Titus L, Hair G, et al. Lumbar spine fusion by local gene therapy with a cDNA encoding a novel osteoinductive protein (LMP-1). *Spine* 1998;23:2486–2492.
7. Boden SD, Zdeblick TA, Sandhu HS, et al. The use of rhBMP-2 in interbody fusion cages. *Spine* 2000;25: 376–381.

8. Buck BE, Malinen TI, Brown MD. Bone transplantation and the human immunodeficiency virus. An estimate of the risk of acquired immunodeficiency syndrome (AIDS). *Clin Orthop* 1989;240:129–136.
9. Burchardt H. The biology of bone graft repair. *Clin Orthop* 1983;174:28–42.
10. Cavagna R, Daculsi G, Bouler JM. Macroporous calcium phosphate ceramic: a prospective study of 106 cases in lumbar spinal fusion. *J Long-Term Effects Med Implants* 1999;9:403–412.
11. Chapman MW, Bucholz R, Cornell C. Treatment of acute fractures with a collagen-calcium phosphate graft material: a randomized clinical trial. *J Bone Joint Surg Am* 1997;79:495–502.
12. Connolly JF, Guse R, Tiedman J, et al. Autologous marrow injection as a substitute for operative grafting of tibial nonunions. *Clin Orthop* 1991;266:259–270.
13. Constantz BR, Ison IC, Fulmer MT, et al. Skeletal repair by in situ formation of the mineral phase of bone. *Science* 1995;267:1796–1799.
14. Cornell CN. Osteoconductive materials and their role as substitutes for autogenous bone grafts. *Orthop Clin North Am* 1999;30:591–598.
15. Cornell CN, Lane JM, Chapman M, et al. Multicenter trial of Collagraft as bone graft substitute. *J Orthop Trauma* 1991;5:1–8.
16. Cunningham BW, Shimamoto N, Sefter JC, et al. *Posterolateral spinal arthrodesis using osteogenic protein-1: an in-vivo time course study using a canine model.* Presented at the 15th annual meeting of the North American Spine Society, New Orleans, October 25–28, 2000.
17. Dodd CAF, Fergusson CM, Freedman L, et al. Allograft versus autograft bone in scoliosis surgery. *J Bone Joint Surg Br* 1988;70:431–434.
18. Enneking WF, Eady JL, Burchardt H. Autologous cortical bone grafts in the reconstruction of segmental skeletal defects. *J Bone Joint Surg [Am]* 1980;62:1039–1058.
19. Erbe EM, Marx JG, Clineff TD, et al. Potential of an ultraporous β-tricalcium phosphate synthetic cancellous bone void filler and bone marrow aspirate composite graft. *Eur Spine J* 2001;10:S141–S146.
20. Fischgrund JS, Mackay M, Herkowitz HN, et al. 1997 Volvo Award in Clinical Studies. Degenerative lumbar spondylolisthesis with spinal stenosis: a prospective, randomized study comparing decompressive laminectomy and arthrodesis with and without spinal instrumentation. *Spine* 1997;22:2807–2812.
21. Fleming JE Jr, Cornell CN, Muschler GF. Bone cells and matrices in orthopedic tissue engineering. *Orthop Clin North Am* 2000;31:357–374.
22. Gazdag AR, Lane JM, Glaser D, et al. Alternatives to autogenous bone graft: efficacy and indications. *J Am Acad Orthop Surg* 1995;3:1–8.
23. Glowacki J, Mulliken JB. Demineralized bone implants. *Clin Plast Surg* 1985;12:233.
24. Interpore Cross. Autologous Growth Factors™ (AGF™). The original growth factors. Available at *http://www.interporecross.com/product_agf.html*. Accessed April 5, 2002.
25. Isobe M, Yamazaki Y, Oida S, et al. Bone morphogenetic protein encapsulated with a biodegradable and biocompatible polymer. *J Biomed Mater Res* 1996;32:433–438.
26. Jorgenson SS, Lowe TG, France J, et al. A prospective analysis of autograft vs. allograft in posterolateral fusion in the same patient. A minimum one-year follow-up in 144 patients. *Spine* 1994;19:2048–2053.
27. Keating JF, McQueen MM. Substitutes for autologous bone graft in orthopaedic trauma. *J Bone Joint Surg Br* 2001;83:3–8.
28. Khan SN, Tomin E, Lane JM. Clinical applications of bone graft substitutes. *Tissue Eng Orthop Surg* 2000;31:389–398.
29. Linovitz RJ, Peppers TA. The use of an advanced formulation of beta-tricalcium phosphate as a bone extender in interbody lumbar fusion. *Orthopedics* 2002;25(5 Suppl):S585–S589.
30. Ludwig SC, Boden SD. Osteoinductive bone graft substitutes for spinal fusion. A basic science summary. *Orthop Clin North Am* 1999;30:635–644.
31. Magin MN, Delling G. Improved lumbar vertebral interbody fusion using rhOP-1. A comparison of autogenous bone graft, bovine hydroxylapatite (Bio-Oss), and BMP-7 (rhOP-1) in sheep. *Spine* 2001;26:469–478.
32. Malinen TI, Brown MD. Bone allografts in spine surgery. *Clin Orthop* 1981;154:68–73.
33. May VR Jr, Mauck WR. Exploration of the spine for pseudoarthrosis following spinal fusion in the treatment of scoliosis. *Clin Orthop* 1967;53:115–122.
34. Meadows GR, Crimmins S, LeCea J. Adjunctive use of ultraporous β-TCP bone void filler in spinal arthrodesis. *Orthopedics* 2002;25(5Suppl):S579–S584.
35. Miyamoto S, Takaoka K, Okada T, et al. Evaluation of polylactic acid homopolymers as carriers for bone morphogenetic protein. *Clin Orthop* 1992;278:274–285.
36. Miyamoto S, Takaoka K, Okada T, et al. Polylactic acid-polyethylene glycol block copolymer. A new biodegradable synthetic carrier for bone morphogenetic protein. *Clin Orthop* 1993;294:333–343.
37. Muschler GF, Hyodo A, Manning T, et al. Evaluation of human bone morphogenetic protein 2 in a canine spinal fusion model. *Clin Orthop* 1994;35:279–284.
38. Nakashima M. Induction of dentine in amputated pulp of dogs by recombinant human bone morphogenetic protein-2 and -4 with collagen matrix. *Arch Oral Biol* 1994;39:1085–1099.
39. Nishida K, Gilbertson LG, Robbins PD, et al. Potential applications of gene therapy to the treatment of intervertebral disc disorders. *Clin Orthop* 2000;379[Suppl]:S234–S241.
40. Oikarinen J. Experimental spinal fusion with decalcified bone matrix and deep frozen allogenic bone in rabbits. *Clin Orthop* 1982;162:210–218.

41. Pals SD, Wilkins RM. Giant cell tumor treated by curettage, cementation, and bone grafting. *Orthopedics* 1992;15:703–708.
42. Passuti N, Daculsi G, Rogez JM, et al. Macroporous calcium phosphate ceramic performance in human spine fusion. *Clin Orthop* 1989;248:169–176.
43. Patel TC, Erulkar JS, Grauer JN, et al. *OP-1 overcomes the inhibitory effect of nicotine on posterolateral lumbar fusion.* Presented at the 15th annual meeting of the North American Spine Society, New Orleans, October 25–28, 2000.
44. Patel TC, Hopkinton MA, Vaccaro AR, et al. *Two-year follow-up of a safety and efficacy study of OP-1 (rhBMP-7) as an adjunct to posterolateral lumber fusion.* Presented at the 16th annual meeting of the North American Spine Society, Seattle, October 31–November 3, 2001.
45. Patel TC, Vaccaro AR, Truumees E, et al. *A safety and efficacy study of OP-1 (rhBMP-7) as an adjunct to posterolateral lumbar fusion.* Presented at the 15th annual meeting of the North American Spine Society, New Orleans, October 25–28, 2000.
46. Pearce RH, Grimmer BJ, Adams ME. Degeneration and the chemical composition of the human lumbar intervertebral disc. *J Orthop Res* 1987;5:198–205.
47. Ransford AO, Morley T, Edgar MA, et al. Synthetic porous ceramic compared with autograft in scoliosis surgery. A prospective, randomised study of 341 patients [published erratum appears in *J Bone Joint Surg Br* 1998 May;80(3):562]. *J Bone Joint Surg Br* 1998;80:13–18.
48. Saito N, Okada T, Toba S, et al. New synthetic absorbable polymers as BMP carriers: plastic properties of poly-D,L-lactic acid-polyethylene glycol block copolymers. *J Biomed Mater Res* 1999;47:104–110.
49. Sandhu HS, Grewal HS, Parvataneni H. Bone grafting for spinal fusion. *Orthop Clin North Am* 1999;30:685–698.
50. Simon SR, ed. *Orthopaedic basic science*, 2nd ed. Rosemont, IL: American Academy of Orthopaedic Surgeons, 1994:284–293.
51. Speck G. *Posterolateral lumbar fusion using OP-1: preliminary results.* Presented at the meeting of the Australian Spine Society, Adelaide, Australia, April 2000.
52. Takaoka K, Koezuka M, Nakahara H. Telopeptide-depleted bovine skin collagen as a carrier for bone morphogenetic protein. *J Orthop Res* 1991;9:902–907.
53. Takaoka K, Nakahara H, Yoshikawa H, et al. Ectopic bone induction on and in porous hydroxyapatite combined with collagen and bone morphogenetic protein. *Clin Orthop* 1988;234:250–254.
54. Thalgott JS, Fritts K, Giuffre JM, et al. Anterior interbody fusion of the cervical spine with coralline hydroxyapatite. *Spine* 1999;24:1295–1299.
55. Thalgott JS, Fritts K, Giuffre JM, et al. The use of coralline hydroxyapatite for interbody spinal fusions. *Spine State Art Rev* 1997;11:325–340.
56. Uludag H, Gao T, Porter TJ, et al. Delivery systems for BMPs: factors contributing to protein retention at an application site. *J Bone Joint Surg Am* 2001;83:S1128–S1135.
57. Younger EM, Chapman MW. Morbidity at bone graft donor sites. *J Orthop Trauma* 1989;3:192–195.
58. Zellin G, Hedner E, Linde A. Bone regeneration by a combination of osteopromotive membranes with different BMP preparations: a review. *Connect Tissue Res* 1996;35:279–284.

15

Inducing Spine Fusion with Osteoinductive Molecules

S. Tim Yoon

Department of Orthopedics, Emory University; and Department of Orthopedics, Atlanta VA Medical Center, Decatur, Georgia

Osteoinductive cytokines are biologic molecules that can induce the formation of bone at orthotopic locations in animals. Since the landmark article published by Urist in 1965 (31), which demonstrated the osteoinductive capacity of demineralized bone matrix (DBM), osteoinductive molecules have been the subject of intense research. The main clinical goal has been to produce a safe and effective substitute for autologous bone graft. Multiple osteoinductive molecules have been identified. The most heavily studied cytokines are bone morphogenetic proteins (BMPs), which are part of the transforming growth factor-β (TGF-β) superfamily. With the onset of molecular cloning techniques, the understanding of these molecules has increased tremendously. Basic science studies have described the chemistry and molecular signaling pathways. Preclinical studies have shown the importance of dosing, carriers, and the biologic milieu. Clinical studies have now demonstrated that BMPs can be used to substitute for autograft bone, realizing the goal of decades of research. This chapter summarizes the most important concepts and research in the use of osteoinductive molecules in spine fusion.

CHEMISTRY OF BONE MORPHOGENETIC PROTEINS

The BMPs are part of the TGF-β family of proteins. Up to 15 BMPs are known (12), and analysis of their protein sequences has revealed significant homology among BMPs and even greater homology between species. The BMPs are soluble, low-molecular-weight, transmembrane glycoproteins that exist as dimers linked by a disulfide bond. The first BMPs were initially identified by their ability to induce the heterotopic formation of bone in standard *in vivo* rodent assays. However, some members of the BMP family do not exhibit this behavior and therefore, by definition, are not osteoinductive. BMPs are important growth and differentiation factors that are necessary for proper embryogenesis. They are also expressed in nonskeletal tissues and involved in the development of nonskeletal tissues, such as renal and neural tissues.

Earlier studies were conducted with BMPs extracted and partially purified from large quantities of demineralized bone. Because a kilogram of cortical bone contains only 1 to 2 μg of BMP, the extraction methods are somewhat cumbersome (27). This extracted BMP contains more than one BMP and minor contaminants of other proteins. Furthermore, because a single chain of BMP can combine with a different BMP to form a heterodimer (e.g., BMP-2 with BMP-7), the composition of the extracted material is even more complex. With the advent of molecular cloning technologies, single BMPs composed only of homodimers are available today. The availability of large quantities of highly characterized recombinant protein has been a necessary step in allowing the widespread evaluation of BMPs in pharmacologic doses.

Interestingly, heterodimers appear to have osteoinductive properties different from those of homodimers. At least two different BMP heterodimers have been shown to be more potent than homodimers. BMP-7/BMP-2 and BMP-2/BMP-6 have been shown to be five to 10 times more potent in inducing cartilage and bone formation than BMP-2 homodimers (16). The identification of a receptor for a heterodimer BMP (BMP-2/BMP-4) in nature further reinforces the concept that heterodimers are part of the normal signaling pathway in nature (23).

PRECLINICAL STUDIES WITH BONE MORPHOGENETIC PROTEINS

Demineralized Bone Matrix

DBM contains some low level of BMP activity. The activity depends on the technique of preparation and sterilization. Morone and Boden (25) demonstrated the effectiveness of DBM in promoting spine fusion in a rabbit model of intertransverse process fusion. In this model, the DBM was effective as a graft extender when combined in up to a 3:1 ratio with autograft. When less than the standard volume of autograft was used, the addition of DBM led to fusion rates comparable with those achieved with the standard amount of autograft alone. However, DBM did not increase the frequency of successful fusion when added to the standard amount of autograft. In another study, in which the same rabbit intertransverse fusion model was used, two fiber-based DBM formulations (flexible sheets and putty) were shown to be substantially more effective than the older, particle-based DBM formulation (gel) (22). This later study demonstrated the importance of osteoconduction as determined by the final three-dimensional structure of the DBM matrix.

Purified Bone Morphogenetic Protein Extract

The first BMP preparation was a partially purified protein extract of bone (31). More recently, Boden et al. (6) demonstrated the efficacy of highly purified bovine BMP (NeOsteo; Sulzer Biologies, Austin, TX, U.S.A.) in rabbit and nonhuman primate models of intertransverse process fusion. They found a dose-dependent response in the rabbit model, which indicated that a threshold concentration and total dose must be overcome before BMP can effectively induce bone formation. In similar experiments in rhesus monkeys, effective spine fusion was achieved with purified BMP in 18 weeks. These experiments highlighted the need for higher doses of BMP in primates than in rodents. Furthermore, the healing time required for primates was significantly longer (18 to 24 weeks).

Recombinant Bone Morphogenetic Protein

Recombinant human BMPs (rhBMPs) have become widely available more recently, and of this group, rhBMP-2 and rhBMP-7 are the two most studied. Preclinical experiments with rhBMP-2 and rhBMP-7 have clearly demonstrated the effectiveness of rhBMPs in spinal fusion. Because of their effectiveness in enhancing spine fusions in animal models, hopes have been high that rhBMP-mediated fusion may be equivalent or superior to fusion with autograft cancellous bone. The key studies are summarized in the next paragraphs.

Schimandle et al. (29) studied rhBMP-2 in a rabbit model of intertransverse process fusion. This model is known to be associated with a significant pseudarthrosis rate and is therefore a challenging environment for bone graft substitutes. The authors were able to show that rhBMP-2, delivered with either a collagen carrier or with autograft bone, was superior to autograft bone alone. The combination of rhBMP-2 with autologous iliac crest bone resulted in 100% fusion, whereas autologous bone alone resulted in 42% fusion. Bone formation was greater and more mature with rhBMP-2. The fusion masses formed with rhBMP-2 were also biomechanically superior to those formed with autologous bone alone at 4 to 5 weeks. Holliger et al. (15) used computed tomography (CT) to study morphologic differences in the fusion mass obtained in rabbit intertransverse process fusion with rhBMP or autograft material. The fusion masses derived from rhBMP-2 had a greater volume and a better attachment to the transverse process than the fusion masses derived from autologous bone alone. Furthermore, these authors showed that the weak point of the fusion mass was generally randomly distributed with rhBMP-2 rather than located at the attachment site to the transverse process, which happened in 11 of 12 instances with autograft. Grauer et al. (13) demonstrated that BMP-7 applied to a collagen sponge could reliably induce spinal fusion in the rabbit model of intertransverse process spine fusion.

The importance of reaching a threshold dose of BMP for a high fusion rate was demonstrated in many different studies. Sandhu et al. (28) studied rhBMP-2 in an adult beagle model of posterolateral fusion. They found that 2,300 μg of rhBMP in an open cell polylactic acid polymer was superior to autograft iliac crest bone graft in achieving a single-level lumbar intertransverse process fusion. They then showed in a later study that exceeding the required threshold concentration of rhBMP-2 did not increase the fusion rate or time to fusion. No significant differences in biomechanical, radiographic, or histologic characteristics of the intertransverse process fusion were noted for the 58- to 2,300-μg doses, nearly a 40-fold difference. Boden et al. (7) studied dose relationship in a nonhuman primate model of intertransverse process spinal fusion. They used a 60% hydroxyapatite–40% tricalcium phospate ceramic block with multiple doses of rhBMP-2 (0, 6, 9, or 12 mg per side). Fusion occurred in all monkeys treated with rhBMP-2; however, a dose-dependent increase in the amount and quality of bone throughout the ceramic carrier was observed based on qualitative assessment.

The effectiveness of rhBMP in promoting anterior interbody fusion has been demonstrated in several studies. Boden et al. (5) studied two different doses in a nonhuman primate model of anterior lumbar interbody fusion (ALIF). They showed that laparoscopic techniques with titanium-threaded cages and collagen soaked in rhBMP-2 could be used to perform successful fusion. The bovine-derived absorbable collagen sponges were soaked in rhBMP-2 at a concentration of either 750 or 1,500 μg/mL. The fusions were evaluated with plain radiography, CT, manual palpation, and histologic analysis. Solid spinal fusion occurred with both doses of rhBMP-2; however, fusion was more rapid with the higher dose. Hecht et al. (14) reported the efficacy of rhBMP-2/collagen sponge with allograft dowel in ALIF at the lumbosacral junction (L7–S1) performed in rhesus macaque. These authors used a single freeze-dried smooth cortical dowel allograft cylinder filled with either autograft bone (control) or an absorbable collagen sponge soaked in rhBMP-2. The three monkeys treated with rhBMP-2 demonstrated radiographic signs of fusion as early as 8 weeks. New bone formation was slower in the control animals, and pseudarthrosis developed in two of the three control animals. Zdeblick et al. (34) studied rhBMP-2 in multiple-level anterior cervical discectomy and fusion in the alpine goat. Three groups of animals showed different fusion rates: titanium intervertebral fusion device [BAK (Bagby and Kuslich) device; Sulzer SpineTech, Minneapolis, MN, U.S.A.] filled with autograft bone (48%), hydroxyapatite-coated BAK device filled with autograft bone (62%), and BAK device filled with rhBMP-2 (95%). Although biomechanical testing did not reveal a statistically significant difference in stiffness between the groups, a tendency toward greater stiffness was noted in the spines in the rhBMP-2 group.

The powerful osteoinductive property of BMP may be able to overcome biologic impediments to fusion and facilitate the use of minimally invasive techniques of spinal fusion. In two separate studies, rhBMP-2 was shown to overcome the inhibitory effect of nicotine and a nonsteroidal antiinflammatory drug in rabbit model of intertransverse process fusion (21,30). In a similar study, rhBMP-7 was effective in overcoming the inhibitory effect of nicotine on spine fusion in a rabbit model of intertransverse process fusion (26). Sandhu et al. (28) showed that with large doses of rhBMP, posterior spinal fusion in the beagle could be performed without decortication. Boden et al. (8) performed video-assisted endoscopic posterolateral fusion in rabbits and monkeys. They found that the procedure could be performed safely even in the face of a laminectomy defect and that the fusion rate was comparable with that after open surgery. Boden et al. (5) also performed laparoscopic ALIF in rhesus macaque. Cunningham et al. (11) studied rhBMP-7 in anterior thoracoscopic fusions in sheep. Four months after surgery, they noted a higher fusion rate and better bone formation with BAK plus rhBMP-7 than with an empty BAK device. These studies support the prospect of less painful and less morbid spinal arthrodesis procedures with faster and stronger fusions.

CLINICAL STUDIES WITH BONE MORPHOGENETIC PROTEINS

Bone Morphogenetic Protein-2

At this time, rhBMP-2 is the only BMP that has been approved by the Food and Drug Administration for clinical use in spine fusion. Specifically, it has been approved for ALIF in the treatment of symptomatic degenerative disc disease delivered at a concentration of 1.5 mg/mL in a collagen sponge placed within a titanium cage. The rhBMP-2 ALIF pilot study was a randomized prospective study in which the 1.5-mg/mL dose (determined by preclinical nonhuman primate studies) with the collagen sponge and cages was used. Fusion occurred in 11 of 11 patients with rhBMP-2 and in two of three patients with autograft as determined by fine-cut CT (10).

The safety and efficacy noted in the pilot study led to the pivotal study in which 143 investigational and 136 control patients with symptomatic single-level disc degeneration were enrolled (24). ALIF was performed in an open fashion to place threaded titanium cages filled with a bovine collagen sponge soaked in rhBMP-2 at a concentration of 1.5 mg/mL in (rhBMP-2) or with autograft (control). More than 90% of the patients underwent a full 2-year follow-up evaluation. Demographically, the two groups were quite similar. The spine fusion rates were similar: 95% (BMP-2) versus 89% at 2 years as determined by thin-cut CT. The Oswestry scores were also similar for both groups, dropping from approximately 55 to 25 during a 2-year period. In the autograft fusion group, however, up to 32% of patients experienced pain at the donor site at 2 years after surgery. Serologic assays of the antibody response to BMP-2 revealed rates of 0.7% (rhBMP-2) and 0.8% (control). Equivalence between the investigational and control groups at 12 months was 99.9%.

A highly similar study of ALIF with allograft bone dowels has been very illuminating (24). ALIF with rhBMP-2–soaked collagen sponge within machined allograft bone dowels demonstrated results clearly superior to those of autograft cancellous bone within allograft bone dowels. The fusion rates were 100% (rhBMP-2) versus 68% (control), and the Oswestry scores were 19 (rhBMP-2) versus 32 (control). The differences in outcome when autograft is used with titanium cages versus allograft bone dowels suggest that the titanium cages induce higher fusion rates and better functional outcomes than the allograft bone dowels. However, it appears that adding rhBMP-2 can overcome the inferiority of the allograft bone dowel.

A posterolateral pilot study with rhBMP-2 at a concentration of 2.0 mg/mL in a biphasic calcium phosphate carrier (10 cc per side) has been performed with three arms: (a) autograft fusion with TSRH instrumentation [autograft/Texas Scottish Rite Hospital (TSRH)], (b) rhBMP-2 fusion with TSRH instrumentation (BMP-2/TSRH), and (c) rhBMP-2 fusion without instrumentation (BMP-2 only) (3). One hundred percent follow-up was achieved at a mean of 17 months postoperatively. Fusion rates, determined with radiography and thin-cut CT at 6, 12, and 24 months, were 40% for autograft/TSRH, 100% for BMP-2/TSRH, and 100% for BMP-2 only. No complications attributable to BMP-2 were noted. Interestingly, the group treated only with BMP-2 had a better functional outcome as determined by the Oswestry Disability Index score, SF-36 (36-item short-form health survey), and pain ratings. This study clearly indicated a higher fusion rate with BMP-7, even in uninstrumented fusions, and suggested that instrumentation may be unnecessary in this group of patients. In another, similar pilot study of posterolateral fusion, in which a slightly lower dose of BMP-2 was used (1.5 mg of BMP-2 per milliliter in a 7-cc volume of biphasic calcium phosphate) (n = 7), a fusion rate of 86% was achieved, suggesting that small changes in the rhBMP-2 concentration and total carrier volume may affect fusion rates (24).

Bone Morphogenetic Protein-7

Although a clinical trial with BMP-7 is ongoing, BMP-7 has not yet been approved by the Food and Drug Administration for routine clinical use in the spine. A safety and efficacy study in humans comparing autograft alone with autograft augmented with BMP-7 putty (3.5 mg of BMP-7 in a collagen carrier) was reported at the annual meeting of the North American Spine Society in 2001 by Patel et al. (32). Union rates at 6 months, measured by radiography, indicated a fusion rate of 75% (9 of 12) for autograft with BMP-7 versus 50% (2 of 4) for autograft only. A statistically significant difference was not achieved between the two groups. This study has been criticized for not having used thin-cut CT and is therefore thought to have applied a much less stringent criterion for fusion than some other BMP studies. An improvement in the Oswestry score of at least 20% was noted in 83% of the autograft with BMP-7 group and in 50% of the autograft-only group. However, these results should be interpreted with caution because of the small number of cases in the autograft-only group (n = 4). Another BMP-7 posterolateral fusion study was reported at the Australian Spine Meeting in 2000 by Speck et al. (32). In this study, patients undergoing decompression and posterolateral lumbar fusion for degenerative spondylolisthesis underwent fusion with autograft bone on one side and BMP-7 putty on the other side. CT evaluation of five patients indicated that the size of the fusion mass at 6 months was larger on average on the BMP-7 putty side than on the autograft side. A pivotal posterolateral fusion study is in progress in the United States.

In Europe, a study of noninstrumented posterolateral fusion at L5–S1 in human patients with L5 spondylolysis and vertebral slip of less than 50% has been published

(17). Twenty patients were randomized to fusion either with autograft bone from the iliac crest (control) or with BMP-7 putty (3.5 mg of BMP-7 in a volume of 3.5 mL per side). Standard radiographic analysis revealed no significant difference in bone formation between the BMP-7 and control groups at 1 year after surgery. Radiostereometric analysis revealed a decrease in translation in the vertical axis in the autograft group in comparison with the BMP-7 group at 1 year after surgery. Clinical results were difficult to compare because standardized outcome measures were not used. The conclusions of the authors were that any differences between the two fusion methods were not significant and that BMP-7 putty therefore did not result in a higher fusion rate than autograft alone.

GENE THERAPY

The use of gene therapy in the treatment of genetic diseases has been impeded by the fact that long-term or permanent expression and high levels of expression are required for clinical effectiveness. The same constraints are not applicable to the orthopedic use of gene therapy (to induce fracture healing or spinal fusion). Transient expression of a sufficient level of gene product to initiate bone formation is all that is necessary. For this reason, gene therapy may be more practical in orthopedics than in other fields. Another advantage of gene therapy in comparison with traditional implantation methods to deliver osteoinductive factors is that cytokines can be delivered continuously for a prolonged time rather than as a single bolus of protein at the time of implantation. The use of gene therapy to induce bone formation holds promise.

Preclinical studies in which human BMP-2 complementary DNA (cDNA) was used to induce bone formation have been performed. Ex vivo gene therapy, in which the ex vivo transfection of cDNA into cells is followed by the implantation of cells, has been successful in several systems. Mesenchymal cells transfected ex vivo with adenovirus-hBMP-2 cDNA have been shown to be capable of forming bone when injected intramuscularly in rodent thighs (19,20). Bone marrow cells transfected ex vivo with hBMP-2 cDNA have been shown to heal femoral defects (18). Percutaneous direct injection of adenovirus-hBMP-2 cDNA into the posterior spine of nude rats induced the formation of bone at different stages of maturity (1). These early studies are promising and show that gene therapy can be used to form bone and that it may lead to better and less invasive methods in the future.

LIM MINERALIZATION PROTEIN

LIM mineralization protein-1 (LMP-1) is an intracellular signaling molecule that initiates bone formation *in vitro* and *in vivo*. The LMP gene was discovered by using a differential display polymerase chain reaction (4). This process involved comparing the RNA from secondary osteoblast cultures stimulated to differentiate by a glucocorticoid with the RNA from unstimulated osteoblast cultures and identifying novel genes. One of the genes found was LMP-1, which has subsequently been shown to be important in osteoblast differentiation. In situ hybridization studies of developing limb buds from mouse embryos has shown that LMP-1 transcripts appear at the time and place of transition from hypertrophic cartilage to primary bone trabeculae during endochondral ossification. LMP-1 transcripts were also seen in areas of membranous bone formation.

LMP-1 is not a secreted factor. It is an intracellular protein that acts by stimulating the synthesis and secretion of other osteoinductive factors. Because LMP-1 is not a secreted factor, a gene therapy approach has been used to induce its intracellular expression. Cells that express LMP-1 can then secrete osteoinductive factors (BMPs are involved) and recruit nearby cells into the osteoinductive cascade. As a result, a relatively small number of cells expressing LMP-1 are needed for effective bone formation, which facilitates gene therapy with conventional vectors (2).

LMP-1 has been shown to be effective in inducing spinal fusion *in vivo*. Boden et al. (9) used a posterior spinal fusion model in nude rats and grafted DBM containing bone marrow cells transfected with LMP-1 cDNA. At 4 weeks, the sites with active LMP-1 cDNA exhibited 100% fusion, whereas no fusion occurred at the sites with the inactive reverse copy of LMP-1 cDNA. Radiography and histology showed virtually no bone induction in the absence of active LMP-1 cDNA. Viggeswarapu at al. (33) showed that LMP-1 is able to induce intertransverse process fusion in immunocompetent rabbits. They performed ex vivo transfection of LMP-1 cDNA into bone marrow or peripheral blood buffy coat cells. These cells were then combined with a collagen/ceramic composite sponge and implanted into the rabbit posterolateral spine. In this pivotal study, fusion occurred in 10 of 10 rabbits treated with cells expressing LMP-1, as tested by manual palpation. Fusion did not occur in any of the control rabbits treated with cells not expressing LMP-1. CT showed that the presence of cells expressing LMP-1 increased the fusion mass density and that the bone formation was mostly confined to the carrier.

CONCLUSIONS

A great deal of progress has been made in understanding the basic science and practical uses of osteoinductive factors. Of the many different osteoinductive factors, BMPs have been most thoroughly investigated. Numerous preclinical studies have shown that these molecules can be used to elicit or enhance bone formation in numerous orthopedic applications. As we have progressed from studies in small animals to experiments in larger animals, we have observed significant increases in dose requirements and time to union. The concentration and volume of the BMP preparation have been shown to be of paramount importance. The role of carriers has been established, further highlighting the importance of the osteoconductive matrix in bone formation. These preclinical studies have led to successful human clinical trials; rhBMP-2–based products are in general clinical use, and other BMPs and preparations are in trial. Clinicians will soon have a wide array of osteoinductive products from which to choose.

REFERENCES

1. Alden TD, Pittman DD, Beres EJ, et al. Percutaneous spinal fusion using bone morphogenetic protein-2 gene therapy. *J Neurosurg* 1999;90:109.
2. Boden SD, Hair GA, Viggeswarapu M, et al. Gene therapy for spine fusion [In Process Citation]. *Clin Orthop* 2000;379(Suppl):S225.
3. Boden SD, Kang J, Sandhu H, et al. 2002 Volvo Award in Clinical Studies. Use of recombinant human bone morphogenetic protein-2 to achieve posterolateral lumbar spine fusion in humans: a prospective, randomized clinical pilot trial. *Spine* 2002;27:2662.
4. Boden SD, Liu Y, Hair GA, et al. LMP-1, an LIM-domain protein, mediates BMP-6 effects on bone formation. *Endocrinology* 1998;139:5125.
5. Boden SD, Martin GJ Jr, Horton WC, et al. Laparoscopic anterior spinal arthrodesis with rhBMP-2 in a titanium interbody threaded cage. *J Spinal Disord* 1998;11:95.
6. Boden SD, Martin GJ, Morone M, et al. The use of coralline hydroxyapatite with bone marrow, autogenous bone graft, or osteoinductive bone protein extract for posterolateral lumbar spine fusion. *Spine* 1999;24:320.
7. Boden SD, Martin GJ Jr, Morone MA, et al. Posterolateral lumbar intertransverse process spine arthrodesis with recombinant human bone morphogenetic protein 2/hydroxyapatite-tricalcium phosphate after laminectomy in the nonhuman primate. *Spine* 1999;24:1179.
8. Boden SD, Moskovitz PA, Morone MA, et al. Video-assisted lateral intertransverse process arthrodesis. Valida-

tion of a new minimally invasive lumbar spinal fusion technique in the rabbit and nonhuman primate (rhesus) models. *Spine* 1996;21:2689.
9. Boden SD, Titus L, Hair G, et al. Lumbar spine fusion by local gene therapy with a cDNA encoding a novel osteoinductive protein (LMP-1). *Spine* 1998;23:2486.
10. Boden SD, Zdeblick TA, Sandhu HS, et al. The use of rhBMP-2 in interbody fusion cages. Definitive evidence of osteoinduction in humans: a preliminary report. *Spine* 2000;25:376.
11. Cunningham BW, Kanayama M, Parker LM, et al. Osteogenic protein versus autologous interbody arthrodesis in the sheep thoracic spine. A comparative endoscopic study using the Bagby and Kuslich interbody fusion device. *Spine* 1999;24:509.
12. Dube JL, Wang P, Elvin J, et al. The bone morphogenetic protein 15 gene is X-linked and expressed in oocytes. *Mol Endocrinol* 1998;12:1809.
13. Grauer JN, Patel TC, Erulkar JS, et al. 2000 Young Investigator Research Award. Evaluation of OP-1 as a graft substitute for intertransverse process lumbar fusion. *Spine* 2001;26:127.
14. Hecht BP, Fischgrund JS, Herkowitz HN, et al. The use of recombinant human bone morphogenetic protein 2 (rhBMP-2) to promote spinal fusion in a nonhuman primate anterior interbody fusion model. *Spine* 1999;24:629.
15. Holliger EH, Trawick RH, Boden SD, et al. Morphology of the lumbar intertransverse process fusion mass in the rabbit model: a comparison between two bone graft materials—rhBMP-2 and autograft. *J Spinal Disord* 1996; 9:125.
16. Israel DI, Nove J, Kerns KM, et al. Heterodimeric bone morphogenetic proteins show enhanced activity in vitro and in vivo. *Growth Factors* 1996;13:291.
17. Johnsson R, Stromqvist B, Aspenberg P. 2002 Volvo Award in Clinical Studies. Randomized radiostereometric study comparing osteogenic protein-1 (BMP-7) and autograft bone in human noninstrumented posterolateral lumbar fusion. *Spine* 2002;27:2654.
18. Lieberman JR, Daluiski A, Stevenson S, et al. The effect of regional gene therapy with bone morphogenetic protein-2–producing bone marrow cells on the repair of segmental femoral defects in rats. *J Bone Joint Surg Am* 1999;81:905.
19. Lieberman JR, Le LQ, Wu L, et al. Regional gene therapy with a BMP-2–producing murine stromal cell line induces heterotopic and orthotopic bone formation in rodents. *J Orthop Res* 1998;16:330.
20. Lou J, Xu F, Merkel K, et al. Gene therapy: adenovirus-mediated human bone morphogenetic protein-2 gene transfer induces mesenchymal progenitor cell proliferation and differentiation in vitro and bone formation in vivo. *J Orthop Res* 1999;17:43.
21. Martin GJ Jr, Boden SD, Titus L. Recombinant human bone morphogenetic protein-2 overcomes the inhibitory effect of ketorolac, a nonsteroidal anti-inflammatory drug (NSAID), on posterolateral lumbar intertransverse process spine fusion. *Spine* 1999;24:2188.
22. Martin GJ Jr, Boden SD, Titus L, et al. New formulations of demineralized bone matrix as a more effective graft alternative in experimental posterolateral lumbar spine arthrodesis. *Spine* 1999;24:637.
23. Mayer H, Scutt AM, Ankenbauer T. Subtle differences in the mitogenic effects of recombinant human bone morphogenetic proteins-2 to -7 on DNA synthesis in primary bone-forming cells and identification of BMP-2/4 receptor. *Calcif Tissue Int* 1996;58:249.
24. McKay B, Sandhu HS. Use of recombinant human bone morphogenetic protein-2 in spinal fusion applications. *Spine* 2002;27:S66.
25. Morone MA, Boden SD. Experimental posterolateral lumbar spinal fusion with a demineralized bone matrix gel. *Spine* 1998;23:159.
26. Patel TC, Erulkar JS, Grauer JN, et al. Osteogenic protein-1 overcomes the inhibitory effect of nicotine on posterolateral lumbar fusion. *Spine* 2001;26:1656.
27. Riley EH, Lane JM, Urist MR, et al. Bone morphogenetic protein-2: biology and applications. *Clin Orthop* 1996; 324:39.
28. Sandhu HS, Kanim LE, Kabo JM, et al. Evaluation of rhBMP-2 with an OPLA carrier in a canine posterolateral (transverse process) spinal fusion model. *Spine* 1995;20:2669.
29. Schimandle JH, Boden SD, Hutton WC. Experimental spinal fusion with recombinant human bone morphogenetic protein-2. *Spine* 1995;20:1326.
30. Silcox DH III, Boden SD, Schimandle JH, et al. Reversing the inhibitory effect of nicotine on spinal fusion using an osteoinductive protein extract. *Spine* 1998;23:291.
31. Urist MR. Bone formation by autoinduction. *Science* 1965;150:893.
32. Vaccaro AR, Anderson DG, Toth CA. Recombinant human osteogenic protein-1 (bone morphogenetic protein-7) as an osteoinductive agent in spinal fusion. *Spine* 2002;27:S59.
33. Viggeswarapu M, Boden SD, Liu Y, et al. Adenoviral delivery of LIM mineralization protein-1 (LMP-1) induces de novo bone formation in vitro and in vivo. *J Bone Joint Surg Am* 2001; 83:364.
34. Zdeblick TA, Ghanayem AJ, Rapoff AJ, et al. Cervical interbody tension cages. An animal model with and without bone morphogenetic protein. *Spine* 1998;23:758–765.

16
Intradiscal Electrothermal Therapy

Gunnar B. J. Andersson

Department of Orthopedic Surgery, Rush Medical College; Department of Orthopedic Surgery, Rush–Presbyterian–St. Luke's Medical Center, Chicago, Illinois

Several chapters in this book attest to the difficulty of diagnosing and treating patients with degenerative disc problems. One reason is that disc degeneration is a normal part of the aging process and occurs with and without symptoms. Another is the general difficulty in diagnosing the pathoanatomic basis for back pain. A third is the complexity of the motion segment itself. Although many of the joints in the body have sliding surfaces that can be replaced, this is not the case with the intervertebral disc. Also, the motion segment is a three-joint complex in which replacement of one joint may not resolve pathology occurring in the other two.

The complexity and magnitude of the problem have led to a search for a less invasive treatment alternative than the fusion procedure, which is the most commonly used surgical procedure for degenerative disc changes, or the more recently introduced nucleoplasty and disc replacement. Intradiscal electrothermal therapy (IDET) is one such method, in which a catheter is inserted percutaneously into a intervertebral disc. The catheter is a thermal resistive coil attached to a heat generator.

The purpose of this chapter is to describe the procedure, present the mechanisms by which it may work, and review the published results.

INTRADISCAL ELECTROTHERMAL THERAPY PROCEDURE

The procedure is performed under sterile conditions, ideally in an operating room. An image intensifier (C-arm) and a radiolucent table are required. It is important to perform the procedure with the patient under conscious sedation. My personal preference is to place the patient prone on the operating table; however, others perform the procedure with the patient lying on the side or in a slightly oblique prone posture. After the level or levels to be treated have been confirmed, adequate anteroposterior fluoroscopic visualization is obtained. To simplify subsequent needle insertion, it is important that both endplates of the involved disc be visualized, which typically requires angulation of the image intensifier. Once the disc is clearly visualized, the image intensifier is rotated such that the superior articular process is seen in the midpoint of the disc. The direction of the insertion needle is then indicated by the direction of the x-ray beam, and the image intensifier can be used as an external directional guide. After the skin and muscles in the direction of the needle insertion have been anesthetized, a 17-gauge needle is introduced into the disc under fluoroscopic control. The insertion is just anterior to the superior articular

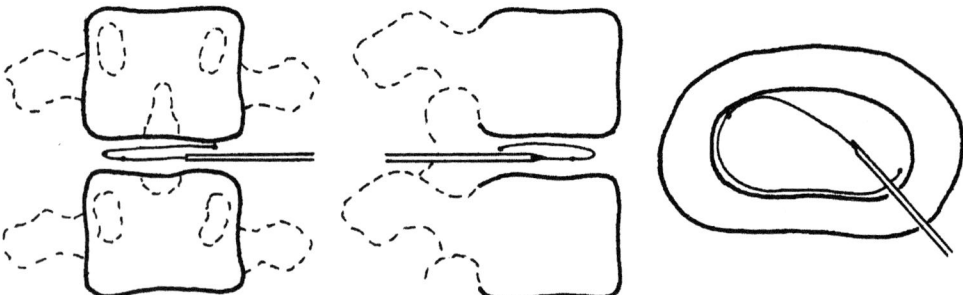

FIG. 16.1. The heating element of the catheter, which is made visible on the radiographic images by markers, should cover both posterolateral corners and the posterior area of the annulus.

process. It is important that the patient be conscious, so that any needle contact with a nerve root is immediately appreciated and the direction of the needle insertion direction can be corrected. Once the annulus has been penetrated, the needle position is verified in the anteroposterior and lateral directions. If necessary, the needle is advanced until it begins to enter the nucleus. The stylet of the introducer needle is removed, and the flexible catheter with a temperature-controlled thermal resistive coil is passed through the needle. Once the catheter is inside the disc, the image intensifier can be used to visualize its position. When the catheter is advanced, the external layers of the annulus deflect the electrode, which typically finds a circumferential course inside the disc. The ideal position is where the heating element of the catheter, which is made visible on the radiographic images by markers, covers both posterolateral corners and the posterior area of the annulus (Fig. 16.1). Care must be taken to ensure that the entire heating portion of the catheter, which is marked, is inside the disc because the introducer needle is itself heat-conductive.

The catheter is now attached to the heat generator, which automatically raises the temperature in 1° increments every 30 seconds from an initial temperature of 65°C to a final temperature of 90°C. Once the 90° temperature has been reached, it is maintained for 5 minutes. The equipment then automatically shuts down. A typical therapeutic session lasts 15 to 17 minutes. It is recommended that 1 g of cefazolin (Ancef) or similar antibiotic be injected into the disc at the end of the procedure for infection prophylaxis.

After completion of the procedure, patients are observed for an hour or as necessary to ensure that they are fully awake and that any procedure-related pain is under control. They are then discharged, typically with oral pain medication.

MECHANISMS OF ACTION

The idea underlying the IDET procedure is that heat will coagulate nociceptors and modulate collagen. The degree to which this happens has not been fully evaluated. Heat can be generated by many methods. Before a thermal resistive coil was applied in IDET, laser and radiofrequency techniques were most often used. Temperature control and precision were the reasons for the new development. Ashley et al. (1) measured the temperature distribution and found that within 10 mm or so of the probe, the temperatures exceeded the 42° to 45° considered necessary to destroy nociceptors (11,12). The maximum disc temperature was 68°C, and the average outer annular temperature was 41.9°C

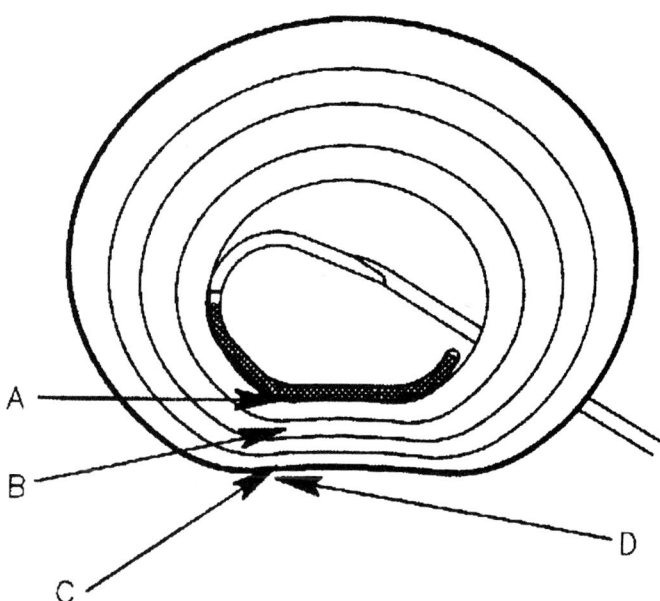

FIG. 16.2. Typical distribution profile: Spine CATH Intradiscal Catheter (Oratec Interventions, Menlo Park, CA, U.S.A.) when catheter temperature = 90°C. *A:* Tissue adjacent to catheter = 68.5°C; *B:* center of annulus wall = 60°C; *C:* outer annulus wall = 42°C; *D:* epidural space = 38°C.

(Fig. 16.2). Houpt et al. (4) studied temperatures generated by way of radiofrequency heating at various distances from a probe placed in the middle of the disc. This method, which is different from the thermal resistive coil used in the IDET procedure, did not result in sufficiently high temperatures in the annulus, but temperatures exceeding 40° were found within 11 mm of the probe. Kleinstueck et al. (5), using a thermal resistive coil, found that the temperature decreased very rapidly with distance from the probe.

Collagen is also affected by heat. Collagen cross-links are broken, and collagen denaturation and shrinkage result from heating (3,13). The effect depends on the temperature and the duration of heating. Shah et al. (10) used histology to evaluate the response to the heat of the IDET catheter in a cadaver model. They observed collagen fiber denaturation in the posterior annulus fibrosus. Kleinstueck et al. (5), on the other hand, did not find significant effects on collagen. These should not be expected in tests performed immediately after the procedure. Unfortunately, long-term effects are yet to be determined. Other studies have identified total reductions in disc volume of between 10% and 16%.

To date, the evidence does not allow a complete understanding of the mechanisms of action. Future studies aimed at clarifying these would be helpful.

SELECTION OF PATIENTS

In contrast to most other intradiscal therapies, the IDET procedure is not intended to treat patients with disc herniation, but rather those with discogenic back pain. Patients with frank disc herniation are not appropriate candidates for this procedure, and the procedure is not competitive with microdiscectomy or arthroscopic discectomy.

The ideal patient is one in whom the disc is considered to be the source of pain and who has failed extensive nonoperative attempts at treatment. Such patients, who otherwise would be offered a fusion or a disc replacement, can be offered the IDET procedure as an alternative. The best results appear to be in patients who have a reasonably well-preserved disc space (collapse of less than 50%) and one or two painful levels on discography. The diagnostic workup typically shows degenerative disc changes on magnetic resonance imaging (MRI) with one or more annular tears. Small contained herniations are acceptable if they do not significantly impinge on the nerve roots and result in radicular pain. Discography should show concordant pain at low-pressure or low-volume injection of the affected level(s). A negative control disc should be included in discography. To avoid obstruction of catheter positioning by contrast, discography should be performed at least 2 days before the IDET procedure.

Patients with stenosis are not candidates for IDET. A severely collapsed disc is technically difficult with respect to needle insertion and catheter advancement in the presence of fissures and cracks. This may be one reason why results are not as good in this group of patients.

RESULTS

Most clinical studies of the IDET procedure are prospective but not randomized (14). Saal and Saal (8,9), who were involved in the development of the IDET procedure, reported results after 1 and 2 years. The 2-year study included 55 patients who had all failed a 6-month course of comprehensive nonoperative care consisting of education, physical therapy, activity modification, antiinflammatory medications, and steroid injections. All patients had normal neurologic examination findings and no evidence of a compressive lesion on MRI. All had positive results on discography. Outcomes were determined with a visual analog scale (VAS) and the Short Form 36 (SF-36). With both, statistically significant improvement was noted. For the entire group, the VAS score changed on average by 3.2 points (of 10), the SF-36 physical function score on average by 20 points (of 100), and the SF-36 bodily pain score on average by 17.8 points (of 100). When a seven-point change between the pretreatment and posttreatment SF-36 scores was used as a measure of success, the procedure was considered successful in 71% of the patients. No complications were reported. The results improved slightly between 1 and 2 years.

Derby et al. (2) reported a 62% success rate overall. Outcomes were successful in 76% of the patients with preserved disc height and no prior surgery. Wetzel et al. (14) performed a multicenter prospective controlled cohort study of 75 patients. All had failed nonoperative treatment and had positive results on discography. All were considered candidates for fusion and were offered the IDET procedure as an alternative. During a 1-year period, the mean change in the VAS score was from 6 to 3.6. About 15% of the patients were considered treatment failures and typically ended up undergoing a fusion procedure.

Karasek and Bogduk (6) enrolled 35 patients in a study; 17 of them had no insurance coverage and therefore were considered a "convenience control group." Although this is not a randomization, it allowed the investigators to follow both groups and determine differences. A VAS score, return to work, use of opiates, and the Oswestry Disability Questionnaire were used to measure outcome. The VAS score in the IDET group had improved at 12 months from 8 to 3, with minor improvement seen in the group without treatment.

A randomized prospective double-blinded study was performed in 55 patients (7). To date, only the 6-month results have been reported. Significant improvement was noted in the IDET group in comparison with the placebo group on both the VAS and the SF-36.

POSTOPERATIVE CARE

Postoperative care is an integral part of the treatment. It is important to recognize that patients rarely respond instantaneously to the procedure. On the contrary, it is not uncommon that the typical back pain increases slightly following the procedure; it then subsides gradually during the first few days. During this period, patients are advised to walk as tolerated but to avoid lifting and stressful activities such as frequent bending or twisting. Many practitioners of the IDET procedure recommend that a corset be worn at this time. Because heating initially weakens the collagen, activities such as lifting, loaded flexion–extension movements, and twisting should be limited for 2 months or so. Although walking can be unlimited, jogging and other sports activities are discouraged during this period. After 8 to 12 weeks, the patients must undergo physical therapy. Initially, this should focus at first on conditioning and stabilization exercises, then strengthening and coordination exercises can be added gradually. Most patients experience a gradual improvement during several months.

CONCLUSIONS

The IDET procedure is an intermediate treatment for patients with degenerative painful discs, falling between nonoperative treatment and fusion or disc replacement surgery. It is sufficiently complex and involved that it should never be undertaken without previous attempts at nonoperative treatment for an extended period of time. When a patient comes to consider surgery as inevitable to relieve pain and improve quality of life, the IDET procedure can be offered as an alternative. If IDET is successful, as it appears to be in about 70% of patients, a fusion or disc replacement may not be necessary. This is an outpatient procedure causing minimal pain and discomfort to the patient and with few reported complications. If, as is inevitable in some patients, the procedure fails to resolve the problem, a fusion or replacement operation can be performed with no added difficulty. The difficult question in these cases is whether or not the disc is in fact the source of the patient's pain. As discussed elsewhere in this book, no perfect diagnostic methods are available to answer this question. The exclusion of other sources, the presence of degenerative changes on MRI, and the confirmation of concordant pain on discography appear to be our best diagnostic combination currently. Because we still obtain false-negative and false-positive results, future research should focus on improving our diagnostic methods. In the meantime, the IDET procedure is a viable alternative in selected cases.

REFERENCES

1. Ashley JE, Gharpuray VM, Saal JS, et al. Temperature distribution in the intervertebral disc: a comparison of intranuclear radiofrequency needle to a novel heating catheter. In: *Proceedings of the 1999 Bioengineering Conference*. BED, 1999:42:77.
2. Derby R, Eck B, Chen Y, et al. Intradiscal electrothermal annuloplasty (IDET): a novel approach for treating chronic discogenic back pain. *Neuromodulation* 2000;3:69–75.
3. Hecht P, Hayashi K, Cooley AJ, et al. The thermal effect of monopolar radiofrequency energy on the properties of joint capsule. An in vivo histologic study using a sheep model. *Am J Sports Med* 1998;26:808–814.
4. Houpt JC, Conner ES, McFarland EW. Experimental study of temperature distributions and thermal transport during radiofrequency current therapy of the intervertebral disc. *Spine* 1996;21:1808–1812; discussion 1812–1813.
5. Karasek M, Bogduk N. Twelve-month follow-up of a controlled trial of intradiscal thermal annuloplasty for back pain due to internal disc disruption. *Spine* 2000;25:2601–2607.
6. Kleinstueck FS, Diederich CJ, Nau WH, et al. Acute biomechanical and histological effects of intradiscal electrothermal therapy on human lumbar discs. *Spine* 2001;26:2198–2207.

7. Pauza K, Howell S, Dreyfuss P, et al. *A randomized double-blind placebo controlled trial evaluating the efficacy of intradiscal electrotherm anuloplasty (IDET) for the treatment of chronic discogenic low back pain: 6-month outcomes.* Presented at the 10th annual meeting of the International Spinal Injection Society, Austin, TX, 2002.
8. Saal JA, Saal J S. Management of chronic discogenic low back pain with a thermal intradiscal catheter. *Spine* 2000;25:382–388.
9. Saal JA, Saal JS. Intradiscal electrothermal treatment for chronic low back pain: prospective outcome study with a minimum 2-year follow-up. *Spine* 2002;9:966–974.
10. Shah RV, Lutz GE, Lee J, et al. Intradiscal electrothermal therapy: a preliminary histologic study. *Arch Phys Med Rehabil* 2001;82:1230–1237.
11. Stronbehn JW. Temperature distributions from interstitial radiofrequency hyperthermia systems: theoretical predictions. *Int J Radiat Oncol Biol Phys* 1983;9:1655–1667.
12. Troussier B, Lebas JF, Chirossel JP, et al. Percutaneous intradiscal radio-frequency thermocoagulation: a cadaveric study. *Spine* 1995;20:1713–1718.
13. Wall MS, Deng XH, Torzilli P, et al. Thermal modulation of collagen. *J Shoulder Elbow Surg* 1999;8:339–344.
14. Wetzel FT, Anderson GBJ, Peloza J, et al. *Intradiscal electrothermal therapy (IDET) to treat discogenic low back pain: preliminary results of a multicenter prospective cohort study.* Presented at the 15th annual meeting of the North American Spine Society, New Orleans, October 25–28, 2000.

17

Anterior Lumbar Interbody Fusion Versus Posterior Lumbar Interbody Fusion for Degenerative Disc Disease

*†Jean-Charles Le Huec, *†Stéphane Aunoble, and ‡Thomas A. Zdeblick

*Department of Orthopedic Surgery, Centre Hospitalier Universitaire Pellegrin Bordeaux;
†Spine Unit, Centre Hospitalier Universitaire Pellegrin, Bordeaux, France; and
‡Department of Orthopedics and Rehabilitation, University of Wisconsin,
Madison, Wisconsin

Treating patients with low back pain (LBP) poses many challenges to the physician. One of the greatest difficulties is to make an accurate diagnosis that can effectively dictate treatment. Inherent to the process of making an accurate diagnosis is an accepted set of diagnostic categories, criteria, and characterizations. Unfortunately, for disorders of the lumbar spine, these are not always available.

Certainly, some diagnostic entities related to degenerative lumbar conditions are well accepted, including disc herniation or protrusion, spondylolysis, spondylolisthesis, and scoliosis. These conditions have alternately been called *spondylosis*, *degenerative disc disease (DDD)*, *segmental instability*, *internal disc disruption*, *isolated disc resorption*, *dark disc disease*, and *discogenic pain syndrome*. However, a continuum of degenerative conditions of the lumbar spine encompasses all these various terms at various stages.

A basic tenet of the successful treatment of low back disorders is to prescribe treatment only after a diagnosis has been made. Diagnostic methods used include history and physical examination, plain radiography, flexion–extension radiography, magnetic resonance imaging (MRI), computed tomography (CT)/myelography, provocative discography, CT discography, facet injections, and selective nerve root blocks. Certainly, not all of these are required in each patient to make a diagnosis. In many cases, a diagnosis can be made based on the history and the examination and plain radiographic findings alone.

Discogenic pain syndrome can be seen as a continuum of diagnostic categories, all related to various entities involving the intervertebral disc. In general, diagnostic conditions such as annular tear, internal disc derangement, and dark disc disease imply normal findings on the plain radiograph but persistent pain that can be provoked with discography or changes seen on MRI. In DDD, isolated disc resorption, and lumbar spondylosis, changes can be seen on plain radiographs, consisting of disc narrowing and collapse, endplate sclerosis, osteophyte formation, facet degeneration, and intervertebral gas. Segmental instability should refer to translational or rotational instability seen at the intervertebral level. This includes spondylolisthesis, lateral listhesis, rotatory subluxation, and scoliosis. Often, these changes are seen on static radiographs but, occasionally, flexion–extension radiographs may be required to detect them. No good valid criteria exist for sagittal, rotational instability (i.e., angular displacement on a flexion–extension lateral radiograph). In most cases, some type of translational shift is required if a condition is to be considered truly unstable.

It must be kept in mind that all the aforementioned diagnoses can be considered a normal part of the aging process. It has been estimated that by the age of 50 years, 85% of adults show evidence of disc degeneration at autopsy (46,52). Thus, in most cases, these conditions can be considered abnormal only in younger patients.

DEGENERATIVE DISC DISEASE

The changes of DDD begin with early disc desiccation, caused by a decrease in proteoglycan water binding (27). This leads to water loss within the nucleus pulposus. In addition, circumferential tears in the inner and outer annulus appear. With time, the distribution of type I and type II collagen in the annulus is altered, and this change is enhanced by altered mechanical loading (7). Radial annular tears may accelerate the degenerative process. Fissuring within the annulus may occur, with subsequent ingrowth of granulation tissue. With time, narrowing of the disc continues, and osteophytes form at the endplate–annular junction. With increased axial loading, marrow changes occur in the trabecular bone of the vertebral body adjacent to the endplate (36). Eventually, endplate sclerosis results (20). As desiccation and cleft formation continue within the disc, empty spaces or vacuum phenomenon may occur, and radiographic air spaces are seen within the disc. End-stage disc degeneration rarely goes on to autofusion but instead may reach a steady state of bone-on-bone contact at the disc space.

Midline back pain with referred pain over the sacroiliac joints and iliac crest is the most typical pattern of symptoms. Aching of the buttock and posterior thigh during ambulation is common. With continued disc space collapse, neural foraminal narrowing may occur, resulting in root stenosis. This leads at L5–S1 to buttock pain with mild L5 radiculopathy or at L4–5 to lateral and anterior thigh pain with L4 radiculopathy.

All these changes are a normal part of disc maturation during aging (47). However, they are unusual in patients younger than 40 years of age. Crock (11) and Jaffray and O'Brien (19) coined the term *isolated disc resorption* to describe single-level loss of disc height, vertebral sclerosis, osteophyte formation, and vacuum disc space in young patients. In reality, this appears to be a syndrome of precocious disc degeneration. Occasionally, isolated disc resorption may occur at two adjacent disc levels.

DIAGNOSIS

Physical Examination

The physical examination findings in patients with DDD are often nonspecific. Point tenderness of the lumbar spinous processes is unusual. An aching sensation during palpation over the sacral iliac joints is common. Sciatic notch tenderness or a positive straight leg raising test result is not present. The range of motion of the lumbar spine is often restricted secondary to pain. Extension often brings out patient's symptoms and is usually limited to less than 30 degrees. Extension may precipitate buttock pain or leg heaviness.

A careful examination for Waddell signs should be performed (48). An exaggerated response to light touch of the skin, increased pain with axial compression of the head or shoulders, increased pain with unrestricted axial rotation of the body, or LBP with downward distraction on the arms all indicate psychologic overlay and symptom magnification.

The neurologic examination is very important in patients with DDD. An examination of motor strength, sensation, and reflexes reveals no abnormalities in DDD, but abnormalities are found if a canal stenosis is also present. This is the main point to assess, so that patients requiring decompression can be identified. Neurologic signs can be permanent or transient, depending on whether the stenosis is dynamic or permanent.

Radiographic Changes

The plain radiograph is the initial diagnostic test of choice. As mentioned, this usually shows disc narrowing at a single level (most commonly L5–S1), endplate osteophyte formation, endplate sclerosis, and possibly gas formation within the disc space (17,19) (Fig. 17.1). In general, the normal architecture of the surrounding discs is maintained. Flexion–extension radiographs occasionally show increased translation or angulation, or retrolisthesis (20,45). Often, however, segmental motion may be diminished on dynamic radiographs (13).

Radiographic Testing

Computed Tomography/Myelography

CT/myelography will only occasionally confirm the diagnosis of DDD. Myelography may show root sleeve blunting in the foramen secondary to foraminal stenosis. CT may show marginal osteophytes causing mild to moderate lateral recess and foraminal stenosis. CT may also demonstrate endplate sclerosis and disc space vacuum signs.

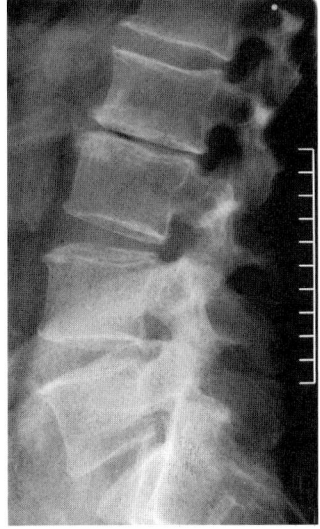
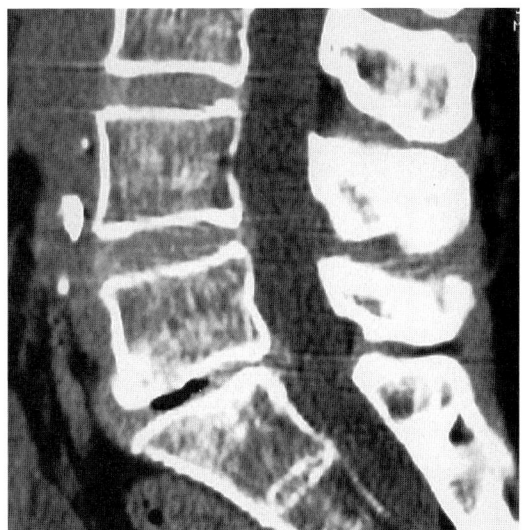

FIG. 17.1. Degenerative disc disease. **A:** Foraminal stenosis and canal stenosis. **B:** Sclerotic endplate with gas formation within the disc.

Magnetic Resonance Imaging

MRI is capable of detecting changes within the nucleus pulposus relative to the nuclear dehydration that occurs with degeneration. This leads to a loss of signal intensity on T2-weighted images. Within a severely degenerate disc in which overall signal intensity is lost, linear areas of high signal intensity on T2-weighted spin echo images may be noted, thought to represent free fluid within cracks or fissures of the degenerate complex (42,46).

Modic et al. (34) described signal intensity changes in the vertebral body marrow adjacent to the endplates of degenerate discs (Fig. 17.2). They described three main forms. Type I changes demonstrate a decreased signal intensity on T1 images and an increased signal intensity on T2 images. These have been identified in approximately 4% of patients with LBP. However, 30% of patients who have previously been treated with chymopapain have type I marrow space changes (32). Modic et al. (31,33) consider chymopapain-treated discs to be a model of acute disc degeneration. Histopathologic sections of discs with type I changes demonstrate disruption and fissuring of the endplate and vascularized fibrous tissue within the adjacent marrow. Thickened bony trabeculae are also seen.

Type II changes appear as increased signal intensity on T1 images and an isointense signal on T2 images. These are seen in approximately 16% of cases. They are always associated with degenerative disc changes on plain radiographs. Discs with type II

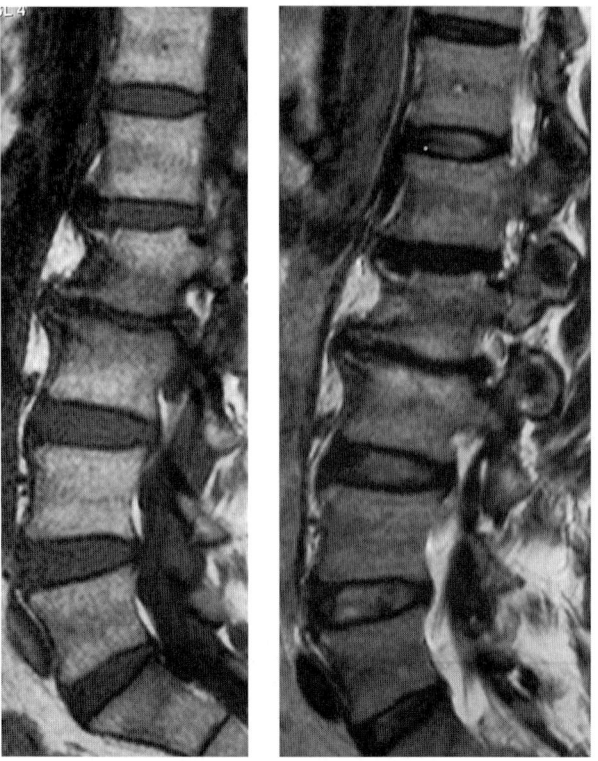

FIG. 17.2. Degenerative disc disease with magnetic resonance imaging changes. Modic type I: hyposignal in T1 **(A)** and hypersignal in T2 **(B)**.

changes show evidence of endplate disruption, with yellow marrow replacement in the adjacent vertebral body. It has been suggested that the increase in lipid content within the marrow spaces is an inflammatory response, indicating a painful disc.

A Modic type III change appears as decreased signal intensity on both T1 and T2 images. This correlates with extensive bony sclerosis on plain radiographs, reflecting the relative absence of marrow elements within the endplate as bony sclerosis advances. Occasionally, Modic type I and type II changes may be confused with discitis. Gadolinium enhancement of discitis should differentiate these conditions (35).

Discography

Appropriately performed provocative discography plays a role in the diagnosis and treatment of patients with DDD, although not as significant a role as in patients with internal disc disruption. DDD can be diagnosed on the basis of plain x-rays films and MR images alone. Discography is used rather to confirm the diagnosis or, more frequently, to rule out degeneration at adjacent disc levels. In a young patient with an isolated degenerate disc at a single level, with appropriate MRI and radiographic changes at that disc and completely normal MRI findings at the adjacent disc, discography is not absolutely indicated. Many of these patients can be treated based on the radiographic and MRI findings alone.

Discography is most useful in two situations involving DDD. In the first, a patient has degenerative disc changes at multiple levels. Often, much more severe disc resorption with endplate sclerosis and bone-on-bone contact is seen at one level, and mild to moderate changes at the adjacent level. Because surgical results are better with single-level fusion than with two- or three-level fusions, the physician should attempt to prove that the more severely involved disc is the symptomatic disc. In such cases, discography of the lower three disc levels is indicated. Surgery may then be based on the results of provocative discography (42,43).

In the second situation, clear-cut radiographic changes of DDD are seen, but equivocal MRI changes are noted at the adjacent disc. In this instance, in which the adjacent disc may show a loss of signal intensity but otherwise normal radiographic findings, provocative discography is indicated to determine whether this disc should be included in a planned fusion.

SURGICAL TREATMENT

In general, in a discussion of the surgical treatment of discogenic pain syndromes, fusion has been the procedure of choice. Although sporadic reports have appeared in the literature of the use of discectomy, percutaneous discectomy, or chymopapain chemonucleolysis to treat discogenic pain syndromes, their efficacy has not been proven. Artificial disc replacement is in its infancy and just beginning to find a proven place in the treatment of disc degeneration. "Restabilization" procedures in which artificial posterior ligaments are used are also new and as yet unproven. At the present time, surgical treatment for axial pain resulting from either a disrupted or degenerate disc should include spinal fusion. Choices at this time include posterolateral fusion with or without instrumentation; posterior lumbar interbody fusion (PLIF) (Fig. 17.3); anterior lumbar interbody fusion (ALIF) (Fig.17.4), combined anterior and posterior fusion (360-degree fusion); and fusion performed by placing interbody cages either anteriorly open, posteriorly, or laparoscopically.

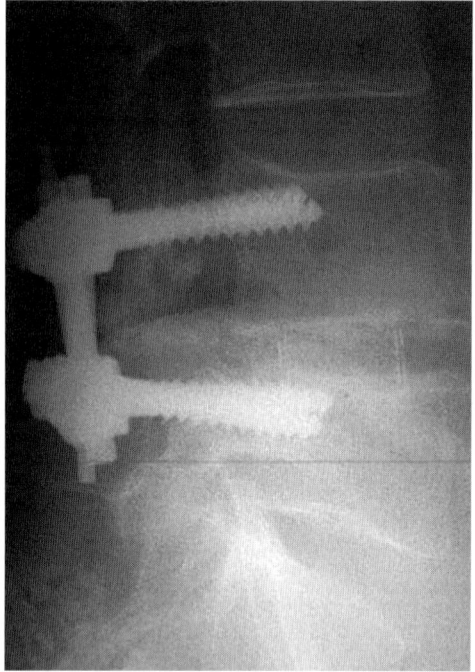
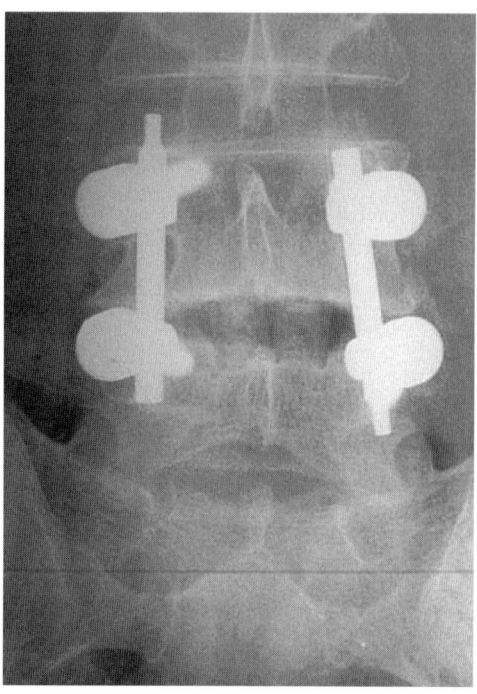

FIG. 17.3. Degenerative disc disease implies disc space narrowing, endplate sclerosis, and osteophyte formation. The posterior lumbar interbody fusion (PLIF) procedure restores disc height, opens the foramen, and allows interbody fusion with posterior stabilization. **A:** Lateral view of PLIF. **B:** Anteroposterior view of PLIF.

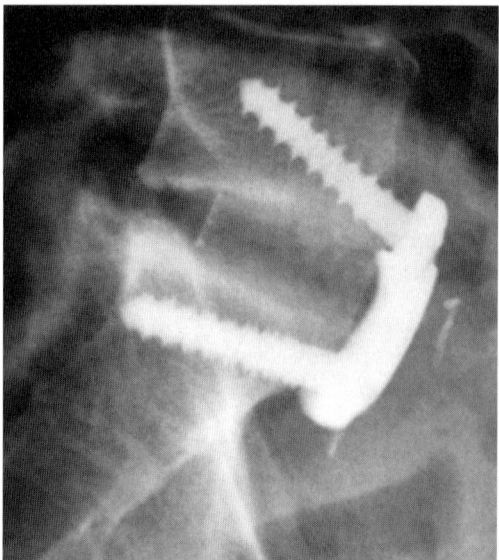
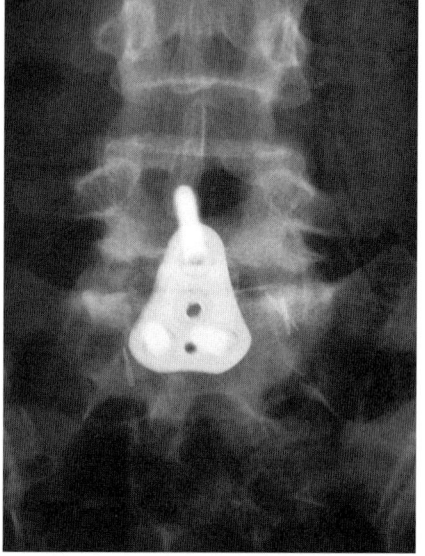

FIG. 17.4. Surgical treatment options for internal disc disruption include anterior lumbar interbody fusion alone. This lateral radiograph **(A)** demonstrates a carbon cage packed with autogenous cancellous bone secured in place with an anterior pyramidal plate **(B)** (Pyramid; Medtronic, Memphis, TN, U.S.A.), which avoids a second posterior approach for stabilization.

In general, the type of fusion that a surgeon chooses to perform should be based on the diagnosis. For instance, in patients with degenerative spondylolisthesis and stenosis, the fusion is preventative—that is, further instability and subluxation are prevented following the decompressive surgical procedure (30,49). Similarly, in degenerative scoliosis, the fusion procedure is usually performed following lumbar decompression for stenosis. In both of these cases, because posterior decompression is indicated, posterolateral fusion with instrumentation becomes the procedure of choice.

However, in the discogenic pain syndromes (internal disc disruption and DDD), the success of the fusion procedure depends on its ability to eliminate the focus of pain within the disc. This is accomplished through either of two mechanisms: complete ablation of the disc or elimination of motion though the disc. Certainly, the most time-honored method of fusion is posterolateral fusion, which is postulated to relieve discogenic pain by eliminating motion through the disc. Posterolateral fusions have been very successful in patients with spinal stenosis. Warner and Simmons (49) presented their results of instrumented posterolateral fusion in nonsmoking patients with degenerative spondylolisthesis. Their fusion rate (90%) and clinical success rate (90%) were similar.

In discogenic pain syndromes, however, this same correlation has not been found. Zucherman et al. (56) examined a series of patients in whom posterolateral pedicle screw fusions were performed for DDD. Although their successful fusion rate was 89%, they achieved clinical success in only 60% of their patients. Similarly, Cowan et al. (9) presented a series of patients undergoing posterolateral fusion augmented with pedicle screws. Fusion was successful in 85%, but clinical success with reduction of back pain was achieved in only 67%. The results of Jackson et al. (18) were less encouraging. Again, although the fusion rate was 87%, only 58% of their patients with DDD experienced pain relief following posterolateral fusion with pedicle screws. Wetzel et al. (51) examined 48 patients with positive discography results and posterolateral lumbar arthrodesis. Only 46% of these patients had a satisfactory clinical result at final follow-up. Zdeblick (53) performed a prospective randomized study of patients undergoing fusions with and without pedicle screw instrumentation. Within this group of patients, a subset had DDD. Successful radiographic fusion was achieved in 93% of this group. However, good or excellent results were achieved clinically in only 64%.

Why should this discrepancy exist? In general, the successful treatment of DDD requires complete immobility of the disc. This is not always possible with a posterolateral fusion, even if rigid pedicle screw instrumentation is used to augment the fusion (40). Weatherley et al. (50) reported five patients with "solid" posterolateral fusions who continued to experience LBP and had positive discography results under the fusion; their pain was relieved by anterior interbody fusion. Lee et al. (24), in an *in vitro* experiment with simulated fusion, have shown that a posterolateral fusion increases the stiffness of the spine 40%. An anterior interbody fusion, however, increases the stiffness 80% and eliminates virtually all motion through the disc space. Zdeblick et al. (55), in a biomechanical study, showed that the most effective means of eliminating motion between two vertebrae is through the disc space rather than through the facets, transverse processes, or spinous processes.

The addition of interbody fusion should increase the clinical success rate (25,29). Lee et al. (24) performed PLIF for internal disc disruption in 62 patients, and with a 94% successful fusion rate (Fig. 17.3), the clinical success rate at relieving back pain was 96%. Other surgeons, however, have not been as successful with the PLIF procedure (5). Brantigan et al. (3,5), using their PLIF and plate operation, achieved only a 56% fusion success rate with freeze-dried bone, which translated into a 60% clinical success rate.

One of the biggest problems associated with posterior approach fusion surgery for discogenic pain syndromes is disruption of the posterior musculature. To perform a posterolateral fusion with or without instrumentation, or indeed to perform a PLIF, one must of necessity strip the musculature of the posterior paraspinals. Muscle stripping and retraction during surgery may lead to ischemia and postoperative fibrosis of the muscles (15). Many of these patients have difficulty becoming fully rehabilitated after fusion surgery. Although their symptoms are relieved and the cases are considered a clinical success, many do not return to full activity or are unable to carry out a full day's work. Often, paraspinal fatigue sets in with either 8-hour work days or heavy lifting. This has been described as "fusion disease." The incidence of fusion disease and its severity are currently unknown.

ALIF was recommended by Crock (10) in his original description of internal disc disruption. An anterior interbody fusion would serve both to ablate the source of pain by complete discectomy and to eliminate motion between the adjacent vertebrae. Crock (11), Goldner et al. (16), and Kozak et al. (21) all reported a high rate of success for anterior interbody fusion with bone grafting alone. Loguidice et al. (28), using ALIF with autogenous bone graft alone, achieved an 80% rate of successful fusion and an 80% clinical success rate. Blumenthal et al. (2), in a similar study, achieved a 73% successful fusion rate and a 74% clinical success rate. Colhoun et al. (8) reported satisfactory clinical results in 88% of a group of nonconsecutive patients undergoing fusion for positive discography results. Newman and Grinstead (37) examined 36 patients with internal disc derangement who were all treated with ALIF. They noted successful clinical results in 86% of their patients and solid fusion in 89%. Gill and Blumenthal (14) found that ALIF alone achieved an 80% fusion rate and a 75% clinical success rate if discography and abnormal MRI findings were correlated. However, when ALIF was used to treat patients with a positive discography result but normal MRI findings, the clinical success rate was only 50%.

Dennis et al. (12) examined a series of patients undergoing ALIF with autogenous iliac crest bone alone. All their patients lost disc height during the healing process, and 30% went on to nonunion. Loguidice (28) similarly found a 34% rate of bone graft collapse, resorption, or both. In general, if ALIF is performed with bone graft alone, a success rate of approximately 70% to 80% can be expected. In 20% to 30% of patients, either pseudarthrosis or significant graft collapse develops and is associated with a poor clinical result.

In an attempt to prevent graft resorption, collapse, and pseudarthrosis, surgeons have combined anterior and posterior surgery. Using pedicle screw instrumentation to prevent graft collapse, surgeons have achieved a high degree of success. Kozak and O'Brien (22) examined 69 patients treated with concomitant anterior and posterior fusion for discographic pain. After an average 2.5-year follow-up, they noted fusion rates of 91% in one- or two-level fusions. They found acceptable clinical results in 80% of their patients. Their success rate dropped, however, when three-level fusions were examined. Linson and Williams (26) described 51 patients treated similarly with combined anterior and posterior fusion. They noted an overall success rate of 80%. O'Brien et al. (39) examined the results of 360-degree combined fusion in 150 patients with 5 years of follow-up. They noted that 86% of their patients were improved and that 60% were "substantially improved" after relief from disabling LBP. Slosar et al. (44) noted a 99% fusion rate after combined instrumented 360-degree fusion. However, an 18% complication rate was related mostly to the anterior approach, spinal hardware, or both. Clinical improvement was observed in 81% of the patients, but only 38% returned to work. Similarly, Albert et al. (1) presented the results of instrumented 360-degree fusion performed for pseudarthrosis. Although the fusion rate was 90%, the clinical success rate was only 69%. Thus, it appears that the use of combined 360-degree fusion increases the fusion rate. However, the same disabilities related to posterior exposure remain, and clinical success rates remain less than ideal.

Overall, when isolated disc disruption or DDD is treated with ALIF alone, a fusion rate of 70% to 80% and a success rate of 70% to 80% can be expected. If ALIF is combined with instrumented 360-degree fusion, the clinical success rate should increase to 80% to 90%, with a 90% to 100% successful fusion rate. These numbers can be compared with those for patients treated with posterolateral instrumented fusion. In these cases, one can expect a fusion rate of 85% to 90%, but a clinical success rate for relief of LBP of only 55% to 60%.

Interbody fusion cages offer the surgeon an alternative approach to fusion for discogenic pain syndromes. Combining the attributes of the anterior approach and complete disc ablation with those of instrumentation should theoretically increase clinical success rates. Brantigan and Steffee (4) developed a carbon fiber cage used with autogenous grafting. Bagby (1a) used an interbody fusion cage to distract, stabilize, and eventually induce arthrodesis in a cervical interbody segment. Kuslich developed a threaded interbody cage. Using open implantation of two Bagby and Kuslich (BAK) devices within a degenerate disc, Kuslich and Dowdle (23) reported a 91% rate of fusion and clinical success in their initial series of patients with 2-year follow-up. Brodke et al. (6) showed that two interbody BAK cages yield stability similar to that of a pedicle screw and PLIF construct. Thus, initial stabilization of the interbody fusion cages is achieved without the morbidity of posterior lateral muscle stripping. However, after initial stability has been obtained with the anterior interbody cage standalone, the ligaments can loosen after some weeks and before the fusion, which leads to pseudarthrosis and recurrence of pain. This biomechanical point was noted by Le Huec et al. (24b), who proposed to stabilize the cage with an anterior plate, thereby avoiding a posterior approach for pedicle screw insertion (Fig. 17.4).

Interest in laparoscopically assisted spinal procedures has increased dramatically. The first reported laparoscopic procedure on the spine was a lumbar discectomy at L5–S1 performed by Obenchain (38). Zucherman et al. (57) were the first to perform instrumented interbody fusion of the spine laparoscopically (Fig. 17.5). These proce-

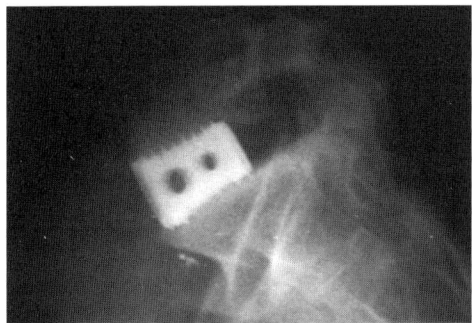
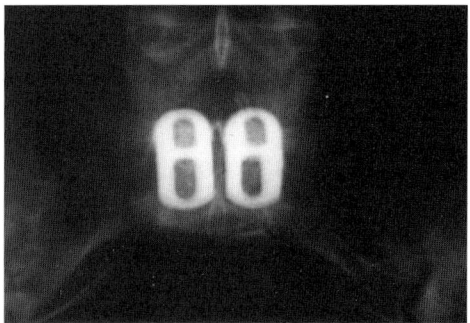

FIG. 17.5. Radiograph demonstrates lordotic tapered titanium cages (Novus L-T; Medtronic, Memphis, TN, U.S.A.) placed laparoscopically at the L5–S1 interspace. This allows immediate fixation and long-term arthrodesis combined with the benefits of early patient mobilization and a lack of posterior muscle disruption. **A:** Lateral view. **B:** Anteroposterior view.

dures were carried out at separate centers. Zucherman et al. (57) published their early experience of 17 patients with a 12-month follow-up who had undergone either L4–5 or L5–S1 anterior interbody fusion with the BAK device. Instruments have been designed that, when placed laparoscopically, allow distraction of the disc space, centering of the implant, and placement of two threaded titanium cylinders that engage the L5 and Sl endplates. These cylinders are packed with cancellous bone obtained from the anterior iliac crest.

Mahvi and Zdeblick (31) reported their laparoscopic technique and complications in their initial series of patients. With 1 year of follow-up, they have a 100% rate of implant retention without migration. Approximately 90% of the patients have experienced excellent clinical relief from their preoperative LBP.

Zdeblick (54) performed a prospective randomized study comparing the surgical treatment of patients with DDD at L5–S1 (one level). The patients underwent either posterolateral pedicle screw fusion, pedicle screw fusion plus PLIF, or laparoscopic BAK interbody fusion. At a minimum of 1 year of follow-up, a shorter operating time, less blood loss, and dramatically shorter hospital stays were noted in the patients with laparoscopically placed interbody fusion cages. On average, patients were discharged home 1.8 days after surgery. Radiographically solid fusions were obtained in 80% of the patients with posterolateral fusions, 91% of those with PLIF, and 100% of those with interbody fusion cages. Return to work was dramatically accelerated in the laparoscopic group. Overall, 67% of the patients with pedicle screw fusions, 64% of those with PLIF, and 85% of those with laparoscopic BAK cages returned to work. These are certainly encouraging numbers in this short-term follow-up.

Overall, the treatment of discogenic pain syndromes is evolving. As more information is gathered regarding less invasive fusion techniques, actual pain relief after fusion can be analyzed without the confounding variables of "fusion disease." The early results of laparoscopically placed interbody fusion cages have been encouraging. Long-term follow-up will be necessary to assess this procedure fully.

Based on all the comments made, we propose the following indications:

1. ALIF is a good technique for posttraumatic kyphosis, iatrogenic lumbar kyphosis, failed posterior fusion, and painful DDD with or without deformity. Its advantages are well-known: excellent rate of fusion through the weight-bearing part of the spine, sparing of back muscles, and reduced blood loss. Disadvantages are the training curve required to learn the approach, the lack of canal decompression, and hypogastric plexus injury at L5–S1 (0.8%) (41). Our experience has been to perform ALIF through a retroperitoneal mini-open video-assisted approach with one or two cages anteroposteriorly plus plate (Pyramid; Medtronic, Memphis, TN, U.S.A.) at L5–S1, and with one cage laterally plus plate (Xantus/Butterfly; Medtronic) at L4–5 or L3–4. Therefore, a second procedure to stabilize the spine after the anterior cage insertion is not required (Fig. 17.4).

2. PLIF is indicated when neurologic decompression is required for spinal canal or foraminal stenosis with primary or secondary instability or deformity. The main advantage is the ability to perform decompression and stabilization through the same approach. Disadvantages are wide exposure with muscle damage, epidural fibrosis, and neurologic compromise. The transverse lumbar interbody fusion (TLIF) technique is an alternative to decrease scar tissue, but the surgeon must take care not to injure the ganglion and root, and this technique is indicated only with a large disc. Evoked potential control during the procedure is a good precaution.

CONCLUSIONS

Pathophysiology, symptom presentation, etiology, diagnostic criteria, and treatment alternatives have been reviewed. This information is by no means meant to be absolute. The diagnosis and treatment of discogenic pain syndromes are evolving rapidly. The overriding concern for the treating physician is proper patient selection. The vast majority of patients with discogenic pain do not require surgical treatment. Fusion surgery should be reserved for patients who are highly motivated, carefully selected, and without psychologic magnification of their symptoms. An indication for the PLIF or ALIF technique is the presence of permanent neurologic signs.

REFERENCES

1. Albert TJ, Pinto M, Denis F. Management of symptomatic pseudarthrosis with anteroposterior fusion. *Spine* 2000;25:123–129.
1a. Bagby G. Arthrodesis by the distraction-compression methods using stainless steel implant. *Orthopedics* 1988; 11:931–934.
2. Blumenthal SL, Baker J, Dossett A, et al. The role of anterior lumbar fusion for internal disc disruption. *Spine* 1988;13:566–569.
3. Brantigan JW. Pseudarthrosis rate after allograft posterior lumbar interbody fusion with pedicle screw and plate fixation. *Spine* 1994;19:1271–1280.
4. Brantigan JW, Steffee AD. A carbon fiber implant to aid interbody lumbar fusion: two-year clinical results in the first 26 patients. *Spine* 1993;18:2106–2117.
5. Brantigan JW, Steffee AD, Keppler L, et al. Posterior lumbar interbody fusion technique using the Variable Screw Placement spinal fixation system. *Spine* 1992;6:175–200.
6. Brodke DS, Dick JC, Zdeblick TA, et al. *Biomechanical comparison of posterior lumbar interbody fusion including a new threaded titanium cage.* Presented at the eighth annual meeting of the North American Spine Society, San Diego, October 15, 1993.
7. Brown MD. The pathophysiology of disc disease. Symposium on disease of the intervertebral disc. *Orthop Clin North Am* 1971;2:359–370.
8. Colhoun E, McCall IW, Williams L, et al. Provocation discography as a guide to planning operations on the spine. *J Bone Joint Surg Br* 1988;70:267–271.
9. Cowan S, Agren K Wright A. *Results of spinal fusion using pedicle screw fixation.* Presented at the ninth annual meeting of the North American Spine Society, Minneapolis, October 21, 1994.
10. Crock HV. A reappraisal of intervertebral disc lesions. *Med J Aust* 1970;1:983–989.
11. Crock HV. Internal disc disruption. A challenge to disc prolapse fifty years on. *Spine* 1986;11:650–653.
12. Dennis S, Watkins R, Landaker S, et al. Comparison of disc space heights after anterior lumbar interbody fusion. *Spine* 1989;18:876–878.
13. Frymoyer JW, Selby DK. Segmental instability. Rationale for treatment. *Spine* 1985;10:280–286.
14. Gill K, Blumenthal SL. Functional results after anterior lumbar fusion at L5–S1 in patients with normal and abnormal MRI scans. *Spine* 1992;17:940–942.
15. Gill K, Blumenthal SL. Posterior lumbar interbody fusion: a 2-year follow-up of 238 patients. *Acta Orthop Scand* 1993;64:108–110.
16. Goldner J, Urbaniak J, McCollum D. Anterior disc excision and interbody spinal fusion for chronic low back pain. *Orthop Clin North Am* 1971;2:544–568.
17. Haughton VM. Imaging of the spine. *Radiology* 1988;166:297–301.
18. Jackson RK, Boston A, Edge AJ. Lateral mass fusion: a prospective study of a consecutive series with long-term follow-up. *Spine* 1985;10:828–832.
19. Jaffray D, O'Brien JP. Isolated intervertebral disc resorption. A source of mechanical and inflammatory back pain? *Spine* 1986;11:397–401.
20. Knutsson F. The instability associated with disc degeneration in the lumbar spine. *Acta Radiol* 1944;25:593–609.
21. Kozak JA, Heilman AE, O'Brien JP. Anterior lumbar fusion options: technique and graft materials. *Clin Orthop* 1994;300:45–51.
22. Kozak JA, O'Brien JP. Simultaneous combined anterior and posterior fusion: an independent analysis of a treatment for the disabled low back pain patient. *Spine* 1990;15:322–328.
23. Kuslich SD, Dowdle JA. *Two-year follow-up results of an interbody fusion device.* Presented at the ninth annual meeting of the North American Spine Society, Minneapolis, October 19, 1994.
24. Lee CK, Vessa P, Lee JK. Chronic disabling low back pain syndrome caused by internal disc derangements. *Spine* 1995;20:356–361.
24b. Le Huec JC, Liu M, Skalli W, et al. Lumbar lateral interbody cage with plate augmentation : in vitro biomechanical analysis. *Eur Spine J* 2002;11:130–136

25. Lin PK, Cautilli RA, Joyce W. Posterior lumbar interbody fusion. *Clin Orthop* 1983;180:165–168.
26. Linson MA, Williams H. Anterior and combined anteroposterior fusion for lumbar disc pain: a preliminary study. *Spine* 1991;16:143–145.
27. Lipson SJ, Muir H. Proteoglycans in experimental intervertebral disc degeneration. *Spine* 1984;6:194–210.
28. Loguidice VA, Johnson RG, Guyer RD, et al. Anterior lumbar interbody fusion. *Spine* 1988;13:366–369.
29. Ma GW. Posterior lumbar interbody fusion with specialized instruments. *Clin Orthop* 1985;195:57–63.
30. MacNab I. Spondylolisthesis with an intact neural arch—the so-called pseudospondylolisthesis. *J Bone Joint Surg Br* 1950;32:325–333.
31. Mahvi DM, Zdeblick TA. A prospective study of laparoscopic spinal fusion. *Ann Surg* 1996;224:85–90.
32. Masatyk TJ, Boumphrey F, Modic MT, et al. Effects of chemonucleolysis demonstrated by MR imaging. *J Comput Assist Tomogr* 1986;10:917–923.
33. Modic MT, Masaryk TJ, Ross JS. *Magnetic resonance imaging of the spine*. Chicago: Year Book, 1989:280.
34. Modic MT, Steinberg PM, Ross JS, et al. Degenerative disc disease: assessment of changes in vertebral body marrow with MR imaging. *Radiology* 1988;166:193–199.
35. Modic MT, Feiglin DK, Piraino DW, et al. Vertebral osteomyelitis: assessment using MR. *Radiology* 1985;157:157–166.
36. Naylor A. Intervertebral disc prolapse and degeneration: the biomechanical and biophysical approach. *Spine* 1976;1:108–114.
37. Newman MK Grinstead GL. Anterior lumbar interbody fusion for internal disc disruption. *Spine* 1992;17:831–833.
38. Obenchain TG. Laparoscopic lumbar discectomy: case report. *J Laparoendosc Surg* 1991;1:145–149.
39. O'Brien JP, Dawson MHO, Heard CW, et al. Simultaneous combined anterior and posterior fusion: a surgical solution for failed spinal surgery with a brief review of the first 150 patients. *Clin Orthop* 1986;203:191–195.
40. Rolander SD. Motion of the spine with special reference to stabilizing effect of posterior fusion. *Acta Orthop Scand Suppl* 1966;90:1–144.
41. Sasso R, Kenneth Burkus J, Le Huec JC. Retrograde ejaculation after anterior lumbar interbody fusion: transperitoneal vs retroperitoneal exposure. *Spine* 2003;28:1023–1026.
42. Schneiderman G, Flannigan B, Kingston S, et al. MRI in the diagnosis of disc degeneration. Correlation with discography. *Spine* 1987;12:276–281.
43. Simmons EK, Segil CM. An evaluation of discography in the localization of symptomatic levels in discogenic disease of the spine. *Clin Orthop* 1975;108:57–69.
44. Slosar PJ, Reynolds JB, Goldthwaite N, et al. *Combined anterior and posterior lateral lumbar fusions*. Presented at the ninth annual meeting of the North American Spine Society, Minneapolis, October 20, 1994.
45. Stokes LAF, Frymoyer JW. Segmental motion and instability. *Spine* 1987;12:688–691.
46. Tertti K, Paajanen K, Laato M, et al. Disc degeneration in magnetic resonance imaging: a comparative biochemical histologic and radiologic study in cadaver spines. *Spine* 1991;16:629–634.
47. Torgerson WR, Dotter WE. Comparative roentgenographic study of the asymptomatic and symptomatic lumbar spine. *J Bone Joint Surg Am* 1976;58:850–853.
48. Waddell G, McCulloch JA, Kummel E, et al. Non-organic physical signs in low back pain. *Spine* 1980;5:117–125.
49. Warner SJ, Simmons ED. *Comparison of surgical techniques for the treatment of degenerative spondylolisthesis*. Presented at the ninth annual meeting of the North American Spine Society, Minneapolis, October 20, 1994.
50. Weatherley CR, Prickett CF, O'Brien JP. Discogenic pain persisting despite solid posterior fusion. *J Bone Joint Surg Br* 1986;68:142–143.
51. Wetzel FT, LaRocca SH, Lowery GL, et al. The treatment of lumbar spinal pain syndromes diagnosed by discography. *Spine* 1994;19:792–800.
52. Yu SW, Haughton VK Sether LA, et al. Comparison of MR and discography in detecting radial tears of the annulus. A post-mortem study. *AJNR Am J Neuroradiol* 1989;10:1077–1081.
53. Zdeblick TA. A prospective, randomized study of lumbar fusion: preliminary results. *Spine* 1993;18:983–991.
54. Zdeblick TA. *A prospective randomized study of the surgical treatment of L5–S1 degenerative disc disease*. Presented at the 10th annual meeting of the North American Spine Society, Washington, DC, October 20, 1995.
55. Zdeblick TA, Smith GR, Warden KE, et al. Two-point fixation of the lumbar spine. Differential stability in rotation. *Spine* 1991;16[6 Suppl]:S298–S301.
56. Zucherman J, Hsu K, Picetti G, et al. Clinical efficacy of spinal instrumentation in lumbar degenerative disc disease. *Spine* 1992;17:834–837.
57. Zucherman JF, Zdeblick TA, Bailey SA, et al. Instrumented laparoscopic spinal fusion: preliminary results. *Spine* 1995;20:2029–2035.

18

Posterolateral Fusion

*‡Norbert Passuti, †Joël Delécrin, *‡Mostafa Romih, and *‡Dominique Brossard

*Department of Orthopedic Surgery, Nantes University; †Clinic of Orthopedic Surgery, Centre Hospitalier Universitaire Hôtel Dieu; and ‡Department of Orthopedic Surgery, Nantes Hospital, Nantes, France

Lumbar fusion is a commonly performed operative procedure for the treatment of low back pain (LBP), but the indications, techniques, and results remain controversial and unclear. The description of the pain can be analyzed, but most important are associated factors, such as socioeconomic status, compensation status, initial psychologic distress, and duration of symptoms. In France, for example, a work accident is a very bad situation in regard to the outcome.

This situation is frequent because in industrialized societies, the lifetime prevalence of back pain is 70%. The incidence in the United States is 15% to 20% per year, and the rate of operations increased by 200% between 1979 and 1987, so the cost of diagnosis and treatment are a major health care issue. Spinal fusion should be performed only after a specific pathoanatomic condition has been identified as the cause of the patient's symptoms. The indications for lumbar fusion have been expanded in an attempt to control pain attributed to abnormal or unstable motion between one vertebra and an adjacent vertebra, or pain resulting from mechanical degeneration of a disc. After fusion, most investigators have used nonstandardized criteria to include patients who underwent surgery for various diagnoses and whose outcomes were assessed with nonvalidated methods. For example, Howe and Frymoyer (7) used 14 different outcome assessments in a group of more than 200 patients who underwent lumbar surgery. The proportion of "successes" was significantly influenced by the outcome measure used, ranging from 90% to 60%.

ETIOLOGY OF LOW BACK PAIN

The etiology must be well analyzed, and the degeneration of facet joints as a cause of LBP has been postulated since 1922. The facet joints can be infiltrated with anesthetic, but disappointing results have been reported with use of selective injection as a therapeutic modality. In a prospective study of Lovely and Rastogni (13), 28 of 91 patients with chronic LBP who experienced at least 70% relief of symptoms after facet blocks were subsequently managed with a posterolateral fusion. The symptoms resolved in more than two thirds of the patients postoperatively. Therefore, facet blocks can solve some lumbar pain problems, but retrospective studies have not confirmed the value of facet block in predicting the success of lumbar arthrodesis.

Some authors believe that a degenerate disc is the most likely source of chronic, disabling LBP. Diagnostic modalities such as discography and magnetic resonance imaging (MRI)

and operative procedures such as disc excision and interbody arthrodesis have been used extensively, but studies have also demonstrated that a degenerate disc may not be painful. Moreover, it has been shown that the density of sensory nerves and neuropeptides in cartilage endplate and underlying cancellous bone is increased in patients with degenerative disc disease, and these structures may transmit pain. Segmental instability induces lumbar pain, and Kirkaldy-Willis and Farfan (8) concluded that degeneration of the lumbar spine occurs in three phases: dysfunction, instability, and restabilization. The natural history of instability was studied radiographically by Sato and Kikuchi (19), who reported restabilization in 20% of 50 patients after a minimum 10-year follow-up.

Clinical assessments and dynamic roentgenography must define the diagnosis of segmental instability, but the greatest debate about the use of diagnostic studies to evaluate LBP concerns provocative discography. The pain provoked during discography can be useful to identify precise indications for fusion (Figs. 18.1, 18.2).

Colhoun et al. (3) retrospectively reviewed the outcomes of 137 patients with LBP who had undergone spinal fusion. Wick discography had demonstrated abnormal morphologic characteristics and reproduced symptoms. At a mean of 3.6 years, 121 (88%) of the patients had a successful result, compared with only 13 (52%) of 25 who had undergone an arthrodesis without reproduction of the typical symptoms. Milette and Melanson (16) reported that discography was associated with only a 5% rate of false-positive results in a study of 320 normal discs. Derby et al. (4), in a study of 96 patients, reported that those with highly sensitive discs appeared to have significantly better long-term outcomes with interbody/combined fusion than with intertransverse fusion. Therefore, this study supports the view that patients with chronic back pain and sensitive discs who undergo surgery that includes an interbody fusion fare significantly better than patients who undergo intertransverse fusion only and patients who have no surgery.

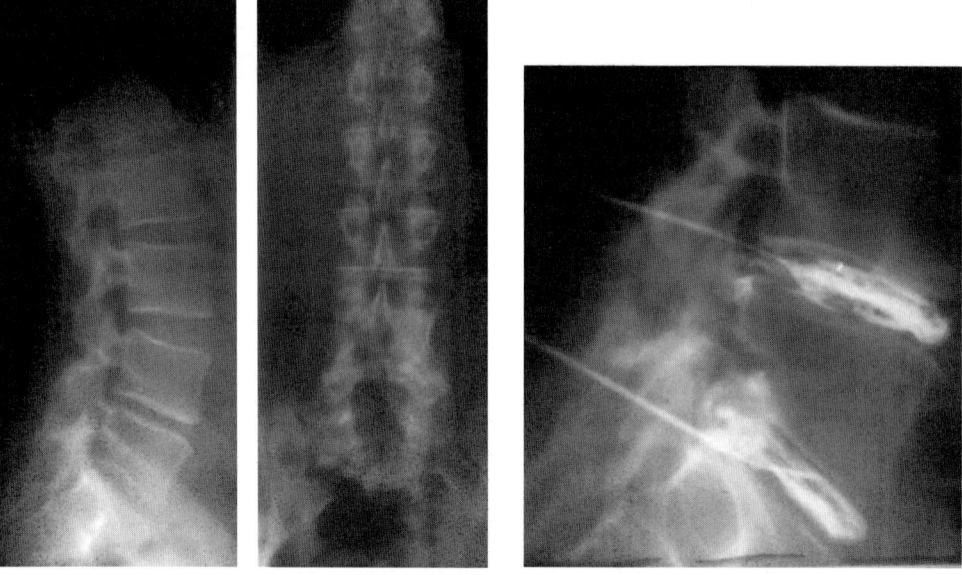

FIG. 18.1. Provocative discography to define an indication for fusion. **A:** A 45-year-old man had undergone surgical discectomy at two levels 5 years previously. **B:** Two years later, he underwent laminectomy at levels L4 and L5.

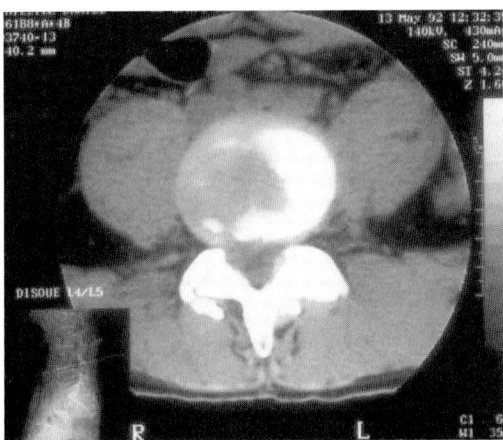 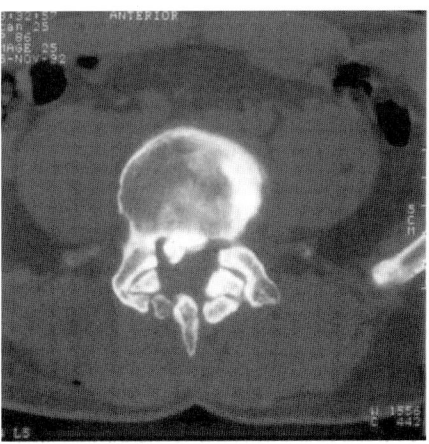

FIG. 18.2. Discography combined with computed tomography revealed selective pain **(A)** and root pain **(B)**. We decided to perform a lumbar fusion (L4–L5–S1).

MRI findings can be compared with the results of discography to avoid disc injection. The development of MRI has provided a noninvasive method for evaluating the morphologic characteristics of the disc. Schneiderman and Flannigon (20) retrospectively studied 101 discs in 32 patients and found a 99% association between the MRI findings and those on discography. Newman and Grinstead (17) reported success in 31 (86%) of 36 patients 2 years after an anterior lumbar fusion performed because of abnormal findings on discography and MRI. Therefore, the Modic signal on MRI is more reliable than discography to define an indication for lumbar fusion (Fig. 18.3).

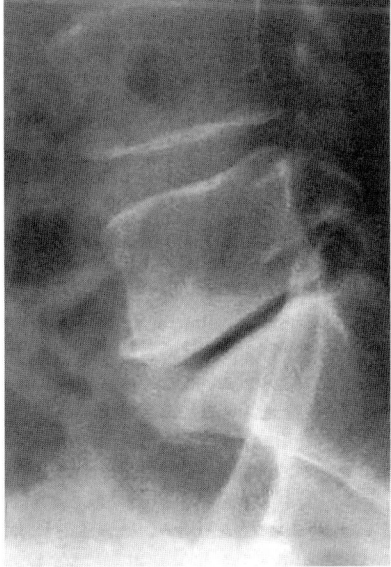 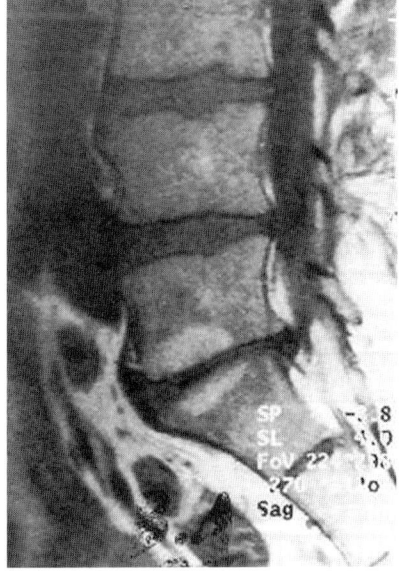

FIG. 18.3. A: A patient who presented with chronic low back pain and loss of height of the L5–S1 disc. **B:** Typical aspect of a Modic type I lesion on magnetic resonance image.

OPERATIVE TREATMENT

Indications for Fusion

The decision to perform a fusion is a difficult one. The patient's pain must be correlated with the results of functional analysis, discography, and now MRI. We use a trial of immobilization with a pantaloon cast, as described by Rask and Dall (18) in 45 patients with LBP. They demonstrated clearly that the pantaloon cast is an effective tool for identifying those patients with chronic LBP who might benefit from a spinal stabilization procedure, and this is a good test for selecting patients for arthrodesis. Temporary external transpedicular fixation of the lumbar spine can be a useful tool in selecting candidates for fusion, but Bednar (1) have reported a poor predictive value with neurologic complications and infection, and on the basis of this analysis, external spinal skeletal fixation should not be used to predict pain relief after lumbar fusion. Therefore, after complete nonsurgical treatment, including rehabilitation and exercise, we select patients for fusion who have responded favorably to immobilization tests.

Results of Posterolateral Fusion

Posterolateral arthrodesis with autogenous bone graft and internal fixation has been most commonly performed. In cases of noninstrumented fusion, the average rate of nonunion is 32%, so adjunctive spinal instrumentation increases the rate of fusion, and in patients managed with pedicle screw instrumentation, consolidation of the fusion tends to be more rapid with more frequent maintenance of spinal alignment and better sagittal balance.

In a metaanalysis of the literature from 1970 through 1993, Mardjetko et al. (15) reported the results of a review of 25 articles. These indicated that posterolateral spinal fusion rates are enhanced by spinal instrumentation ($P = 0.08$), with no significant differences detectable between control devices and pedicle screw devices.

The results of fusion for LBP are not well defined, but a multicenter randomized controlled trial has compared lumbar fusion with nonsurgical treatment (5). This study confirmed that lumbar fusion in a well-informed and selected group of patients with severe LBP can diminish pain and decrease disability in the surgical group 63%. The surgical group rated much better or better in comparison with 29% in the nonsurgical group. However, back pain was reduced in only of 33%, and the Oswestry score was reduced by 25%. Therefore, lumbar fusion can be used to reduce pain and decrease disability in selected patients.

Complications

Yuan et al. (22) retrospectively analyzed the outcomes of 2,177 patients who underwent pedicle screw fixation. The rates of nerve root, spinal cord, and vascular injuries were low (less than 0.5%), but in the literature, the rate of misplaced pedicle screws ranges between 2% and 5%, and the rate of loosening or breakage between 2% and 6%. However, McAfee et al. (14) reported that in 120 cases, the 10-year predicted survival of spinal fusion with pedicle fixation was 90% solid arthrodesis. Furthermore, in our experience, hardware breakage in the absence of pseudarthrosis is not associated with a poor outcome, and we have observed after more than 5 years of follow-up the spontaneous formation of anterior calcifications, which improve the consolidation.

According to the use of specific instrumentation, one concern is to maintain or restore segmental lordosis inside the fusion, and the correlation with pelvic parameters, as described by Legaye and Duval-Beaupere (12), is fundamental for sagittal balance.

Lazennec et al. (11) retrospectively studied 81 patients who had undergone lumbar fusion. The group of patients with pain after fusion had a relatively vertical sacrum with less sacral tilt and more pelvic tilt. At last follow-up, pelvic tilt was almost twice the normal value. Therefore, it is evident that an appropriate position of the fused vertebrae is of paramount importance to minimize muscle work during maintenance of posture. The main risk is failing to correct or causing excessive pelvic retroversion with a vertical sacrum, which replicates the sitting position. Kumar et al. (10) retrospectively reviewed 83 patients who underwent lumbar fusion for degenerative disc disease. The mean follow-up was 5 years. Patients with a normal sacral incline had a lower incidence of change in the adjacent level than patients in whom this parameter was abnormal. The risk for degeneration in the adjacent segment was high when the sacrum was vertical, so this is an important component of sagittal alignment in patients undergoing lumbar fusion (Fig. 18.4).

The level immediately above the fusion is thought to be at high risk because biomechanics are altered following fusion. Most studies suggesting a high incidence of clinically significant degeneration at the adjacent level have focused only on symptomatic patients and have not studied all patients undergoing fusion. Kumar et al. (9) performed a study with a long-term follow-up of 30 years. A significantly higher incidence of radiographic changes was observed at adjacent levels following lumbar fusion, but these were not accompanied by a significant change in functional outcomes, which were assessed

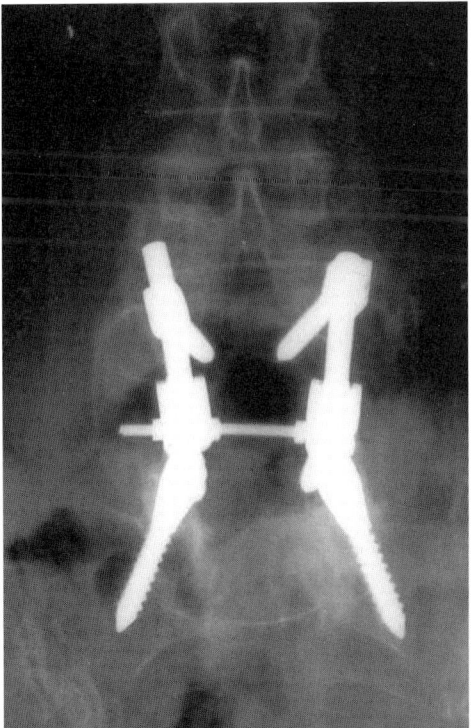 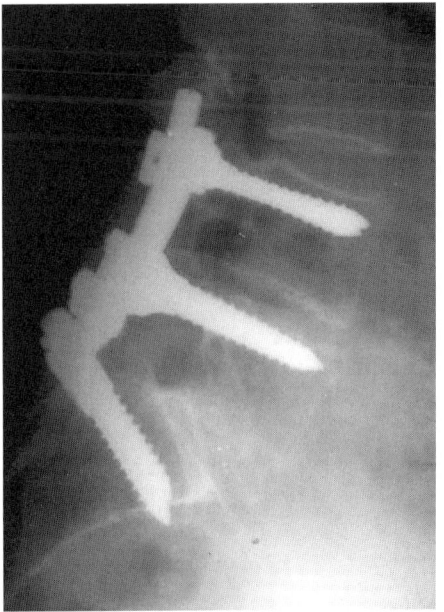

FIG. 18.4. A and B: The clinical result in a 55-year-old woman 8 years after surgery for chronic low back pain is excellent. Images show good sagittal balance, absence of a vertical sacrum, and spontaneous anterior calcifications.

with validated outcome measures and performance tests. This finding was confirmed by Guigui et al. (6), who followed 102 patients undergoing posterolateral fusion for an average of 9 years. Degenerative changes were frequent, with disc space narrowing. Degenerative spondylolisthesis or angular hypermobility was found, but no significant correlation between the radiographic findings and final functional results. Only eight patients required an additional surgical procedure.

Therefore, segmental instrumentation can be used to provide lumbar lordosis, respect the pelvic parameters, and maintain normal sagittal balance. Degenerative changes occurred above the fusion but were not correlated with the clinical and functional results.

NEW CONCEPTS

Some authors have tried to treat degenerative disc disease at the beginning of the natural history. Vital et al. (21) performed a prospective study of 16 patients with chronic LBP and Modic type I lesions. After lumbar fusion with instrumentation and 9 months of follow-up, the Modic I lesions had changed to Modic II lesions and the clinical results were good, so the posterior fusion had accelerated the course of the Modic lesions by arresting mechanical instability. Other authors have described anterior fusion; Chataigner et al. (2) retrospectively reviewed 56 patients who had undergone anterior interbody fusion. The best results were observed in the patients with Modic I changes suggesting degenerative changes. Of five patients with nonunion, Modic II changes were observed in three, who required posterior osteosynthesis.

CONCLUSIONS

Major controversies center around which treatment is best when nonoperative measures have failed. Operative treatment maintains that these patients have no other options. Some improvement as a result of operative treatment occurs in about 75% of patients, but major or complete relief of pain and recovery of function are seen in 50% or fewer. We hope to decrease the problems associated with the surgical approach by using a minimally invasive approach or percutaneous fixation, as described with the Sextan system (Medtronic Sofamor Danek Company, Paris, France). We must also improve the tools used to analyze the initial instability and confirm the exact rate of fusion. However, the most difficult problem continues to be determining the parameters that indicate when fusion should be undertaken.

REFERENCES

1. Bednar DA. Failure of external spinal skeletal fixation to improve predictability of lumbar arthrodesis. *J Bone Joint Surg Am* 2001;83:1656–1659.
2. Chataigner H, Onimus M, Polette A. La chirurgie des discopathies lombaires. *Rev Chir Orthop* 1998;84: 583–589.
3. Colhoun E, McCall IW, Williams L, et al. Provocation discography as a guide to planning operations on the spine. *J Bone Joint Surg Br* 1988;70:267–271.
4. Derby R, Howard MW, et al. The ability of pressure-controlled discography to predict surgical and nonsurgical outcome. *Spine* 1999;24:364–372.
5. Fritzell P, Hägg O, et al. Lumbar fusion versus nonsurgical treatment for chronic low back pain. *Spine* 2001;26: 2521–2534.
6. Guigui P, Lambert P, Lassale B, et al. Evolution à long terme des niveaux adjacents à une arthrose lombaire. *Rev Chir Orthop* 1997;83:685–696.
7. Howe J, Frymoyer JW. The effects of questionnaire design on the determination of end results in lumbar spine surgery. *Spine* 1985;10:804–805.
8. Kirkaldy-Willis WH, Farfan HF. Instability of the lumbar spine. *Clin Orthop* 1982;165:110–123.

9. Kumar MN, Baklanov A, Chopin D. Correlation between sagittal plane changes and adjacent segment degeneration following lumbar spine fusion. *Eur Spin J* 2001;10:314–319.
10. Kumar MN, Jacquot F, Hall H. Long-term follow-up of functional outcomes and radiographic changes at adjacent levels following lumbar spine fusion for degenerative disc disease. *Eur Spine J* 2001;10:309–313.
11. Lazennec JY, Romare S, Arafati N, et al. Sagittal alignment in lumbo-sacral fusion: relations between radiological parameters and pain. *Eur Spine J* 2000;9:47–55.
12. Legaye J, Duval-Beaupere G, et al. Pelvic incidence: a fundamental pelvic parameter for three-dimensional regulation of spinal sagittal curves. *Eur Spine J* 1998;7:99–103.
13. Lovely TJ, Rastogni P. The value of provocative facet blocking as a predictor of success in lumbar spine fusion. *J Spinal Disord* 1997;10:512–517.
14. McAfee PC, Werland DJ, Corlow JJ. Survivorship analysis of pedicle spinal instrumentation. *Spine* 1991;16[Suppl]:S422–S427.
15. Mardjetko S, Connoly PJ, Schott S. Degenerative lumbar spondylolisthesis. A meta-analysis of the literature. *Spine* 1994;19[Suppl 20]:S2256–S3365.
16. Milette PC, Melanson D. A reappraisal of lumbar discography. *J Can Assoc Radiol* 1982;33:176–182.
17. Newman MH, Grinstead GL. Anterior lumbar interbody fusion for internal disc disruption. *Spine* 1992;17:831–833.
18. Rask B, Dall BE. Use of the pantaloon cast for the selection of fusion candidates in the treatment of chronic low back pain. *Clin Orthop* 1993;288:148–157.
19. Sato H, Kikuchi S. The natural history of radiographic instability of the lumbar spine. *Spine* 1993;18:2075–2079.
20. Schneiderman G, Flannigon B, et al. Magnetic resonance imaging in the diagnosis of disc degeneration. Correlation with discography. *Spine* 1987;12:276–81.
21. Vital JM, Azzouz S, et al. The course of Modic 1 signal after lumbar posterior osteosynthesis. *Eur Spine J* 2002;11[Suppl]511.
22. Yuan HA, Garfin SR, et al. A historical cohort study of pedicle screw fixation in thoracic lumbar and sacral spinal fusion. *Spine* 1994;19[Suppl 20]:S2279–S2296.

19

A New Concept in Spinal Stabilization: OptiMesh

Stephen D. Kuslich

Department of Orthopedics, University of Minnesota, Minneapolis, Minnesota; and Spineology Research Group, Spineology Inc., Stillwater, Minnesota

WHAT IS OPTIMESH?

OptiMesh (Spineology Inc., Stillwater, MN, U.S.A.) is a three-dimensional mesh container designed to retain and reinforce granular grafting materials. The OptiMesh system comprises a series of novel techniques, tools, and devices that allow a surgeon to create and fill cavities with compacted granular materials through very small entrance portals. With this system, a surgeon can use minimally invasive surgical techniques to stabilize certain spinal disorders. The space in which the OptiMesh device is implanted can be any cavity already present or newly created in a bone or joint structure. A unique characteristic of our method is the ability to introduce an unfilled mesh container into a body cavity during an installation procedure, then fill it within the body cavity to construct a com-

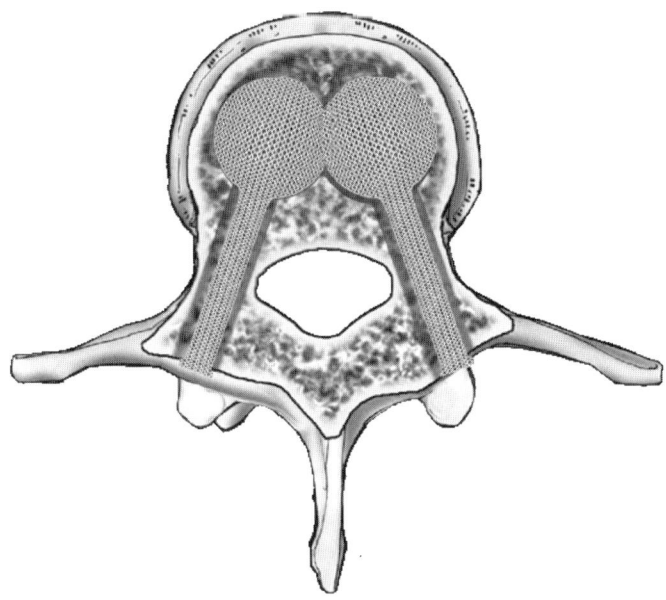

FIG. 19.1. Two OptiMesh containers placed through the pedicles into a vertebral body. The containers can be filled with a bone graft slurry, ceramic granules or beads, or bone cement to elevate and stabilize a fracture. The porosity varies depending on the type of fill material used.

pacted, relatively rigid, yet porous and biocompatible stabilizing structure. Figure 19.1 is a photograph of one form of OptiMesh container (13).

HOW DOES OPTIMESH DIFFER FROM TRADITIONAL SPINAL DEVICES?

Traditional spinal devices are designed to bear or share mechanical loads. OptiMesh technology departs from this strategy. Our devices simply contain and reinforce the graft or graft substitute, allowing the granular fill materials to change phase from liquid-like to solid-like structures. The firm granular pack itself, rather than the device, is responsible for bearing spinal loads. The compacted graft or graft substitute is also responsible for any interspace distraction, restoration of disc height, annulotaxis, or platform reinforcement, thereby improving motion segment stability. Our devices are unlike cages or other fixation devices in that the mesh itself does not function to bear load directly or hold portions of the spine in any particular alignment or position.

Although OptiMesh devices initially function to restrict the migration of bone-grafting materials during implantation, it is important to realize that packed granular materials become extremely self-adherent once a certain packing density has been achieved. Therefore, once the pack becomes firm, it can no longer flow out of the mesh container, even if the entrance portal is left unclosed. The mesh does not have to withstand compression, shear, or bending loads, as spinal interbody cages and screw or rod–plate fixation devices are required to do. The mesh casement must simply be strong in tension to contain and reinforce the graft material. In this respect, OptiMesh differs fundamentally from all previous devices used for interbody or intrabody stabilization (14).

PRECLINICAL TESTING

We have used three different animal models (rabbits, monkeys, and sheep) to complete extensive *in vitro* and *in vivo* testing and determine whether OptiMesh allows unobstructed through-growth and ingrowth. Our test results show that in appropriate circumstances (i.e., when the segment is sufficiently stable and the graft material is optimal), the mesh does not interfere with this process (23).

DEVICES

OptiMesh devices are three-dimensional mesh structures used to contain and reinforce bone-grafting or other bone replacement materials implanted in a body cavity. Our proprietary technology includes any pliable, porous, balloon-like structure, of almost any shape, size, or thickness, and may be constructed by several means, including weaving or braiding of filaments or threads and extrusion of a balloon followed by perforation of the balloon wall. We have used all these techniques to create test models. In theory, the material used in construction can include any biocompatible material that is strong in tension. In addition to bone graft, our group has developed two types of bioceramic beads (combinations of tricalcium phosphate and hydroxyapatite in various proportions) and the tools used to deliver them into the OptiMesh container. *In vitro* and *in vivo* studies have shown that the bead pack stabilizes the intervertebral disc space and allows bony ingrowth both outside and inside the mesh. Combining the bioceramic beads with an osteogenic enhancement material, such as marrow blood or bone morphogenetic protein, enhances bone formation (23).

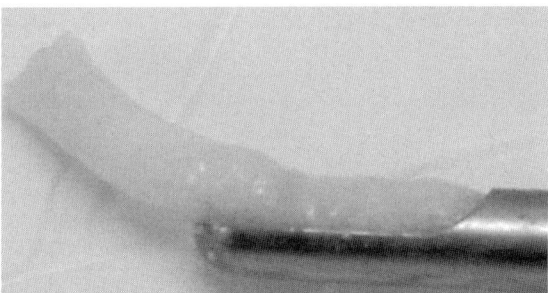

FIG. 19.2. A specially designed fill tube with a ramp at the end causes fill material to be extruded away from the long axis of the injection tube. This deflected material improves the ability of the fill material to distract the disc space, or the vertebral endplates in the case of a vertebral compression fracture.

TOOLS

The tool set includes several key instruments for creating and filling cavities. Our *expanding reamer* allows the surgeon to create a cylindric, elliptic, or spherical cavity within a hard or soft tissue structure; this cavity can be up to 2.5 times larger than the entrance hole through which the tool is placed. For instance, the surgeon can use the tool to enter a biologic structure through a 6-, 8-, or 10-mm hole and then easily and rapidly create a cavity with any diameter up to a maximum of 14, 20, or 25 mm, respectively.

Another unique instrument is the *circumferential reciprocating reamer*. This tool allows the surgeon to evacuate a toroidal (tire-shaped) cavity in bone or joint tissue. The instrument is applied in the disc space (after the nuclear space is first evacuated with the expanding reamer) to create a cavity with a flattened Saturn-like shape (spherical or ovoid with a surrounding rim). A cavity of this shape results when the surgeon removes the degenerate nucleus and inner annulus and a millimeter or two of endplate, leaving the outer annulus intact. This particular shape is ideal for creating an interbody fusion cavity or preparing an open cavity within a vertebral compression fracture.

The third key component of the tools set is the specially designed *injection tube*, which is a long metal cylinder with a thin, rigid wall; the internal wall surface is highly polished. The ideal internal tube dimension was determined by trial and error. An appropriately dimensioned tube allows a piston to move graft material easily through the tube and into the implant or cavity at its distal end. After experimenting with various lengths and diameters, we settled on certain lengths and diameters to optimize the flow of different materials. In addition to square-ended tubes, we developed a design that allows the surgeon to direct bone graft materials laterally from the main axis of the tube. With this feature, the surgeon can direct the bone graft material in the direction required for intervertebral distraction, or to reduce the kyphosis produced by a compression fracture. Figure 19.2 is a photograph of the tip of the diverted fill tube. Note the tendency of the injected graft to deflect away from the long axis of the fill tube. This deflected material is better able to generate distraction forces perpendicular to the long axis of the injection tube.

The naïve notion that one can use an ordinary syringe to fill a narrow tube with morcellized bone graft is quickly disproved during actual experience. The syringe quickly becomes jammed, and if great pressure is applied, it explodes, but the graft material does not flow into the tube. We solved this problem by developing the fourth key component of our tool set—the *injection tube loading tool*. This allows a graft supplier, either the surgeon or the surgeon's assistant, to fill the injection tube with bone graft materials easily and quickly.

MECHANICAL AND BIOLOGIC TESTING

When OptiMesh was used to stabilize a cadaveric spinal motion segment, we found that although the graft-filled container was somewhat less rigid than a metal interbody cage, annulotaxis did occur, and the motion segment was significantly more stable than the intact segment. Other tests indicated that the application of additional posterior stabilization in the form of pedicle fixation systems, transfacet screws, or posterior tension bands could further improve initial stability.

Using a validated rabbit tibial defect model, we demonstrated that the polyester OptiMesh is well tolerated biologically. Implantation of the mesh did not result in an inflammatory response. Rather, it allowed unimpeded bony union around and through the mesh container. We used our OptiMesh system to perform a series of anterior interbody fusions in rhesus monkeys. The histologic appearance at 12 months was remarkably similar to that in the rabbit study. Animal trials of OptiMesh for interbody fusion in the sheep model are now complete. Results varied according to the fill material used and the degree of segmental stability provided by ancillary fixation. These tests indicate that the system is capable, under certain conditions, of inducing stability and bony arthrodesis at 6 months after surgery.

USE OF OPTIMESH IN VERTEBRAL COMPRESSION FRACTURES

Vertebroplasty represents a significant advance in the treatment of vertebral compression fractures (1–8,11,15,17,18). Important technical aspects of the operative technique are well described in the literature (10,12,16,22). In contradistinction to the attitude of benign neglect that characterized the standard management of this entity in prior years, the management of vertebral compression fractures by means of bone cement injection results in immediate and long-term relief of pain in a majority of patients, which improves their function and quality of life. That is the good news.

The bad news is that a small percentage of patients experience serious side effects of the vertebroplasty procedure (9,19,20,21), including paralysis, nerve root impingement, pulmonary embolus, and death. All these complications result from cement leakage outside the area of intended cement placement.

OptiMesh is currently being evaluated for its ability to reduce and stabilize vertebral compression fractures by means of graft or bone cement containment. We found that we could reduce and stabilize laboratory-induced fractures by filling the mesh container with bone graft materials, bone graft substitutes, or bone cement. It appears that a tightly woven mesh container will restrict the potentially injurious extravasation of bone cement. Serendipitously, our expandable reamers (miniaturized) work very well to prepare the initial cavity in osteoporotic vertebral bodies, through either the pedicles or a small puncture portal in the side of the vertebral body, before mesh container installation and inflation. Thus, our system may eliminate the need to perform balloon cavitation before cement injection.

ADDITIONAL LABORATORY AND EARLY CLINICAL EXPERIENCE WITH OPTIMESH

Our research associates used cadaveric spinal segments in a number of experiments to test the ability of OptiMesh containers, filled with a variety of bone grafts and bone cements, to reduce and stabilize osteoporotic compression fractures. We hypothesized that injecting a slurry of cortical bone granules plus demineralized bone matrix into the standard OptiMesh container, or pressure-filling a tightly woven OptiMesh container with bone cement, could elevate and stabilize a compressed vertebral body to its original height before fracture. The early results of laboratory trials are encouraging (Fig. 19.3 A–C).

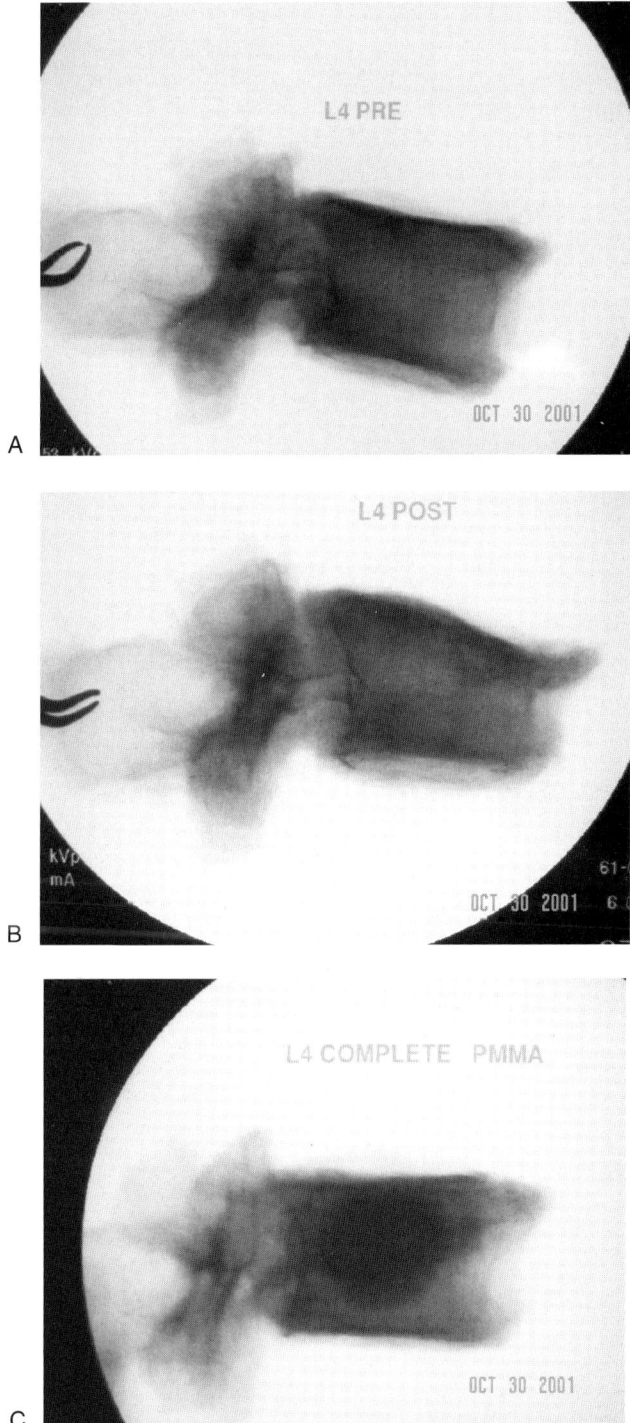

FIG. 19.3. Testing OptiMesh theory in a cadaveric spine. The L4 vertebral body of an 85 year old with osteoporosis. **A:** Before fracture. **B:** After fracture. **C:** After reduction and stabilization with two OptiMesh containers filled with bone cement inserted through the pedicles.

We are currently evaluating a variety of bone cement fill materials and two different types of mesh in the treatment of laboratory-induced vertebral compression fractures in cadaveric spines. Case work in live humans is expected to begin within the next few months. We have experimented with mesh of various degrees of porosity to discover the ideal porosity to reduce the compression fracture by distending the mesh container yet allow just enough "leakage" to lock the implant securely into the surrounding bone. It appears that the ideal mesh porosity depends on specific characteristics of the bone cement (e.g., its viscosity and rate of polymerization).

After qualifying for CE Mark status (required by the European Community), a group of European surgeons began using OptiMesh for interbody stabilization in patients with back pain secondary to degenerative disc disease in October 2002. To date, 70 operations

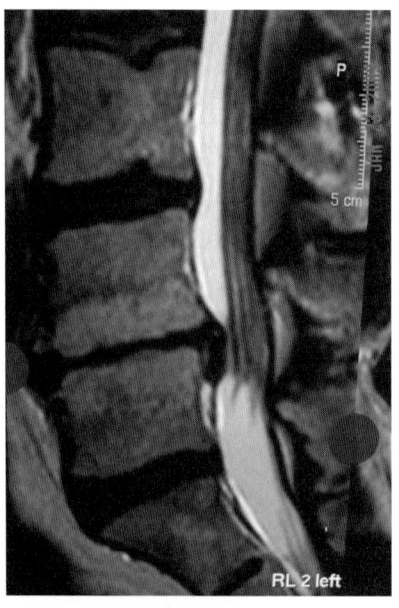
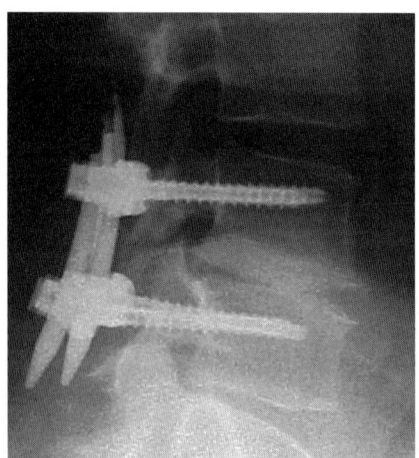
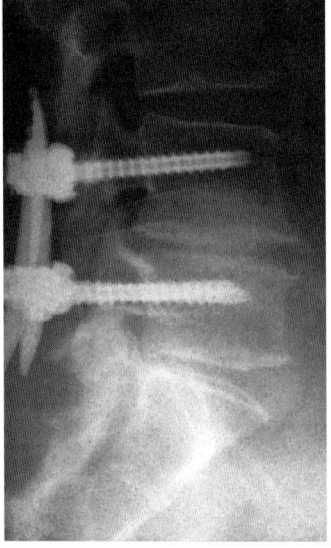

FIG. 19.4. Middle-aged woman with chronic low back pain secondary to degenerative disc disease at L4–5, status post prior partial discectomy for disc herniation. **A:** Preoperative magnetic resonance image. **B:** Six weeks after OptiMesh interbody stabilization with allograft. **C:** Three months postoperatively.

have been completed by 18 different surgeons in Switzerland, Germany, and Italy. These surgeons used a variety of fill materials—autograft, allograft, or allograft plus demineralized bone matrix. To date, no serious side effects or device-related complications have been reported, but the follow-up is too short to draw conclusions about the efficacy of the product. However, we have noted that, as in the preclinical animal experiments, the system appears capable of producing powerful distraction on the annulus. Roentgenographic follow-up at 3 months in a small group of patients suggests that early bony union is probable. The combination of cortical allograft plus demineralized bone matrix appears to be the best injection medium in terms of stability and ease of use.

Figure 19.4 A–C shows the roentgenographic appearance of a typical case of chronic mechanical back pain secondary to degenerative disc disease in a patient previously treated for herniated disc by laminotomy and partial discectomy.

REFERENCES

1. Arnold W. Early surgical treatment of traumatic paraplegia with an external fixation device and diagonal vertebroplasty [in German]. *Unfallchirurg* 1985;88:293–298.
2. Barr JD, Barr MS, Lemley TJ, et al. Percutaneous vertebroplasty for pain relief and spinal stabilization. *Spine* 2000;25:923–928.
3. Bostrom MP, Lane JM. Future directions. Augmentation of osteoporotic vertebral bodies [Review]. *Spine* 1997;22[24 Suppl]:38S–42S.
4. Castel E, Lazennec JY, Chiras J, et al. Acute spinal cord compression due to intraspinal bleeding from a vertebral hemangioma: two case-reports. *Eur Spine J* 1999;8:244–248.
5. Dudeney S, Lieberman I. Percutaneous vertebroplasty in the treatment of osteoporotic vertebral compression fractures: an open prospective study. *J Rheumatol* 2000;27:2526.
6. Einhorn TA. Vertebroplasty: an opportunity to do something really good for patients. *Spine* 2000;25:1051–1052.
7. Galibert P, Deramond H, Rosat P, et al. Preliminary note on the treatment of vertebral angioma by percutaneous acrylic vertebroplasty [in German]. *Neurochirurgie* 1987;33:166–168.
8. Garfin SR, Yuan HA, Reiley MA. New technologies in spine: kyphoplasty and vertebroplasty for the treatment of painful osteoporotic compression fractures. *Spine* 2001;26:1511–1515.
9. Harrington KD. Major neurological complications following percutaneous vertebroplasty with polymethylmethacrylate: a case report. *J Bone Joint Surg Am* 2001;83:1070–1073.
10. Heini PF, Walchli B, Berlemann U. Percutaneous transpedicular vertebroplasty with PMMA: operative technique and early results. A prospective study for the treatment of osteoporotic compression fractures. *Eur Spine J* 2000;9:445–450.
11. Jarvik JG, Deyo RA. Cementing the evidence: time for a randomized trial of vertebroplasty. *AJNR Am J Neuroradiol* 2000;21:1373–1374.
12. Jensen ME, Evans AJ, Mathis JM, et al. Percutaneous polymethylmethacrylate vertebroplasty in the treatment of osteoporotic vertebral body compression fractures: technical aspects. *AJNR Am J Neuroradiol* 1997;18:1897–1904.
13. Kuslich SD. Soft hardware for the spine: OptiMesh—a preview of some novel tools and methods for manipulating and stabilizing bone graft and bone graft substitutes. In: Gunzburg R, Szpalski M, eds. *Lumbar disc herniation*. Philadelphia: Lippincott Williams & Wilkins, 2002:214–221.
14. Kuslich SD. A novel method for microsurgically stabilizing spinal diseases and injuries: "soft hardware for the spine—the OptiMesh system." In: Kaech DL, Jinkins RJ, eds. *Spinal restabilization procedures*. New York: Elsevier Science, 2002:197–204.
15. Levine SA, Perin LA, Hayes D, et al. An evidence-based evaluation of percutaneous vertebroplasty. *Managed Care* 2000;9:56–60, 63.
16. Liebschner MA, Rosenberg WS, Keaveny TM. Effects of bone cement volume and distribution on vertebral stiffness after vertebroplasty. *Spine* 2001;26:1547–1554.
17. Mathis JM, Barr JD, Belkoff SM, et al. Percutaneous vertebroplasty: a developing standard of care for vertebral compression fractures [Review]. *AJNR Am J Neuroradiol* 2001;22:373–381.
18. Murphy KJ, Lin DD. Vertebroplasty: a simple solution to a difficult problem. *J Clin Densitom* 2001;4:189–197.
19. Padovani B, Kasriel O, Brunner P, et al. Pulmonary embolism caused by acrylic cement: a rare complication of percutaneous vertebroplasty. *AJNR Am J Neuroradiol* 1999;20:375–377.
20. Perrin C, Jullien V, Padovani B, et al. Percutaneous vertebroplasty complicated by pulmonary embolus of acrylic cement [in French]. *Rev Mal Respir* 1999;16:215–217.
21. Ratliff J, Nguyen T, Heiss J. Root and spinal cord compression from methylmethacrylate vertebroplasty. *Spine* 2001;26:E300–E302.
22. Wenger M, Markwalder TM. Surgically controlled, transpedicular methyl methacrylate vertebroplasty with fluoroscopic guidance. *Acta Neurochir (Wien)* 1999;141:625–631.
23. Engineering documents. Stillwater, MN: Spineology Inc, 1997–2003.

20

The Graf Ligament System

*‡Norbert Passuti, †Joël Delécrin, *†Mostafa Romih, and *‡Dominique Brossard

*Department of Orthopedic Surgery, Nantes University;
†Clinic of Orthopedic Surgery, Centre Hospitalier Universitaire Hôtel Dieu;
and ‡Department of Orthopedic Surgery, Nantes Hospital, Nantes, France

Instability between two or more lumbar levels, usually caused by degenerative disease, is a characteristically painful disorder. Historically, symptoms of mechanical instability have been treated surgically with spinal fusion in an attempt to modify the movement pattern of an abnormal motion segment. The Graf ligament system was introduced to avoid intervertebral fusion and its various consequences. The ligament attempts to re-create lumbar lordosis and allows limited movement—hence, the concept of "flexible intervertebral stabilization."

CONCEPT OF THE GRAF LIGAMENT

Lumbar Instability

The lumbar instability syndrome is often characterized by recurrent or chronic low back pain with disabling episodes of acute muscle spasm. The pain is described as a vague, heavy ache associated with tingling into the feet and toes in a nondermatomal distribution. Graf (3) proposed various tests to provide a better understanding of instability during bending and flexion–extension. Using roentgenograms and a microcomputer, he was able to measure the shear deformity of a disc. On magnetic resonance images, fatty degeneration in subchondral bone appears to correlate with abnormal movement. This can be demonstrated in the "twist test," in which computed tomography is performed through the facet joint articulation while the patient twists the torso in relation to the legs, as when rolling over in bed. Subluxation of the joint is indicated by the appearance of a void between the articular surfaces of the facet joint. The definitive diagnosis is made when an intraarticular injection of lidocaine and corticosteroid alleviates the pain caused by this twisting motion (Fig. 20.1).

A preoperative functional restoration or self-management program is often helpful, providing educational material and instruction in physical therapy. A positive (pain-free) response to spinal bracing has been used to indicate the presence of pain-producing degenerative changes. Therefore, selective facet injection combined with a pantaloon cast can be used to identify patients who are candidates for surgery.

According to Gardner and Pande (2), the indications for Graf ligamentoplasty can be summarized as follows:

- Lumbar instability syndrome with or without associated lumbar nerve root involvement
- Stabilization of a degenerate and symptomatic disc above or below an existing fusion

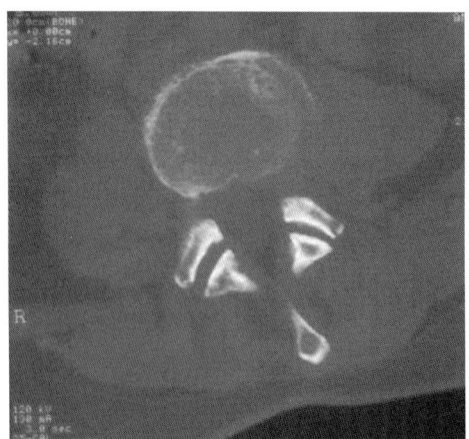 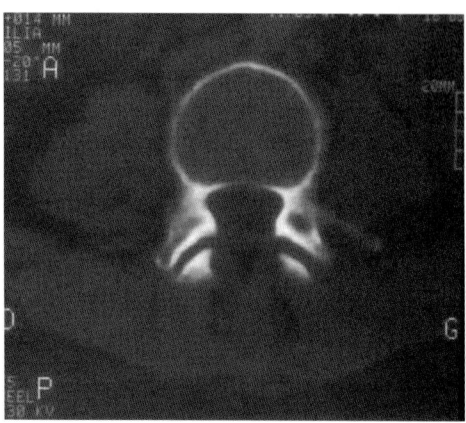

FIG. 20.1. A and B: Example of decoaptation during the "twist test," confirming the gaping accident of the posterior articular facets.

- Stabilization of a symptomatic disc adjacent to a spondylolisthesis, which is repaired at the same time.

However, the Graf band immobilizes the facet joints in a position of full extension; as a consequence, the lateral recess and exit foramen are narrowed to some extent.

Graf Band

The Graf band consists of titanium pedicle screws interconnected with braided polypropylene. The device maintains two adjacent vertebrae in extension. The posterior prestress so generated is calculated to be between 5 to 10 kg and stabilizes the posterior facet joints in extension, minimizing rotatory movement and "distraction" of the facet joints. During the first 2 to 3 months, a progressive viscoelastic adaptation of the remaining disc takes place and a new range of movement of several degrees. However, this has the theoretic disadvantage of overloading the posterior annulus, which is associated with a painful disc. According to some authors (4), application of the Graf ligament transfers the load to the posterior annulus and also produces a significant increase in lateral canal stenosis, especially if any preexisting degenerative change in the facet joints or folding of the ligamentum flavum is present.

Clinical Results

Early results of the Graf ligament were encouraging, as described by Gardner and Pande (2) and Markwalder and Merat (7), although these authors reviewed only 27 patients after 1 year; results were good or excellent in 74% of the patients. As in the initial report by Graf, 120 patients with a follow-up of 6 to 24 months were evaluated; 80% were satisfied, whereas 20% reported the result to be "passable or mediocre" (5). In the series reported by Grevitt at al. (4), excellent or good results were obtained in 72% of the patients, at the cost of a 34% revision rate, and a downward trend in Oswestry Disability Index scores was noted after surgery. It is noteworthy that the most common complication they reported was postoperative radicular pain (24%).

However, mid- to long-term results are different, as described by Rigby at al. (9) in 51 of 69 patients reviewed. After 50 months of follow-up, the authors described an overall reoperation rate of 21%, including seven patients who required a bony fusion procedure. Gardner and Pande (2) reported the first 50 patients who underwent surgery; after 7 years of follow-up, 31 still had the Graf ligament in situ, and excellent and good subjective results were reported in 62%. Only 61% reported significant or total relief of low back pain; the mean Oswestry Disability Index score was 59 preoperatively and 37.7 after 7 years.

RETROSPECTIVE STUDIES WITH COMPARISON OF OTHER SURGICAL METHODS

Hadlow et al. (5) published the results of a retrospective, nonrandomized case control comparison between the Graf ligamentoplasty procedure and instrumented posterolateral fusion. The Graf ligamentoplasty was associated with a worse outcome at 1 year and a significantly higher revision rate at 2 years.

Konno and Kikuchi (6) performed a prospective study of patients with degenerative spondylolisthesis who underwent decompression with or without stabilization by means of the Graf system. Although lumbar Graf stabilization did not prevent the recurrence of leg symptoms, a significant reduction of low back pain was noted at 1- and 3-year follow-up.

Our experience included 30 patients operated on between 1990 and 1995. All patients presented with segmental instability associated with sudden episodes of low back pain and decoaptation on flexion–extension x-ray films. The patients were enrolled very selectively and were offered facet blocks, pantaloon casts, and rehabilitation. We performed only Graf stabilization without any decompression. After 8 years of follow-up, we observed excellent or good results in 65%, but three patients had undergone reoperation; assessment with SpineView software (Surgiview, Paris, France) revealed no or few intervertebral mobility in flexion–extension analysis.

Complications not specific to the Graf system included neurologic problems related to pedicle screw insertion. In the study of Esses et al. (1), the rate ranged from 1.7% to 22.5%. In a review of nearly 5,000 pedicle screws, Lonstein et al. noted malposition in 2.8% of the screws inserted, but only 0.2% of the screws caused nerve root irritation requiring screw revision or removal, as cited by Markwalder and Merat (7).

DISCUSSION AND CONCLUSIONS

Graf ligamentoplasty is quicker, less invasive, and in experienced hands less prone to cause complications than spinal fusion, being a simpler procedure that is less likely to go wrong. Recovery and rehabilitation can proceed more quickly, and most patients are able to resume light work within 6 to 8 weeks. According to many authors, the results of Graf stabilization are inferior to those of fusion or are not sustained; mid- to long-term results have been disappointing in comparison with the published data on spinal fusion (8). Significant spondylolisthesis and severe degenerative disc disease with secondary bone changes are problems requiring spinal fusion. However, flexible stabilization merits consideration when the symptomatic disc can be identified with reasonable certainty, and in young and active patients, we have obtained satisfactory results after the application of strict selection criteria.

SAMPLE CASE

A 52-year-old woman presented with the sudden onset of severe back pain. Instability in flexion and a degenerate disc with arthritis of facet joint were identified (Fig. 20.2 A–E).

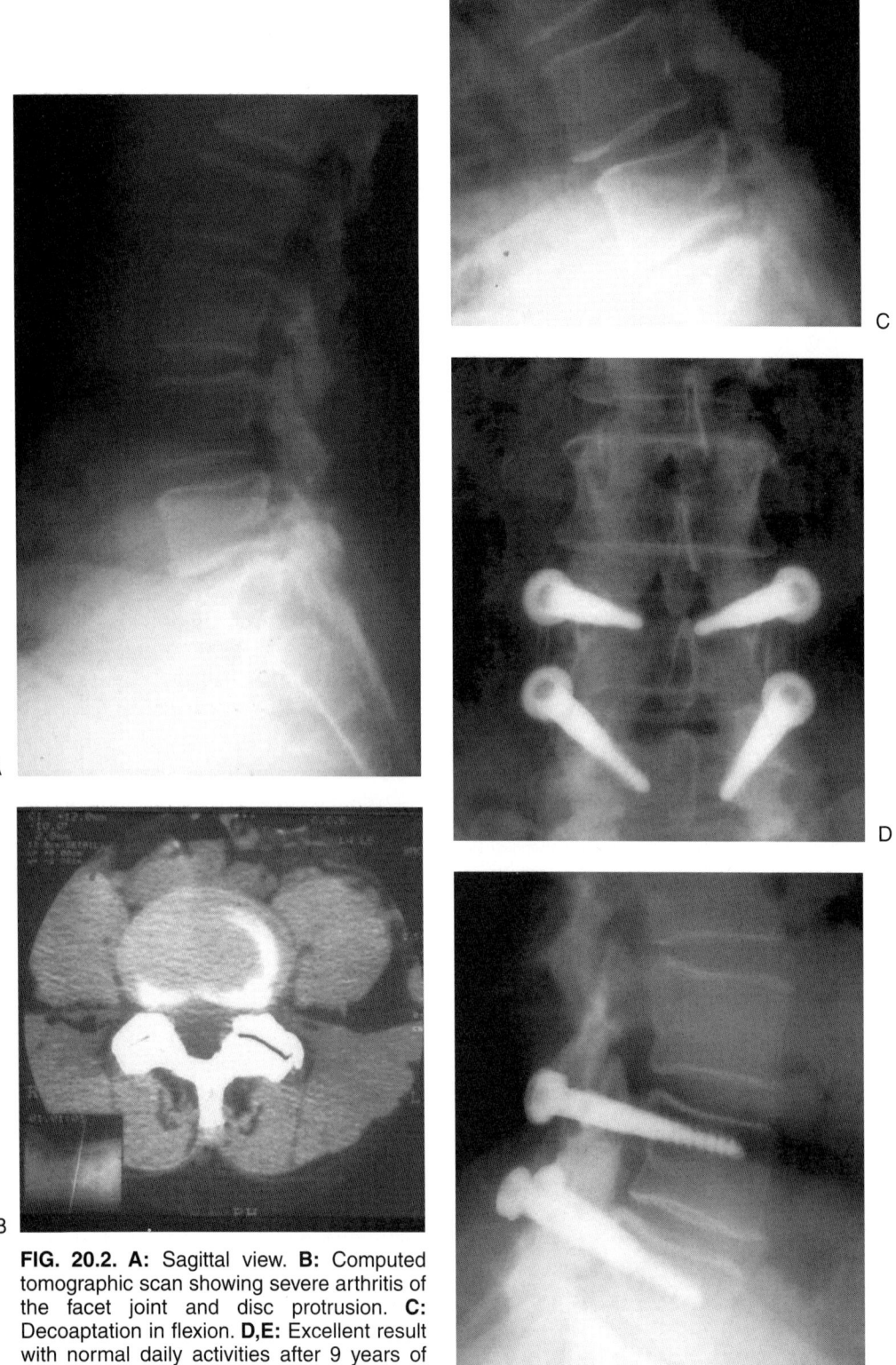

FIG. 20.2. A: Sagittal view. **B:** Computed tomographic scan showing severe arthritis of the facet joint and disc protrusion. **C:** Decoaptation in flexion. **D,E:** Excellent result with normal daily activities after 9 years of follow-up.

COMPUTER-ASSISTED EVALUATION OF INTERVERTEBRAL STABILITY

Purpose and Principles

The accurate and reproducible measurement of intervertebral stability and spinal posture may be one of the major challenges in spinal surgery and biomechanics during the next decade. Indeed, the functional purpose of a restabilization or fusion procedure is to stabilize or fuse spinal segments. Therefore, the best way to measure the efficacy of such procedures objectively, in addition to clinical examination and follow-up, is to quantify their effect on intervertebral motion and spinal posture quickly and reliably.

Software such as SpineView has been developed to address these needs. To be really efficient, computer-aided measurement tools must be analyzed together with the clinical data so that biomechanical parameters can be correlated with clinical information. Two types of analyses are available:

1. Measurements of intervertebral mobility (Fig. 20.3).
   Principles. The vertebrae are contoured semiautomatically within less than 3 minutes. Kinetic parameters (intervertebral range of motion, coordinates of the mean centers of rotation, anteroposterior translation) are then instantaneously computed and exported into the patient file during the relevant clinical examination.
2. Measurements of spinal posture (Fig. 20.4).
   Principles. The vertebral plates are digitized within a few minutes. Postural pelvic and spinal parameters (e.g., sacral slope, lordosis, kyphosis) are then instantaneously computed and exported into the patient file during the relevant clinical examination.

Posterolateral Fusion

These technologies have been used to evaluate spinal motion and posture before and after osteosynthesis.

Before Surgery

Figure 20.5 shows the range of motion for each lumbar segment in a population of 120 patients with degenerative spinal disease (isthmic spondylolisthesis, discopathy without spondylolisthesis, discopathy with spondylolisthesis, disc hernia with previous nucleotomy, disc hernia with previous discectomy, and disc hernia without previous surgery). The red lines show the minimum and maximum values for normal asymptomatic subjects (synthesis of the literature). We see that the pathologic segments are clearly hypomobile. We also see that disease is concentrated near the lumbosacral junction.

After Surgery

We can study the effect of segment fixation in terms of range of motion and function of the type of implant. Figure 20.6 shows that the four types of implant used in this series (frame/wire, dynamic rod, plate, and classic rod) significantly reduce the range of motion 6 months postoperatively. We also see that the greatest range motion in the L4–5 fixed segments is approximately 10 degrees and corresponds to a frame/wire fixation. However, no major differences in stabilization capabilities are seen.

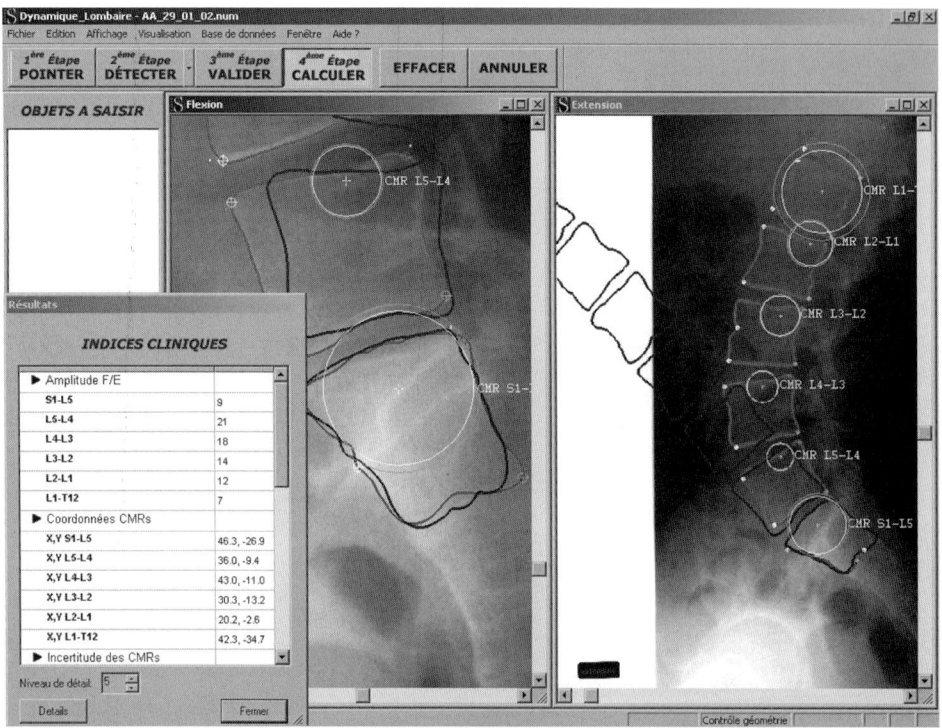
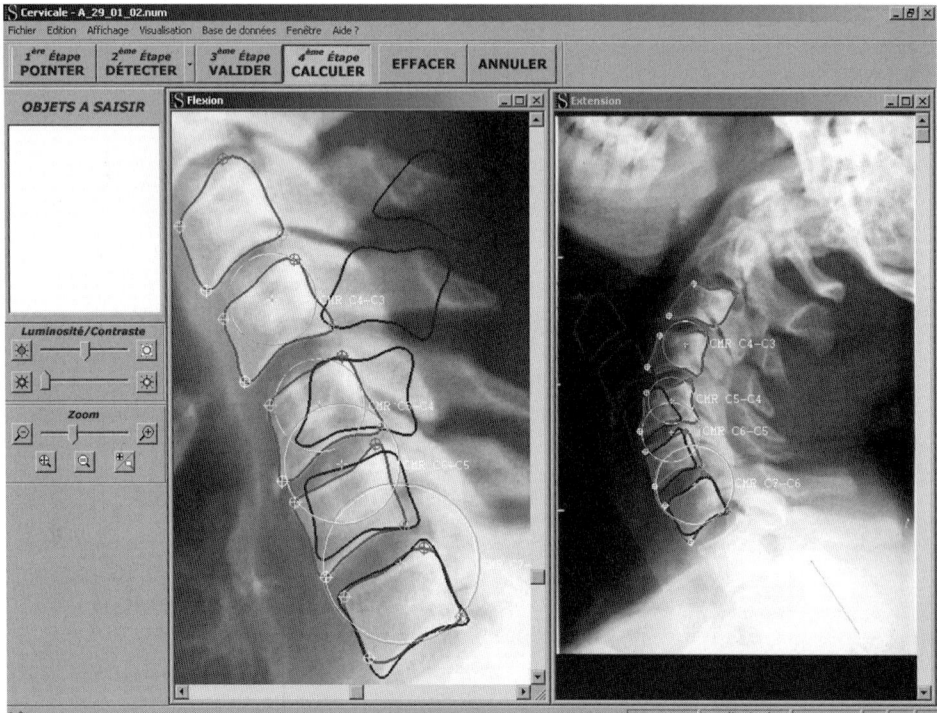

FIG. 20.3. A and B: Measurements of intervertebral mobility.

A B

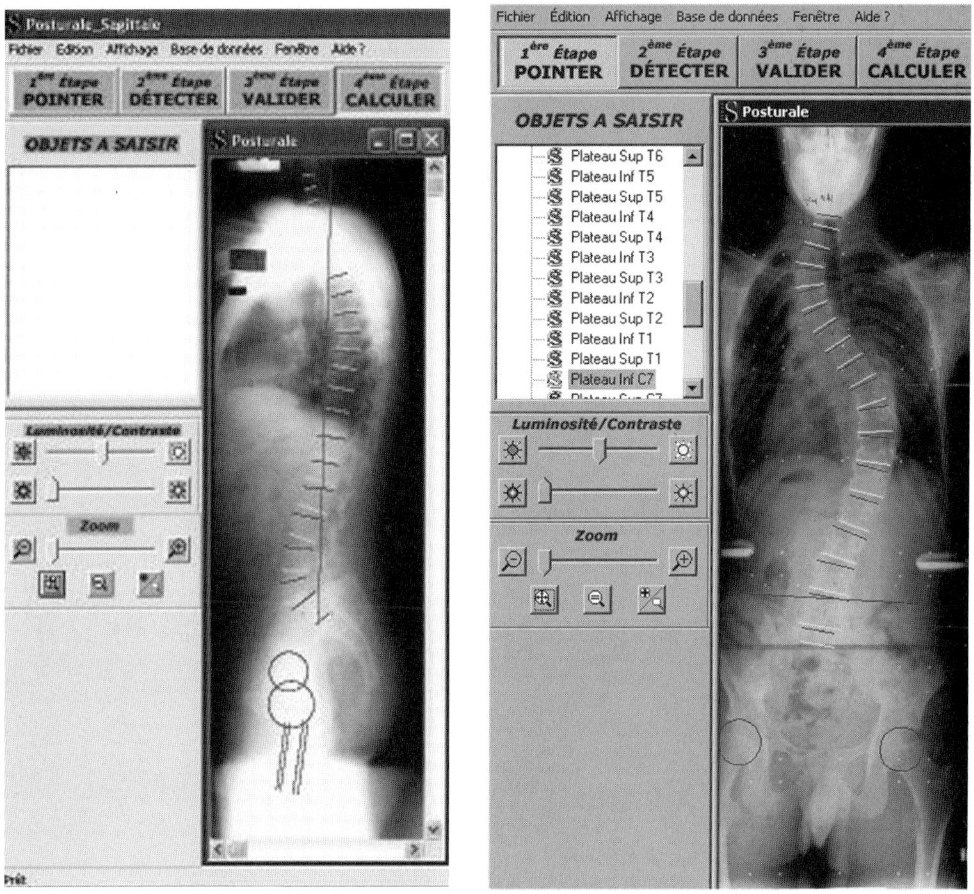

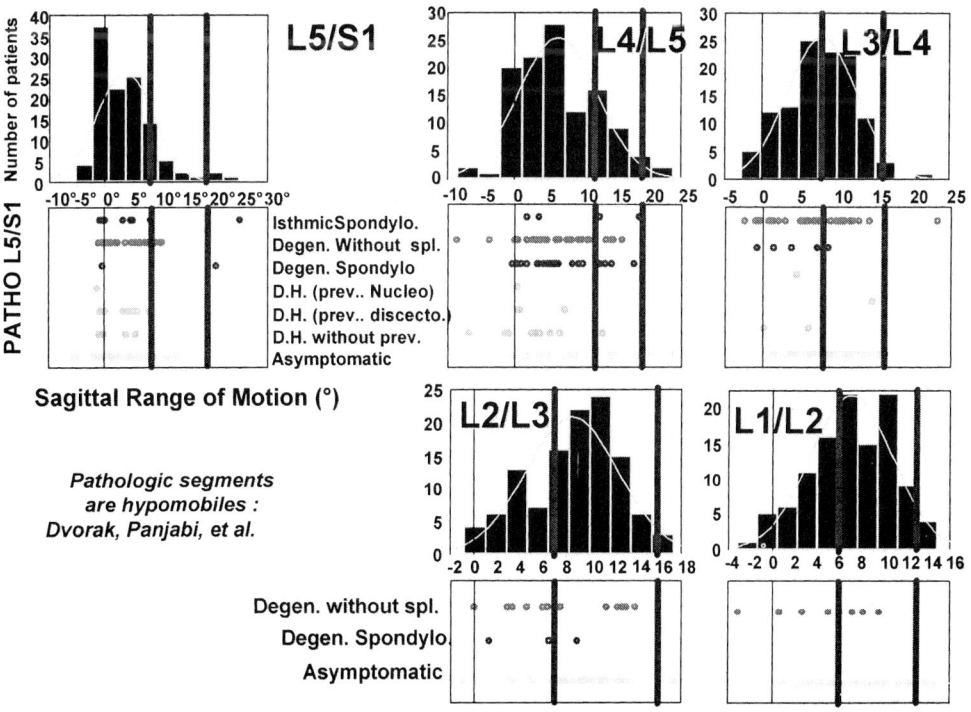

FIG. 20.4. A and B: Measurements of spinal posture.

FIG. 20.5. Range of motion before surgery.

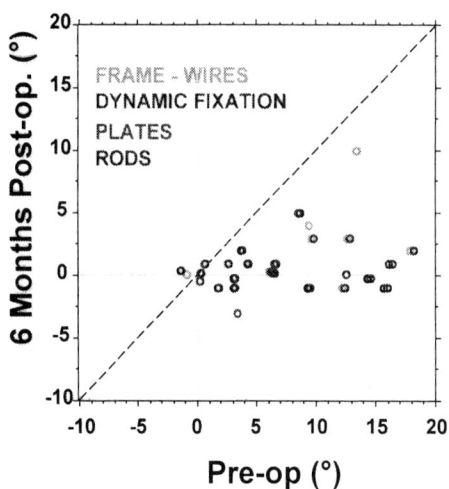

FIG. 20.6. Range of motion after surgery.

Ligamentoplasty

Patient 1 postoperatively (Fig. 20.7):
Woman, 62 years old.
Dysfunction above sacralized L5.
Follow-up, 8 years (good result).
Objective range of motion: L5–S1, 9 degrees; L4–5, 0 degrees; L3–4, 7 degrees.

Figure 20.7 shows the vertebral contours of the flexion picture and the extension picture, with S1 as a reference. We see that the L4–5 instrumented segment is completely

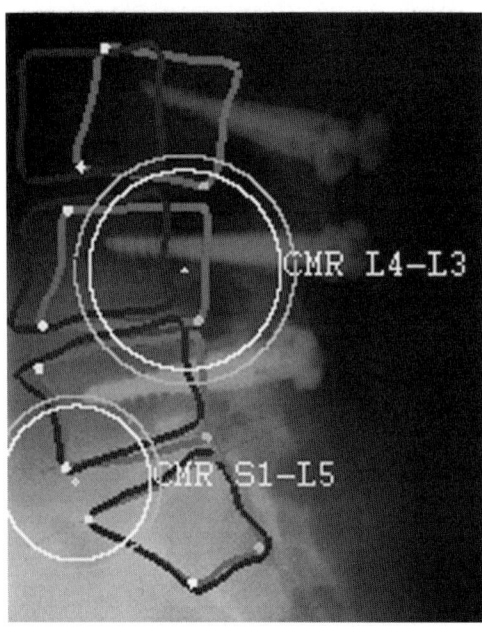

FIG. 20.7. Example of postoperative assessment with flexion–extension test.

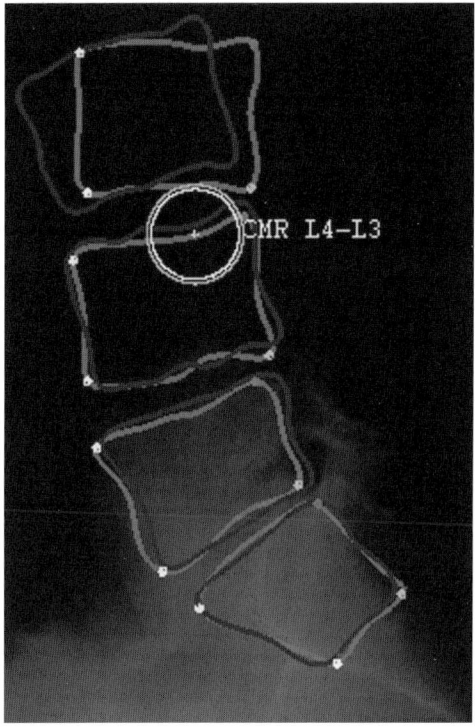

FIG. 20.8. Example of preoperative segmental mobility at level L4–5.

fixed, whereas L5–S1 has a 9-degree range of flexion–extension, with an anterior mean center of rotation (the anterior part of the disc seems abnormally stiff). L3–4, which is also instrumented, still has 7 degrees of mobility.

Patient 2 preoperatively (Fig. 20.8):
Man, 48 years old.
Typical dysfunction L4–5.
Follow-up, 10 years (good result).
Objective range of motion: L5–S1, 0 degrees; L4–5, 3 degrees; L3–4, 13 degrees; L2–3, not in picture.

Figure 20.8 shows the vertebral contours of the flexion picture and the extension picture, with S1 as a reference. L4–5 and L5–S1 have no significant motion, whereas L3–4 is moving normally, with a normally located center of rotation.

REFERENCES

1. Esses SI, Sachs BL, Dreyzin V. Complications associated with the technique of pedicle screw fixation. *Spine* 1993;18:2231–2239.
2. Gardner A, Pande KC. Graf ligamentoplasty: a 7-years follow-up. *Eur Spine J* 2002;11[Suppl 2]:157–163.
3. Graf H. Instabilité vertébrale. Traitement à l'aide d'un système souple. *Rachis* 1992;4;2:123–137.
4. Grevitt MP, Gardner AD, Spilsbury J, et al. The Graf stabilization system: early results in 50 patients. *Eur Spine J* 1995;4:169–175.
5. Hadlow SV, Fagon AB, Hillier TM, et al. The Graf ligamentoplasty procedure. Comparison with posterolateral fusion in the management of low back pain. *Spine* 1998;23:1172–1179.
6. Konno S, Kikuchi S. Prospective study of surgical treatment of degenerative spondylolisthesis. *Spine* 2000;24;12:1533–1137.

7. Markwalder TM, Merat M. The lumbar and lumbosacral facet syndrome. Diagnostic measure, surgical treatment and results in 119 patients. *Acta Neurochir* 1994;124:40–45.
8. Markwalder TM, Dubach R, Braun M. Soft system stabilization of the lumbar spine as an alternative surgical modality to lumbar arthrodesis in the facet syndrome. *Acta Neurochir* 1995;134:1–4.
9. Rigby MC, Selmon GP, Foy MA, et al. Graf ligament stabilization: mid- to long-term follow-up. *Eur Spine J* 2001;10:234–236.

21

Characterization of a Synthetic Bioactive Spinal Interbody Device

Gina M. Nagvajara, James P. Murphy, Theodore D. Clineff, and Erik M. Erbe

Orthovita, Inc., Malvern, Pennsylvania

Degenerative disc disease (DDD) of the cervical spine results in approximately 130,000 cervical fusion surgeries in the United States each year. Conservative therapy usually consists of the intermittent application of heat, bed rest, rehabilitative exercise, and medications to relieve pain, muscle spasm, and inflammation. When this regimen fails to bring relief after a minimum of 6 weeks, cervical discectomy accompanied by spinal fusion through the use of an interbody fusion device (IBFD) may be prescribed. The purpose of the IBFD is to provide stability between two vertebrae during the spinal fusion process. Spinal fusion is considered to be the standard of care in the surgical management of DDD.

Cervical, thoracic, and lumbar spinal fusions have been safely and effectively performed for many years, and the procedure has been extensively documented in the scientific and medical literature. Historically, spinal fusion has been achieved through the use of structural autograft or allograft bone implants. The use of screws and plates to improve stability and prevent implant migration was introduced more than 40 years ago. Advances in technology have led to the development of metal and carbon fiber–reinforced IBFDs for the treatment of DDD. Although frequently used, each of these materials has its own set of limitations with regard to the ideal IBFD.

An ideal IBFD should have the following mechanical and material characteristics:

- Sufficient mechanical strength.
- A modulus of elasticity that allows appropriate load sharing. If the device is too stiff, lack of load sharing may result in graft resorption without ingrowth of new bone; if it is too flexible, macromotion may cause a pseudarthrosis to develop.
- Radiodensity that allows visualization of implant placement and simultaneous direct visualization of the grafted areas.
- Bioactivity that enhances fusion by allowing the implant to become incorporated into the surrounding bone.
- Biocompatibility.

SPINAL IMPLANT MATERIALS

Present-day IBFD materials include tricortical autograft, allograft, titanium, and carbon fiber–reinforced polyetheretherketone (CF/PEEK). In addition, various investigational materials, such as hydroxyapatite/tricalcium phosphate, porous tantalum, and polylactic acid/polyglycolic acid resorbable polymers, are currently being evaluated. Although these materials are promising, none can be considered ideal.

Structural autograft, the current gold standard, theoretically has the ideal stiffness to allow effective load sharing and the ideal radiodensity to allow assessment of the fusion mass. However, the use of autogenous bone exposes the patient to a second surgical procedure, with pain and morbidity at the donor site. Allograft devices also are of ideal stiffness and radiopacity, but they carry the risk for disease transmission, are restricted in terms of variations in shape and size, have suboptimal strength properties that decrease after implantation, and vary in quality because the product is natural. Furthermore, because companies that provide allograft implants obtain their supply from donor tissue banks, supply tends to be limited. Titanium has long been used in orthopedics and can be machined into a variety of shapes and sizes, but it is very stiff and radiodense. CF/PEEK and pure PEEK are less stiff than metals, but implants made of these materials are radiolucent and can be hard to locate on x-ray films without the use of beads. Also, they promote fibrous tissue encapsulation rather than bone bonding.

In the early 1990s, Orthovita (Malvern, PA, U.S.A.) began to develop spinal implant materials and devices that would overcome some of the shortcomings of available materials and devices. Rhakoss Synthetic Bone Spinal Implant is currently undergoing clinical trials.

Rhakoss is a polymer matrix composite of bioactive and nonbioactive fillers. Its mechanical and material properties have been specifically engineered for use in spinal implantation—its compressive strength, tensile strength, and elasticity are very similar to those of cortical bone. The implant survives compressive loads beyond those that occur in the human cervical spine and meets the compressive fatigue requirements of an IBFD. The radiodensity of Rhakoss has been engineered to allow good visualization of the device following implantation and to facilitate the visualization of bone formation at the grafted sites. The components of the material have an extensive history of safe use in medical devices (3–6,8,9,11,12). The implant is synthetic and supplied in a sterile state, and material quality is controlled, so disease transmission is not a risk. Together with a synthetic bone graft, this synthetic construct eliminates the need for autogenous bone harvest.

Radiopacity

The radiopacity of materials intended for medical use is clinically important because roentgenography is frequently applied to measure their placement, function, form, and effectiveness. Fusion is typically assessed radiographically. Autograft bone and allograft bone are currently the most optimal radiodense materials. In contrast, the radiodensity of metals limits the radiographic evaluation of devices made of them (Fig. 21.1).

A new synthetic spinal implant material has been engineered to allow visualization of the device following implantation, in addition to bone formation at the grafted site (Fig. 21.2). Results of a quantitative evaluation of radiopacity of this material indicate an average radiopacity value of 42.9 ±1.0. This value compares favorably with that of human bone, which has a radiopacity between 27 and 51 (2) (Fig. 21.3).

As seen in Figures 21.1 and 21.2, the radiopacity of Rhakoss allows visualization of the implant between adjacent vertebral bodies, in addition to the eventual visualization and assessment of fusion on a medial–lateral radiograph. The similar radiopacity of an implant made of allograft bone and one made of Rhakoss is shown in Figure 21.3, which also illustrates the improved consistency and homogeneity of a synthetic material in comparison with allograft bone.

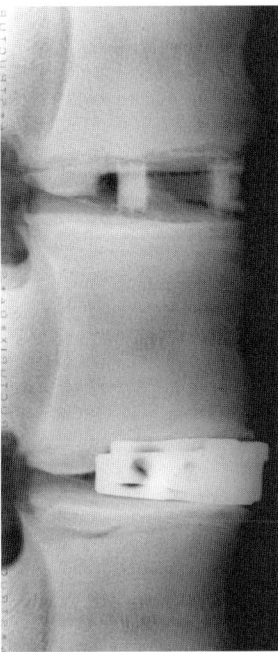

FIG. 21.1. Radiopacity of Rhakoss implant (*top*) and titanium implant (*bottom*).

Mechanical Properties

In addition to optimal radiopacity, spinal implant materials should possess mechanical properties that enable them to withstand the various physiologic loads and motions of the spine. The ideal IBFD should be able to restore disc height, lordosis, and sagittal alignment and to provide stability. Table 21.1 compares some of the mechanical properties of

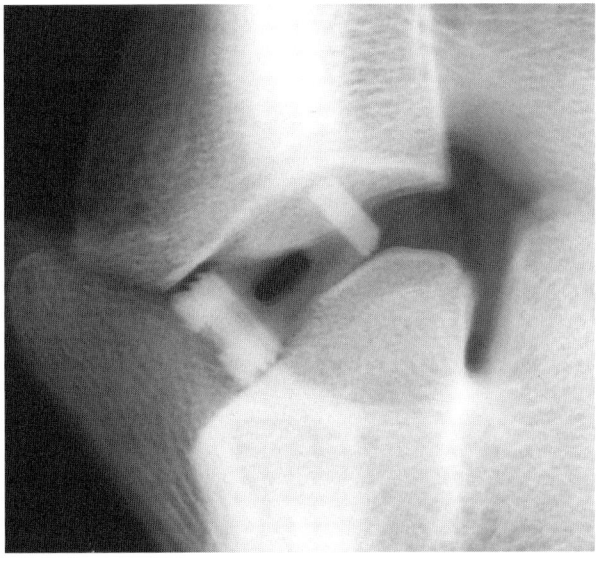

FIG. 21.2. Radiopacity of Rhakoss implant in a sheep spine.

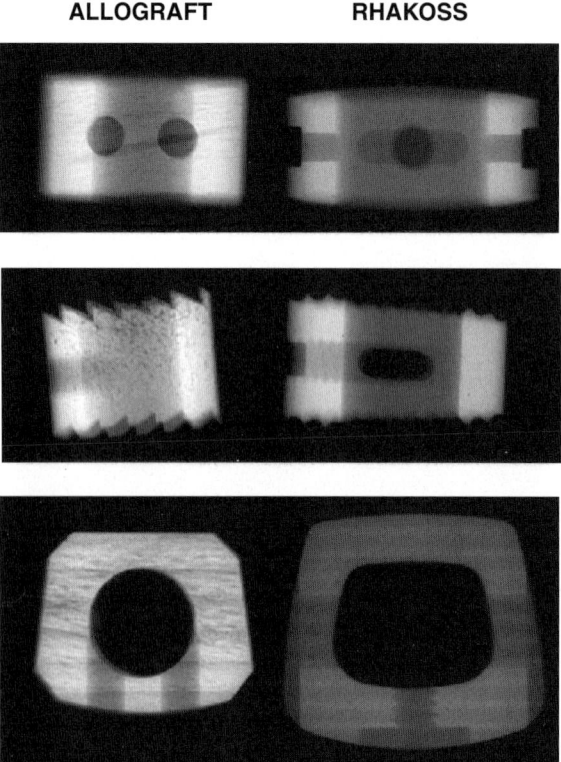

FIG. 21.3. Radiographs of an implant made of allograft bone **(left side)** versus an implant made of Rhakoss **(right side)**.

human cortical bone with those of Rhakoss, titanium, and CF/PEEK, for which data were available.

The mechanical properties of Rhakoss are well matched with those of human cortical bone. It should be noted that the compressive modulus of Rhakoss was engineered to be lower that that of bone to avoid the stress shielding effect.

TABLE 21.1. *Mechanical properties of spinal implant materials*

Property	Human cortical bone literature	Rhakoss[a]	Titanium[a]	CF/PEEK[a]
Compressive strength (MPa)	167–215 (1)	239.2 ± 14.4	—	262
Compressive modulus (GPa)	14.7–19.7 (1)	8.0 ± 1.0	—	—
Compressive yield strength (MPa)	121–182 (1)	177.5 ± 20.7	860	240
Tensile strength (MPa)	70–140 (1)	85.2 ± 10.2	860	225
Tensile elastic modulus (GPa)	10.9–14.8 (1)	15.8 ± 1.8	—	—
Three-point flexural strength (MPa)	103–238 (1)	112.4 ± 8.1	—	355
Shear by punch tool (MPa)	51.6 (10)	69.5 ± 8.7	—	—
Compressive fatigue strength (10^6 cycles) (MPa)	<100 (7)	180 ± 5	300	—
Tensile fatigue strength (10^6 cycles) (MPa)	49 (14)	45 ± 5	—	—

[a]Rhakoss values were obtained by following the ASTM standard for each test parameter. Titanium values are for Ti-6Al-4V (grade 5), extra-low intersititial, annealed; CF/PEEK values are for Victrex PEEK 150CA30, 30% carbon fiber reinforced (13).

ASTM, American Society for Testing and Materials; CF/PEEK, carbon fiber–filled polyetheretherketone.

BIOACTIVITY: A CASE STUDY

Bioactivity can be defined as the ability of a material to interact chemically with, and bond to, surrounding bone. A unique characteristic of Rhakoss is its ability to bond directly with bone. *In vitro*, this property can be measured by quantitatively analyzing the ability of Rhakoss to form a calcium phosphate layer on its surface when immersed in simulated body fluid.

Thin discs and implants of Rhakoss were placed in simulated body fluid at 37°C for up to 50 days. Each sample was evaluated at various time periods. Nondestructive Fourier transform infrared spectroscopy (FTIR) was used to note spectral similarities between hydroxyapatite and the deposited layer on Rhakoss, and scanning electron microscopy/energy dispersive spectroscopy (SEM/EDS) was used to note the appearance of calcium phosphate deposition, determine the thickness of the calcium phosphate layer, and detect the presence of calcium and phosphorus and reduced sodium levels at a bioactive filler.

Early results of FTIR showed few spectral changes in the material. The day 6 sample showed the same type of strong organic absorption as the day 0 sample. However, as early as day 14, the sample exhibited a surface coating of calcium phosphate, which thickened with time. By day 50, spectra taken at various locations on the material showed only inorganic phosphate absorbencies, and none of the organic bands seen in the early samples (days 0 and 6). The depth of penetration for this FTIR technique is 2 µm. This indicates that the thickness of the calcium phosphate growth is *at least* 2 µm. The day 50 spectra were compared with several reference spectra standards of calcium phosphates. The best spectral match for both samples was hydroxyapatite (Fig. 21.4). The close match indicates that hydroxyapatite is the calcium phosphate species growing on the sample surface. The primary hydroxyapatite band seen occurs at approximately 1014 cm^{-1}. This band demonstrates a more resolved hydroxyapatite shoulder at 955 cm^{-1}, pointing to a mature species.

Based on SEM, the material demonstrated a calcium phosphate crystal as early as 6 days, confirmed by EDS analysis. In the day 6 sample, growth was limited to a few bioac-

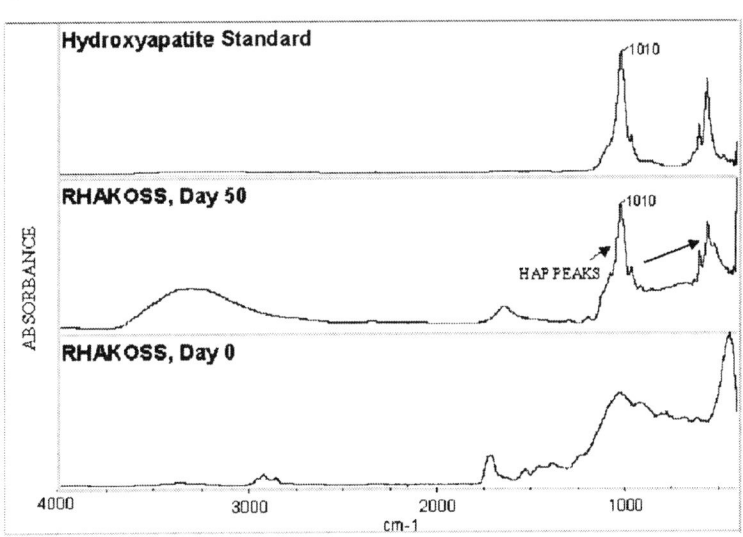

FIG. 21.4. Fourier transform infrared spectroscopy showing a close match of Rhakoss with hydroxyapatite by day 50.

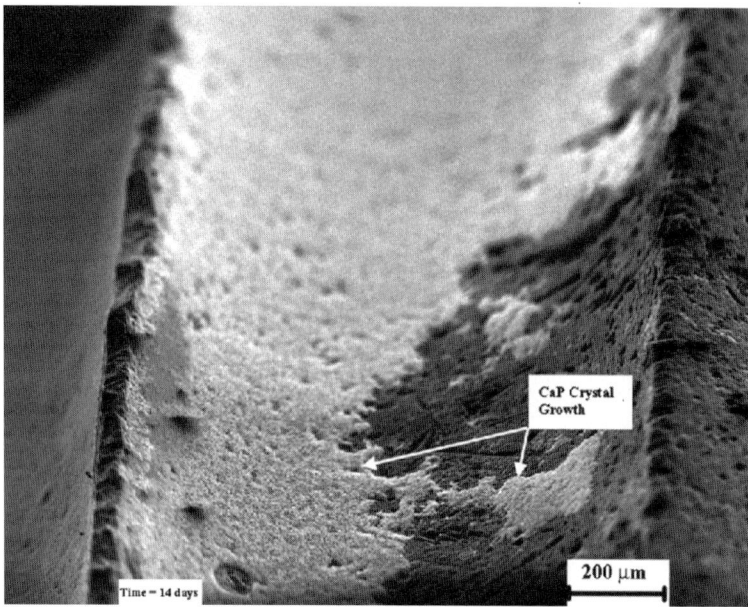

FIG. 21.5. Scanning electron microscopy showing calcium phosphate layer on the surface of the Rhakoss implant by day 14.

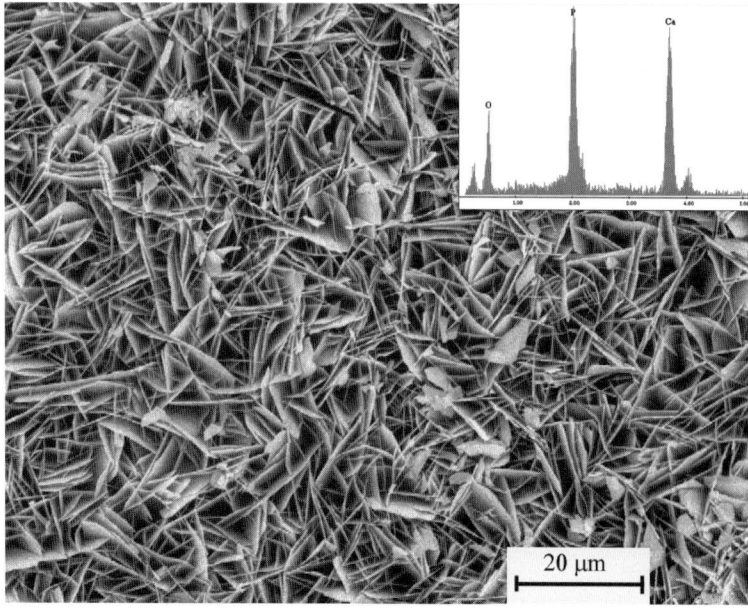

FIG. 21.6. Calcium phosphate layer formed on the surface of Rhakoss *in vitro* in simulated body fluid. Energy dispersive spectroscopy **(inset)** reveals that the calcium and phosphate composition of this layer resembles that of hydroxyapatite.

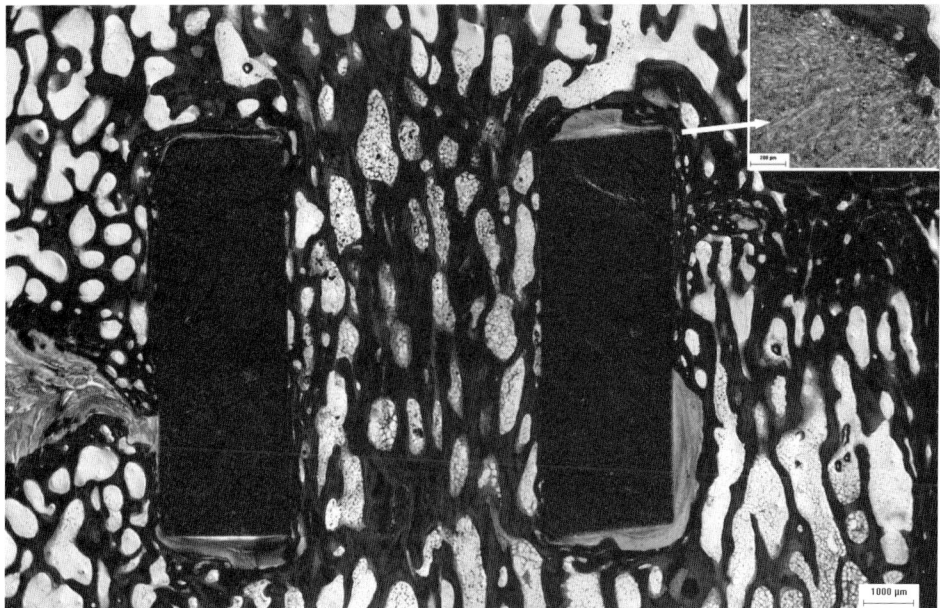

FIG. 21.7. Histologic section of a Rhakoss spinal implant shows bone bonding and fusion through the center of the implant (original magnification ×75). **Inset:** High-magnification image shows incorporation of bone implant.

tive fillers. The day 14 sample showed a layer of calcium phosphate (Fig. 21.5), and by day 50, the material exhibited a thicker, denser layer of calcium phosphate. Again, this layer covered the entire surface of the composite.

The calcium phosphate crystals were mature, with the appearance of stacked plates. The calcium phosphate was determined to have a thickness of approximately 10 µm and was interdigitated with bioactive fillers at the surface of the composite. Figure 21.6 illustrates the calcium phosphate crystals on the surface of Rhakoss. The evaluation of cross-sectional samples allowed an accurate measurement of the thickness of the calcium phosphate. Also, the calcium phosphate layer was evaluated for interdigitation with the composite. Several observations of calcium phosphate migrating into bioactive ceramic fillers at the surface were made. Based on these results, Rhakoss can be described as bioactive.

The bioactive nature of Rhakoss has also been observed *in vivo*. Figure 21.7 shows bone bonding adjacent to, and through the center of, a specifically designed Rhakoss spinal implant for the lumbar region of a sheep at 1 year.

CONCLUSION

Spinal fusion is the main treatment option for patients with back pain who do not experience relief after conservative therapy. In current fusion procedures, materials are used that are less than optimal in terms of the ideal IBFD.

A new material for interbody fusion has been developed with favorable mechanical properties and a radiodensity engineered for the evaluation of spinal fusion and implant placement. It is biologically capable of bonding to host bone and is biocompatible.

REFERENCES

1. An Y, et al. *Mechanical testing of bone*. Boca Raton, FL: CRC Press, 2000.
2. Brantigan JW, et al. Compression strength of donor bone for posterior lumbar interbody fusion. *Spine* 1993;18:1213–1221.
3. Brantigan JW, et al. Interbody lumbar fusion using a carbon fiber cage implant versus allograft bone. An investigational study in the Spanish goat. *Spine* 1994;19:1436–1444.
4. Corvelli AA, et al. Characterization of a PEEK composite segmental bone replacement implant. *J Materials Sci* 1999;34:2421–2431.
5. Costamagna G, et al. Hydrophilic hydromer-coated polyurethane stents versus uncoated stents in malignant biliary obstruction: a randomized trial. *Gastrointest Endosc* 2000;51:8–11.
6. Narva KK, et al. Clinical survey of acrylic resin removable denture repairs with glass-fiber reinforcement. *Int J Prosthod* 2001;14:219–224.
7. Pattin CA, et al. Cyclic mechanical degradation. *J Biomech* 1996;29:69–79.
8. Schulte M, et al. Anterior cervical fusion using preserved bone allografts. *Transplant Proc* 1976;8[2 Suppl 1]:73–76.
9. Shaudig U, et al. The polyurethane nasolacrimal duct stent for lower tear duct obstruction: long-term success rate and complication. *Graefes Arch Clin Exp Ophthalmol* 2000;238:733–737.
10. Turner CH, et al. Shear strength and fatigue properties of human cortical bone determined from pure shear tests. *Calcif Tissue Int* 2001;69:373–378.
11. Vallittu PK. Glass fiber reinforcement in repaired acrylic resin removable dentures: preliminary results of a clinical study. *Quintessence Int* 1997;28:39–44.
12. Van Den Hazel SJ, et al. A randomized trial of polyurethane and silicone percutaneous endoscopic gastrostomy catheters. *Aliment Pharmacol Ther* 2000;14:1273–1277.
13. www.matweb.com.
14. Zioupos P, et al. Fatigue test of bone and antler. *J Biomech* 1996;29:989–1002.

22

K-Centrum, a "Zero-Profile" Anterior Spinal Intramedullary Rod Fixation System: Preclinical Testing and Clinical Experience

*Matthew D. Garner and *†Stephen D. Kuslich

*Spineology Inc., Stillwater, Minnesota; and †Department of Orthopedics, University of Minnesota, Minneapolis, Minnesota

Our group has developed a new fixation system for the anterior spine, the *K-Centrum Anterior Spinal Fixation System*. The device provides stable fixation without bulky metal lying near the great vessels. The unique position of the linkage rod creates a load-sharing construct with the interposed bone graft that is designed to reduce metal fatigue and stimulate fusion.

BACKGROUND

The thoracolumbar spine is particularly susceptible to fractures and tumor metastasis as a consequence of the mechanics at the thoracolumbar junction and the dissemination of cancer cells via the vascular and lymphatic drainage of the thorax (4,11). Advances in spinal instrumentation have increased surgeon acceptance of a single-stage anterior procedure to address compression of the spinal cord by either bone fragments or an expanding tumor. This pathology-directed anterior approach is argued to result in a more complete decompression with less risk for further injury to the cord (9,16).

The anterior–posterior procedure, or 360-degree fusion, can yield high fusion rates when used to treat lumbar degenerative disc disease (DDD) (12,19). This combined approach, however, results in relatively long operative times and significant blood loss (5,18), and patient repositioning can be burdensome to operating room personnel. Complete excision of a diseased disc and placement of a load-bearing graft are easier via an anterior approach, but the psoas muscle or pelvic crest may restrict safe implantation of vertebral body screws in a coronal plane. For this reason, the use of currently available anterior fixators is generally limited to L3 and above.

Wenger developed the first anterior spinal fixation system to treat scoliosis in the thoracolumbar spine in 1953 (8,17). Humphries, in 1961, described the application of instrumentation directly to the ventral aspect of the spine to use compression forces and the large area or "interposition" between the graft and the vertebrae (13). Dwyer and Newton (7) attached a cable to a single screw in each vertebral body and applied the system to the convex side of a scoliotic curve. Hall and Micheli (10) and Zielke and Pellin (24) improved on this system by replacing the cable with a single rod. In the early 1980s, Dunn (6) developed one of many large, bulky anterior fixators that was quite stable. Like other anterior fixators, the Dunn device was intended for placement on the lateral aspect of the spine, and when placed too far anteriorly, it caused erosion of the aorta and death in several patients (14). The device was removed from the market. This problem of injury to the great vessels stimulated the development of devices that afford similar stability to the spine but at the same time are lower in profile (15).

K-CENTRUM ANTERIOR SPINAL FIXATION SYSTEM

The K-Centrum is the first anterior fixator that combines the following features:

- *Zero profile.* This feature permits safe implantation into the ventral spine from a lateral, oblique, or even direct midsagittal approach, with less concern for intraoperative and postoperative nerve, soft tissue, or vessel irritation (Fig. 22.1).
- *Bone ingrowth anchors.* Unlike the commonly used small-diameter solid screws and bolts (3), these anchors become firmly incorporated into the vertebral body during the first few weeks or months following surgery. When the anchor is correctly sized for a vertebral body, it engages the dense subchondral bone of the endplates above and below, in addition to the cortical face. The result is a "tricortical" hold on each vertebral body (Fig. 22.2).
- *Single, nonround rod.* The rod is placed near the central axis of the spine. The amount of metal interfering with the vascularization of a graft from surrounding tissues or preventing visualization of the graft on plain x-ray films is minimal.

The assembly consists of two vertebral body bone anchors, a linkage rod, set screws, and locking caps (Fig. 22.3). The system can be adapted for use with a variety of load-sharing grafting techniques:

- Autograft struts
- Bone cement
- Manufactured allograft or ceramic spacers
- Mesh cages filled with autograft, allograft, or ceramic bone substitutes
- Expandable vertebral body replacement devices.

The K-Centrum has received Food and Drug Administration (FDA) and CE Mark clearance for the treatment of tumors, fractures, DDD, pseudarthrosis, spinal stenosis, spondylolisthesis, and spinal deformities. It is approved for implantation in T6 to L5 and can span one or two motion segments. Osteoporosis is a relative contraindication that may limit the effectiveness of spinal instrumentation. Additional posterior fixation may be warranted in cases with three-column spinal instability.

BENCH TESTING

Quasistatic and cyclic load testing of the K-Centrum followed American Society for Testing and Materials (ASTM) F 1717-96 (1), the standard for testing anterior fixation devices. The K-Centrum straight rod was compared with the Z-Plate Thoraco-Lumbar device (Medtronic Sofamor Danek; Memphis, TN, U.S.A.) and the K-Centrum rod bent to 10 degrees. The devices were secured in blocks of ultra–high molecular weight polyethylene (UHMWPE) simulating the vertebral bodies and were tested with no interposed

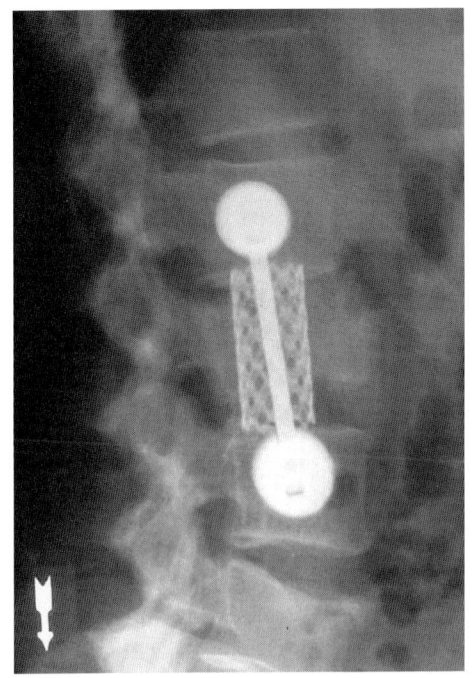
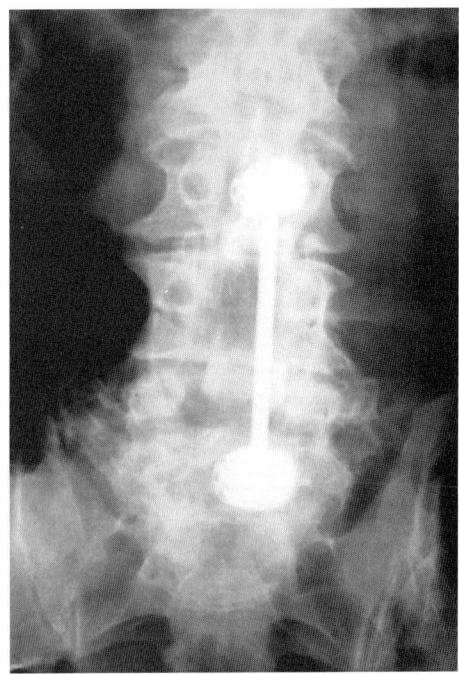
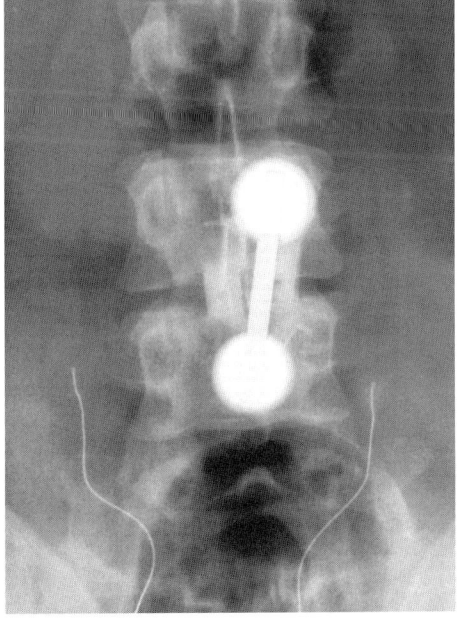

FIG. 22.1. Implant options for K-Centrum system lateral **(A)**, oblique **(B)**, and midsagittal **(C)**. Note that the upper anchor has purposely been displaced laterally to avoid severe retraction of the vena cava. Note easy visualization of interposing graft in all three cases because of the paucity of metal in the area between the anchors.

graft–that is, the test represented a complete, unsupported corpectomy. Test data were also considered in light of the FDA review guidance document for anterior fixators (2).

Figure 22.4 is a summary of ASTM testing (20). These results show that the mechanical performance of the K-Centrum exceeds FDA minimum requirements and is comparable with that of the Z-Plate.

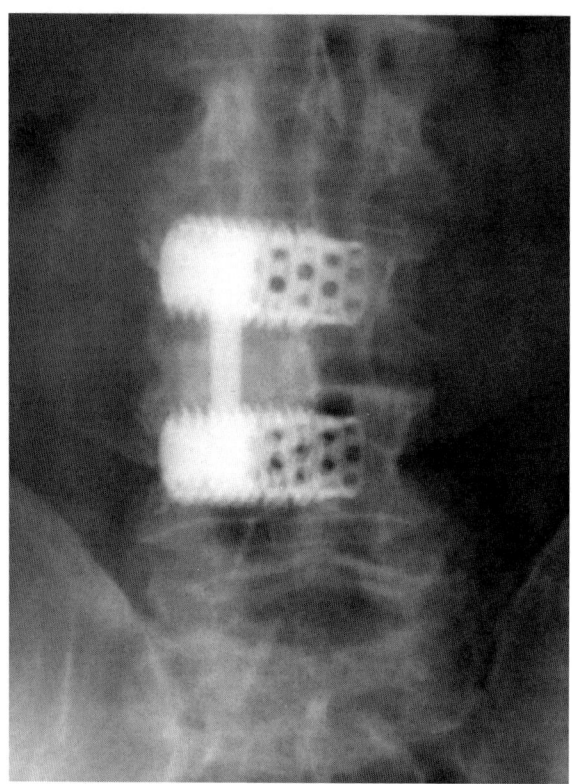

FIG. 22.2. Tricortical hold of vertebral bodies with K-Centrum bone anchors.

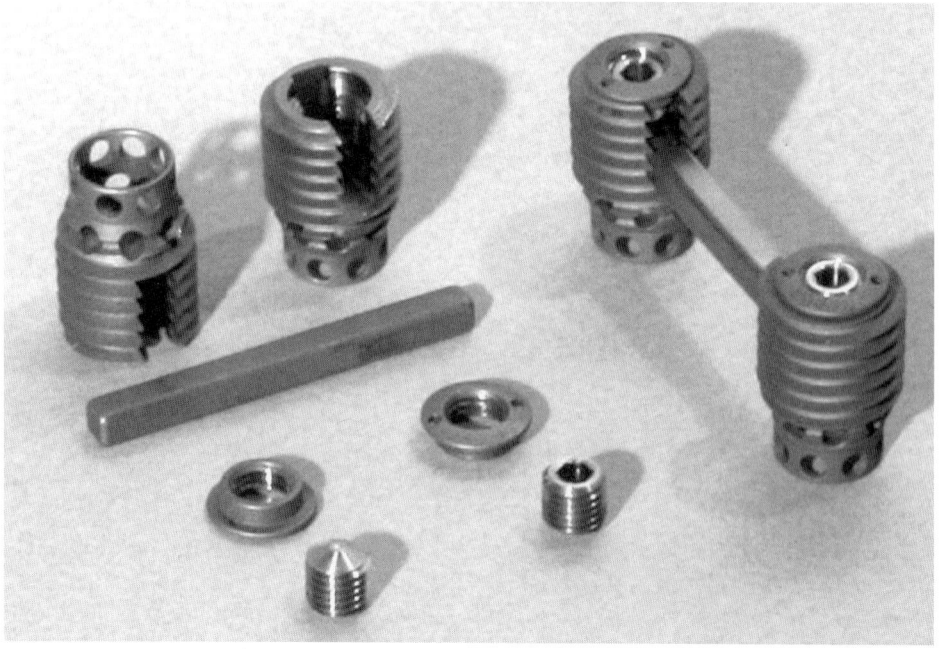

FIG. 22.3. K-Centrum components.

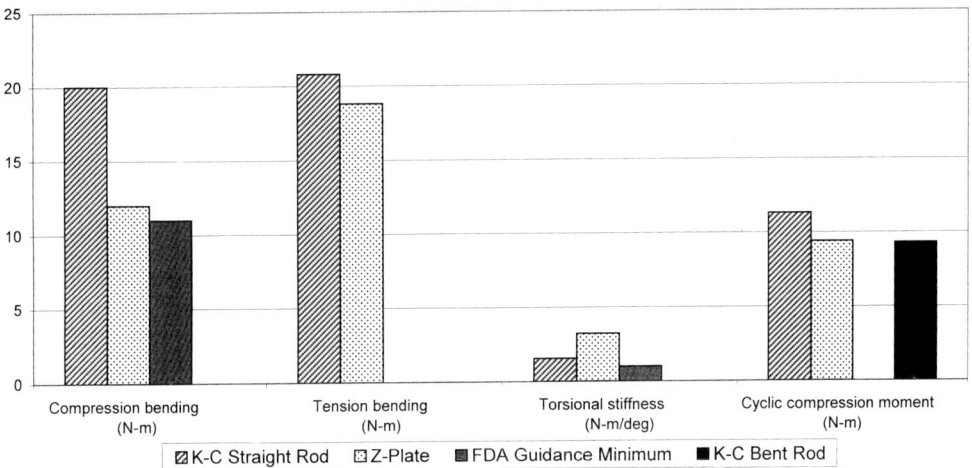

FIG. 22.4. American Society for Testing and Materials bench testing: comparison of K-Centrum (*K-C*) straight rod and bent rod with the Z-Plate.

IN VITRO TESTING

The model used to compare anterior devices for corpectomy constructs consisted of a calf spine; five-vertebrae segments were mounted in a biaxial test fixture (EnduraTec, Minneapolis, MN, U.S.A.). The partially constrained fixture permitted rotation and slight translation out of plane, and eccentric compressive loads were applied to cause bending in each plane. A fixed axis was used in axial rotation testing. The following loads were applied: axial compression to 500 N (Newtons) of flexion–extension, lateral bending to 8 N-m (Newton-meters), and axial rotation to 10 N-m under an axial compressive preload of 110 N. After the intact spine had been tested, a corpectomy was performed, with the posterior elements left intact. The spines were then implanted with the K-Centrum device or Z-Plate; a slotted wooden dowel was used to simulate a structural graft in both cases.

For comparison, the K-Centrum construct for the treatment of lumbar DDD was tested. This model consisted of a four-segment calf spine, with a free disc left above and below the implant construct. A 40-mm rod was used instead of the longer (80 to 90 mm) rods used to test the corpectomy model. Again, a slotted wooden dowel was used to simulate a femoral ring allograft.

Figure 22.5 shows the normalized stiffness results for all three implant constructs (23), which are quite comparable in overall performance. Because of its position on the left side of the spine, the Z-Plate tends to be stiffer when bending to the left. The lateral stiffness of the K-Centrum is approximately the same whether it is bending to the left or right, so that loads tend to be transferred to the graft and the spinal column more symmetrically. In the shorter K-Centrum single-motion segment model, torsional stiffness is fully restored.

Additional testing to evaluate the bone–implant interface showed that the K-Centrum anchor pullout strength is comparable with that of systems in which two convergent screws with bicortical purchase are used (22). Load cells placed between the corpectomy strut graft and the endplate during *in vitro* testing indicate that the bone graft feels additive load with axial compression and bending (21). The bone graft is not "stress-shielded," even though the linkage rod is near the axis of rotation.

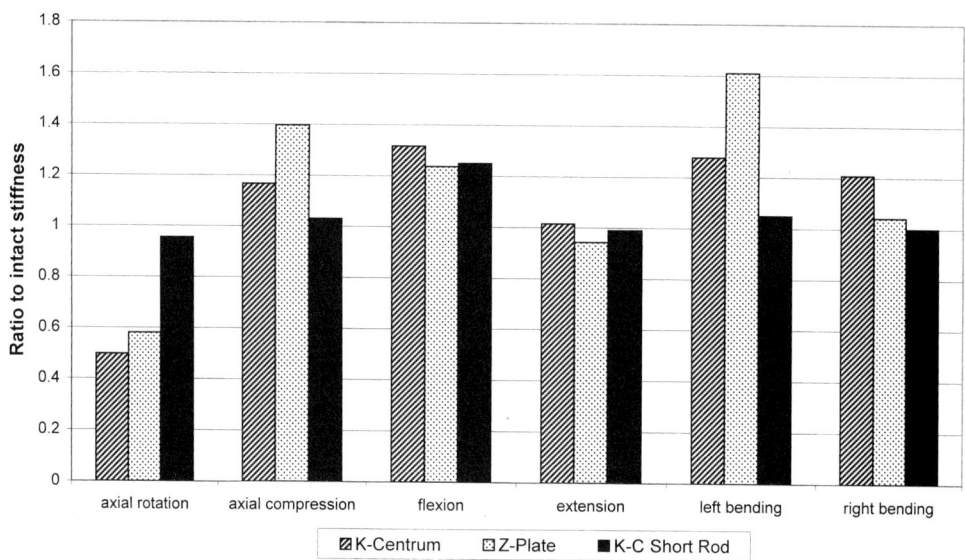

FIG. 22.5. *In vitro* testing. Normalized stiffness results for K-Centrum (*K-C*) corpectomy model, Z-Plate corpectomy model, and K-C single-level model.

TECHNIQUE

The K-Centrum can be applied to the front or side of the vertebral bodies. The incision varies according to the approach, level of pathology, and number of segments involved. When pathology in the thoracic and upper lumbar regions is treated, a lateral thoracotomy or thoracolumbar approach with rib resection is preferred. For L3–L5, a retroperitoneal direct anterior or slightly oblique abdominal approach is used. The great vessels should be adequately protected during implantation.

A system of sophisticated tools allows the surgeon to obtain parallel anchor alignment, distraction and realignment of the spine, and compression of the graft. Intraoperative fluoroscopy is used to monitor alignment of the first anchor relative to the endplates. The alignment tools direct parallel placement and depth of the second anchor.

When fractures resulting from trauma are treated, a complete or partial corpectomy can be performed before or after the placement of both anchors. A load-sharing graft [e.g., iliac crest autograft, femoral ring allograft, mesh cage with autograft, or polymethylmethacrylate (PMMA)] is inserted into the corpectomy defect. The distance between anchor trough ends is measured to determine rod length, which should be 2 to 3 mm short of the actual trough distance to allow room for compression of the construct. The compression tool is used to close the gap at the endplate–bone graft interface and load the graft before the set screws are locked.

Standard interbody grafting techniques with structural autograft or allograft can be used in the treatment of single-level pathology (i.e., DDD or spondylolisthesis). If a femoral ring allograft is used, a slot is cut with a powered burr before the rod is inserted. A simple jig is attached to both anchors to define the bending angle for the rod. This allows placement of the anchors parallel to the endplates with maintenance of lordosis after the construct has been locked. Properly fitted bone grafts that stretch the annulus and manipulation of the operating table can assist in distracting and compressing the construct before the set screws and locking caps are applied.

CLINICAL RESULTS

The original 52 patients (21 women and 31 men) in whom the K-Centrum was implanted ranged in age from 20 to 72 years (mean, 47.6 years). The primary indications were tumor (seven cases), fracture (17 cases), DDD (23 cases), pseudarthrosis (two cases), and vertebral body collapse following osteomyelitis (three cases). Three disc levels were fused in two patients, two levels in 27 patients, and one level in 23 patients. In general, PMMA was used for fill material in the patients with tumor, whereas bone graft (allograft, autograft, or both) was used in the patients with fracture or DDD. Metal mesh cages were used for corpectomy replacements in 19 cases. The K-Centrum was implanted laterally in 33 cases, anteriorly (midsagittal) in 15 cases, and obliquely in four cases. In seven cases, additional posterior spinal fixation was used because of either severe osteoporosis or three-column spinal instability, both of which are contraindications for the use of the system.

The clinical results have been positive, with good relief of preoperative pain and early ambulation and rehabilitation except in patients with concomitant medical conditions. No deaths, instances of surgery-induced paralysis, or cases of deep infection have occurred. In one case, the K-Centrum hardware was removed during repair of a pseudoarthrosis 1 year postoperatively. In this case, the system was implanted without a load-sharing structural graft. In four patients with severe osteoporosis, subsidence of the bone anchors was noted during follow-up. A mesh cage was used as the structural component of the corpus reconstruction in all four cases, which leaves a relatively small support surface at the cage–endplate interface. Three of these patients underwent augmentation with pedicle fixation without further sequelae. The fourth patient was a 72-year-old man with a 20-year history of chronic obstructive pulmonary disease and oral steroid use in whom sudden collapse of L1 resulted in 90% canal compromise and paraplegia. He underwent anterior decompression and stabilization with the K-Centrum and a mesh cage filled with autograft for corpus reconstruction. Approximately 2 weeks postoperatively, the patient fell, and his back pain recurred. Roentgenography revealed collapse of the construct into the neighboring disc spaces. The patient was returned to the operating room for posterior instrumentation, which repositioned the K-Centrum back within the vertebral bodies. At 1-year follow-up, roentgenography revealed solid anterior and posterior fusion.

CLINICAL CASE EXAMPLES

Case 1

A 48-year-old woman, a teaching assistant, presented with severe anemia, progressive back pain of 3 months' duration, and quadriparesis on examination. Blood analysis and magnetic resonance imaging (MRI) confirmed a diagnosis of multiple myeloma and collapse of the L1 vertebral body with 30% canal compromise secondary to tumor. She underwent L1 corpectomy and anterior column reconstruction with the K-Centrum and PMMA in the corpectomy defect. The left extremity weakness resolved immediately postoperatively. Ambulation and rehabilitation were started on postoperative day 2, and she returned to work before her 3-month postoperative follow-up visit. One year postoperatively, roentgenography showed no lucency around the vertebral body anchors, healing bone around the cement, and maintenance of alignment (Fig. 22.6).

Case 2

A 20-year-old man, a window washer, fell 20 feet from a scaffold. He experienced immediate paraplegia, which resolved after approximately 10 minutes. He was able to

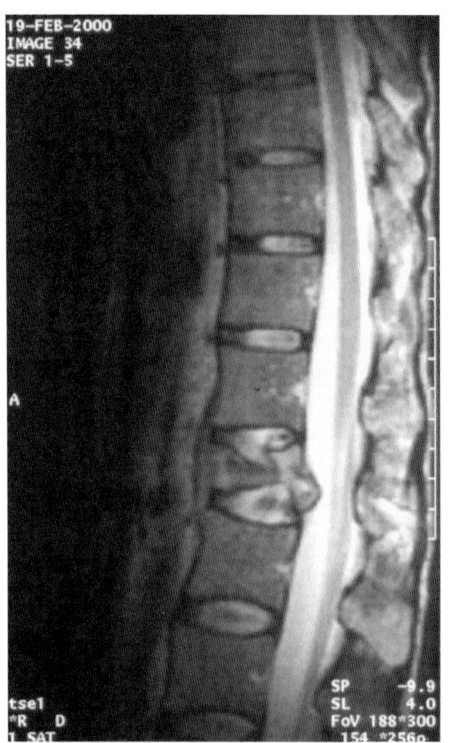
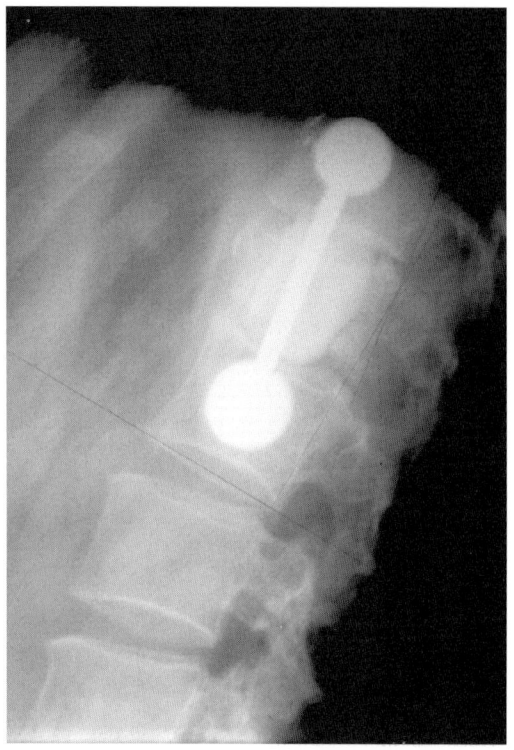
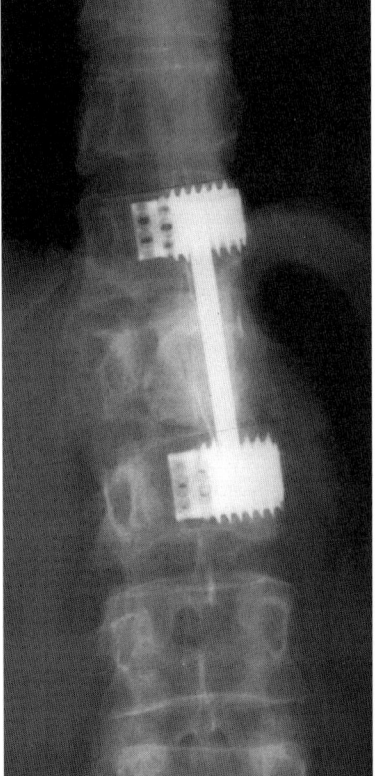

FIG. 22.6. Case 1. **A:** L1 tumor on preoperative magnetic resonance image. **B:** Lateral view 12 months postoperatively. **C:** Anteroposterior view 12 months postoperatively.

ambulate shortly thereafter with severe back pain and some residual numbness in both lower extremities. MRI revealed an L2 burst fracture with 80% canal compromise. He underwent an L2 hemicorpectomy and anterior column reconstruction with the K-Centrum and a mesh cage filled with autograft. He was able to ambulate wearing a thoracolumbo-sacral-orthosis (TLSO) No. 6 on postoperative day 2. He was released to seden-

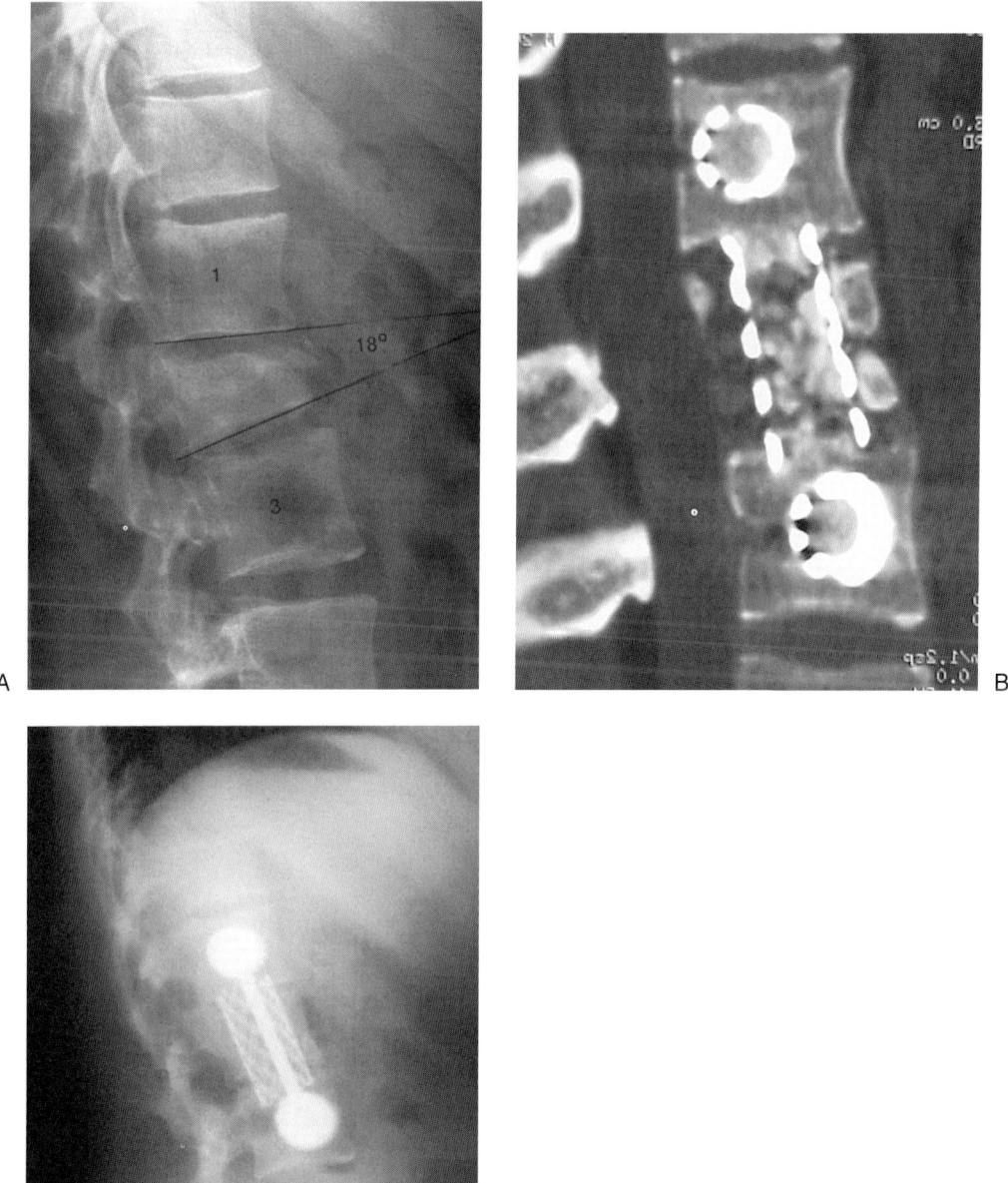

FIG. 22.7. Case 2. **A:** L2 burst fracture preoperatively. **B:** Sagittal computed tomographic scan at 7 months. **C:** Lateral view at 12 months.

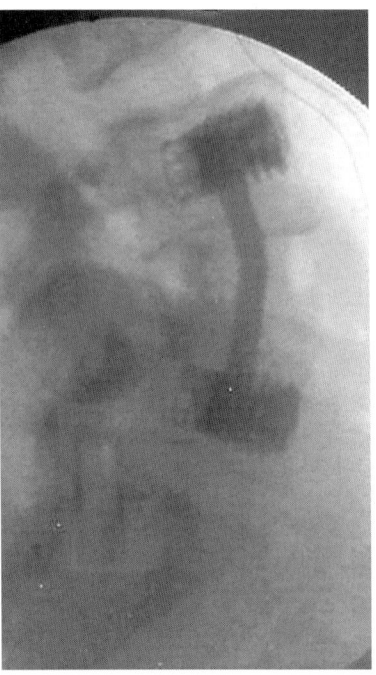

FIG. 22.8. Case 3. L4–5 fusion for degenerative disc disease.

tary work after his 3-month follow-up but because of his occupation did not return to full work until after his 6-month postoperative visit. Despite mild residual left extremity numbness, he has returned to vigorous activities and aggressive sports, including basketball and racquetball. One-year postoperative roentgenography and computed tomography revealed no lucency around the vertebral body anchors, fusion across the hemicorpectomy site, and no loss of correction (Fig. 22.7).

Case 3

A 29-year-old woman had a 2-year history of chronic low back pain. MRI and discography confirmed L4–5 discogenic pain. She underwent midsagittal placement of the K-Centrum with a horseshoe femoral graft (Tutogen Medical, Clifton, NJ, U.S.A.) at L4–5. The K-Centrum rod was bent to maintain lumbar lordosis, as seen in the immediate postoperative lateral x-ray film (Fig. 22.8). She reported good relief of her preoperative low back pain at the 3-month follow-up visit.

CONCLUSIONS

The K-Centrum is a new anterior thoracolumbar fixation system. It is the first true "zero-profile" intramedullary rod system for spinal stabilization. Clinical results show that the K-Centrum Anterior Spinal Fixation System, in combination with a load-sharing construct, is effective in the reconstruction of vertebral body fractures and tumors and in the treatment of DDD of the thoracolumbar spine. As is the case with all other anterior fixation systems, we do not suggest its use as a stand-alone system in cases of severe osteoporosis.

REFERENCES

1. *ASTM F 1717-96, standard test method for static and fatigue for spinal implant constructs in a corpectomy model.* West Conshohocken, PA: American Society for Testing and Materials, 1996.
2. *Device considerations for spinal fixation device systems* (19930820). Washington, DC: Orthopedic Devices Branch (ORDB), Office of Device Evaluation (ODE), Center for Devices and Radiologic Health (CDRH), Food and Drug Administration (FDA), 1993.
3. Ashman RB, Birch JG, Bone LB, et al. Mechanical testing of spinal instrumentation. *Clin Orthop* 1988; 227:113–125.
4. Breeze SW, Doherty BJ, Noble PS, et al. A biomechanical study of anterior thoracolumbar screw fixation. *Spine* 1998;23:1829–1831.
5. Christensen FB, Hansen ES, Eiskjaer SP, et al. Circumferential lumbar spinal fusion with Brantigan cage versus posterolateral fusion with titanium Cotrel-Dubousset instrumentation: a prospective, randomized clinical study of 146 patients. *Spine* 2002;27:2674–2683.
6. Dunn HK. Anterior stabilization of thoracolumbar injuries. *Clin Orthop* 1984;189:116–124.
7. Dwyer AF, Newton NC. An anterior approach to scoliosis–a preliminary report. *Clin Orthop* 1969;62:192–202.
8. Ghanayem AJ, Zdeblick TA. Anterior instrumention in the management of thoracolumbar burst fractures. *Clin Orthop Rel Res* 1997;335:89–100.
9. Haas N, Blauth M, Tscherne H. Anterior plating in thoracolumbar spine injuries: indication, technique, and results. *Spine* 1991;16:S100–S111.
10. Hall JE, Micheli LJ. *The use of modified Dwyer instrumentation in anterior stabilization of the spine.* Presented at the annual meetings of the Scoliosis Research Society, Hong Kong, October 1977, and Montreal, September 1981.
11. Harrington KD. Current concepts review. Metastatic disease of the spine. *J Bone J Surg Am* 1986;68:1110–1115.
12. Hee HT, Castro FP, Majd ME, et al. Anterior/posterior lumbar fusion versus transforaminal lumbar interbody fusion: analysis of complications and predictive factors. *J Spinal Disord* 2001;14:533–540.
13. Humphries AW, Hawk WA, Berndt AL. Anterior interbody fusion of the lumbar vertebrae: a surgical technique. *Surg Clin North Am* 1961;41:1685–1700.
14. Jendrisak MD. Spontaneous abdominal aortic rupture from erosion by a lumbar fixation device: a case report. *Surgery* 1986;99:631–633.
15. Jenis LG, An HS. Anterior thoracolumbar instrumentation for tumor or trauma. *Semin Spine Surg* 1997;9:250–259.
16. Kostuik JP. Anterior fixation for burst fractures of the thoracic and lumbar spine with or without neurological involvement. *Spine* 1988;13:286–293.
17. Kostuik JP. Anterior Kostuik-Harrington distraction systems. In: An HS, Cotler JM, eds. *Spinal Instrumentation.* Baltimore: Williams & Wilkins, 1992:359–377.
18. Schofferman J, Slosar P, Reynolds J, et al. A prospective randomized comparison of 270 fusions to 360 fusions (circumferential fusions). *Spine* 2001;26:E207–E212.
19. Slosar PJ, Reynolds JB, Schofferman J, et al. Patient satisfaction after circumferential lumbar fusion. *Spine* 2000;25:722–726.
20. Test Report, DOC #21-059 (2/99) and #21-133 (5/02). Stillwater, MN: Spineology, Inc.
21. Test Report, DOC #21-071 (5/99). Stillwater, MN: Spineology, Inc.
22. Test Report, DOC #21-079 (9/99). Stillwater, MN: Spineology, Inc.
23. Test Report, DOC #24-003 A (12/00) and #21-099 (11/00). Stillwater, MN: Spineology, Inc.
24. Zielke K, Pellin B. New Instrumente und Implantate zur Erganzung des Harrington Systems. *Z Orthop Chir* 1976;114:534.

23

Dynamic Neutralization System for the Spine in Degenerative Disc Disease

*Thomas M. Stoll, †Gilles G. Dubois, and ‡Othmar Schwarzenbach

*Department of Orthopedic Spine Surgery, Bethesda Spital, Basel, Switzerland;
†Department of Neurosurgery, Clinique de l'Union, St. Jean, France;
and ‡Das Ruckenzentrum, Thun, Switzerland

The term *degenerative disc disease (DDD)* addresses mainly lumbar discogenic pain. This pain syndrome is also referred to as *axial low back pain (LBP)* or *mechanical LBP*. The vagueness of the terms expresses some of the difficulties involved in understanding the syndrome, which occurs so frequently. From a scientific point of view, the term *DDD* is not used correctly because it currently denotes a syndrome of LBP. However, every stage of spinal degenerative disease involves disc degeneration. Early stages are symptomatic annular tears, more advanced stages may be disc herniation or instability with involvement of the facet joints, and later stages include degenerative stenosis and degenerative deformities such as degenerative spondylolisthesis and scoliosis.

Degeneration of the motion segment of the spine most probably begins primarily with degeneration of the disc. Degeneration of the disc with dehydration of the nucleus and disc lesions such as tears and rim lesions affect the mechanical properties of the disc and correlate with a decrease in joint stiffness, as biomechanical studies have confirmed (10,35). Segmental motion increases as disc degeneration progresses, and this process coincides with degeneration of the facet joints, contributing to increased segmental motion by a reduction of control over the motion pattern. An excessive or pathologic motion pattern—segmental instability, also called *dysstability*—is established. These findings support the concept of Kirkaldy-Willis and Farfan (17). In the individual life cycle, degenerative spondylosis frequently develops into instability, as these authors have well depicted with their concept of three phases of degenerative spondylosis: (a) dysfunction, (b) unstable phase, and (c) restabilization. It is only in the late stages of degeneration that the segment may undergo spontaneous restabilization by fusion. This concept is supported by Husson et al. (16).

Lumbar pain is caused by mechanical and chemical factors. Instability is the mechanical component. Abnormal and excessive motion patterns strain all the physiologic stabilizing structures—annulus, joint capsules, ligaments, and muscles. Excessively strained tissues of the segment generate pain (24). Physiologically, nociceptors are present mainly in the annulus and may be stimulated (19). However, in the course of degenerative disease, ingrowing repair tissue with additional neuroreceptors causes further sensitization. In addition to mechanical overloading, chemical processes increase the generation of pain when metabolites of the nucleus leak through annular tears and rim lesions and act as inflammatory agents in surrounding tissues. An additional site where pain is generated may be the endplate. In a normal disc, internal pressure is uniform; the distribution of pressure is even because the intact nucleus behaves like a fluid. Consequently, the pressure on the endplate is also uniform. As nuclear degeneration increases, the distribution of pressure becomes irregular, and peak high loads occur at the endplates. These may lead to endplate lesions, and it is hypothesized that ingrowth of nociceptive tissue occurs (2). In addition to discogenic pain, segmental pain may be generated in osteoarthritic facet joints, some ligaments, and muscles with reactive spasms (24).

Immobilization can stop the production of segmental pain, as has been shown with various treatment modalities. Restabilization can be achieved by muscle training (internal bracing), external bracing, and surgical procedures such as fusion. The concept of surgical restabilization by nonfusion instrumentation has generated considerable interest (3,4,13,16,27). Discogenic pain is addressed by disc replacement, nucleus replacement, and stabilization with pedicle systems. Interspinous instrumentation aims primarily at neurocompressive syndromes (32). Thus, spinal instrumentation has always addressed some form of instability.

In most cases, discogenic pain can be managed with conservative measures, although in a few selected patients, a surgical procedure is required. Currently, a fusion procedure is typically associated with inherent disadvantages, causing considerable morbidity and possibly contributing to future degeneration in adjacent segments. Mobile stabilization would be advantageous, allowing more physiologic function.

The *dy*namic *ne*utralization *sys*tem (DYNESYS) for the spine is a nonfusion pedicle screw system that stabilizes the lumbar spine (4,5,8,33). It is designed for single- or multiple-segment use. It is intended to treat pathologic conditions associated with some form of segmental instability and its various sequelae. DYNESYS was developed based on familiarity and experience with conventional rigid pedicle systems. It establishes a mobile load transfer and controls motion of the segment in all planes while inducing stability. It substitutes physiologic tissue restraints and so approximates the unstable motion pattern to a normal pattern. The bilateral implant system controls motion in all planes. Stability with controlled segmental motion is established, achieving a more physiologic condition than can be accomplished by fusion of such a segment. In combination with decompressive procedures, the system reestablishes stability or prevents iatrogenic instability. Some of the disadvantages of fusion may be minimized, such as the transition syndrome, caused by overloading adjacent segments (18,30), and increased invasiveness. The system can be applied by a medial approach or by the paraspinal approach (Wiltse approach) (36).

A multicenter study was performed with the primary objective of demonstrating the safety and efficacy of this novel posterior instrumentation system. The study reflects the first clinical experience with the DYNESYS implant based on a prospective protocol and including frequent indications for surgery for which conventional procedures would otherwise have been applied. This chapter describes the subgroup of patients who underwent surgery for predominantly discogenic pain.

PATIENTS AND METHODS

A prospective multicenter study with a minimum follow-up of 1 year was performed to evaluate the safety and efficacy of DYNESYS in the treatment of degenerative lumbar pathology (33). The study included a subgroup of 20 patients treated for degenerative disc disease (DDD).

Patients

The study included 20 consecutive patients who underwent surgery with DYNESYS instrumentation performed by the three authors. At two centers (T.S., O.S.), the patients in the subgroup were part of the first consecutive series of patients treated with DYNESYS.

Patient Selection and Inclusion Criteria

Patients with DDD were selected for the procedure who had neurogenic, radicular pain and/or chronic LBP resistant to any conservative treatment and who presented with some form of instability for which stabilization was judged to be beneficial. Most of these patients would have undergone fusion if DYNESYS had not been available.

Nine (45%) of the patients had previously undergone lumbar surgery. In three patients, the index operation was a revision operation.

The average age at operation was 41.9 years (range, 26.8 to 56.9 years). Eleven (55%) of the patients were men, and nine (45%) were women.

Preoperative Assessment

The preoperative assessment included a history, physical examination, neurologic assessment, and imaging studies. Imaging included anteroposterior, lateral, and dynamic lateral roentgenography in addition to at least one other modality (myelography, magnetic resonance imaging, computed tomography, discography). The scoring system of Prolo et al. (26) was used. Patients answered the Oswestry Low Back Pain Questionnaire [Oswestry Disability Index (ODI)] (7) and two numeric pain score questionnaires (15)—one for axial LBP and one for leg pain.

Assessment at Follow-up

The assessment at follow-up was performed by independent examiners. It included the same protocol as the preoperative assessment except for imaging studies other than roentgenography.

Surgical Technique

Surgery was performed by a midline approach and instrumentation by the surgical technique for DYNESYS, with the pedicle screw position at the conventional (Magerl) site. Postoperative bracing was applied only in exceptional cases.

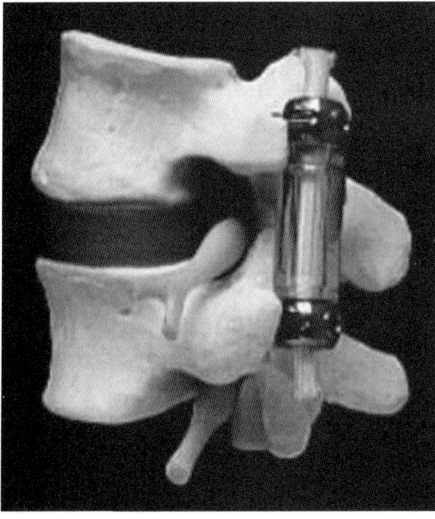 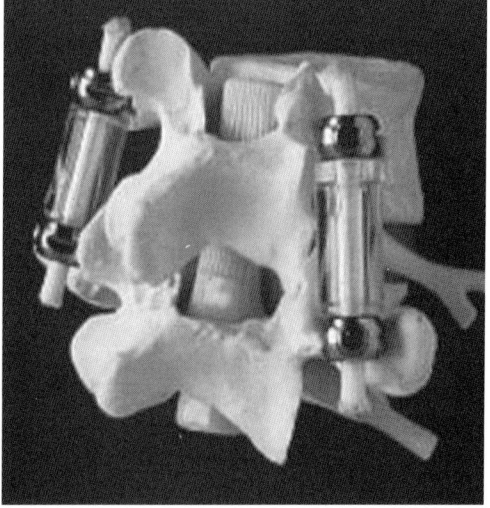

FIG. 23.1. Photographs of a single-segment dynamic neutralization system (DYNESYS) on a spine model.

TABLE 23.1. *Instrumented segments*

	No.	Percentage (%)
Number of levels treated		
One	13	65
Two	3	15
Three	3	15
Four	1	5
Distribution of levels treated[a]		
L1–2	1	5
L2–3	2	10
L3–4	4	20
L4–5	10	50
L5–S1	3	15

[a]Highest level treated in patients treated at multiple levels.

Implants

The DYNESYS system is composed of titanium alloy (Protasul 100) pedicle screws, polyester [Sulene-PET (polyethylene terephthalate)] cords, and Sulene-PCU (polycarbonaturethane) spacers (Centerpulse, Winterthur, Switzerland). The surface of the screw is sand-blasted. The screws anchor the DYNESYS system in the pedicle and in the vertebral body. The modular spacer is cut intraoperatively to the appropriate size to fit between the pedicle screw heads. The stabilizing cord connects the pedicle screw heads via the hollow core of the spacer and holds the spacer in place. Its preload provides a uniform system rigidity. The stabilizing cord carries tensile forces, and the spacers resist compressive forces. The inherent stability of the whole construct also resists bending and shear forces (Fig. 23.1).

Biomechanical Testing

All components underwent various biomechanical and biologic tests. These included fatigue testing of the whole construct for distraction and compression during 10 million cycles. The nonmetallic parts were further tested for biocompatibility.

In most of the cases (65.0%), single-segment instrumentation was performed (Table 23.1). The segment most frequently instrumented was L4–5. When indicated, a direct decompression was also performed at the instrumented levels (Table 23.2).

RESULTS

Of the 20 patients, 18 were available for follow-up. Two were not included because they underwent reoperations 5.8 and 9.1 months after the index operation for adjacent segment problems. Implant removal and a fusion procedure were performed. The mean operation time was 121 minutes (range, 60 to 205 minutes). The mean follow-up time was 43.2 months (range, 12.8 to 61.4 months).

TABLE 23.2. *Additional procedures*

Additional procedure	No.	Percentage (%)
Direct decompression	5	25
Nucleotomy	1	5
Neurolysis	1	5
Implant removal	1	5
Interspinous ligamentoplasty (adjacent)	2	10

TABLE 23.3. Prolo functional status

Functional score	Preoperative		Follow-up	
	No.	Percentage (%)	No.	Percentage (%)
Total incapacity	7	39	1	5.5
Back pain mild to moderate, able to perform all daily tasks of living	7	39	4	22
Low level of pain, able to perform all activities except sports	4	22	5	28
No pain, but patient has had one or more occurrences of back pain	—	—	6	33
No recurrent episodes of back pain, all previous sports and social activities	—	—	2	11

Eighteen patients available at follow-up.

Complications occurred in two cases. In one, a screw was incorrectly placed, but no clinical consequences developed and no revision operation was necessary. The other complication was a thromboembolic event.

In this subgroup of patients with DDD, no radiologic signs of screw loosening were detected at follow-up. In concordance with the literature, a positive sign was defined as halo formation around the screws or screw migration.

Low back pain was assessed with a numeric pain scale on which 1 indicated absence of pain and 10 represented a maximum level of pain. The LBP scores improved significantly from a mean of 7.7 (3 to 10) at baseline to a mean of 3.1 (1 to 9) at follow-up. The scores for leg pain were 6.0 (1 to 10) at baseline and 1.7 (1 to 4) at follow-up. A decrease in the pain score of 2 points, indicating a clinically significant reduction of pain, was noted in 83.5% of the patients. The improvement was statistically significant (back pain and leg pain, $P < 0.001$).

The functional (Table 23.3) and economic (Table 23.4) status of the patients improved significantly ($P < 0.01$).

The ODI score is interpreted as follows (7): 0% to 20%, minimal disability; 20% to 40%, moderate disability; 40% to 60%, severe disability; 60% to 80%, crippled; 80% to 100%, either bed-bound or exaggerating symptoms.

The mean preoperative ODI score was 59.2% (12% to 92%), which indicates severe disability in the average patient. At follow-up, the mean score was 24.2% (0% to 62%). This improvement is also highly significant ($P < 0.001$).

CASE PRESENTATION

See Figures 23.2 and 23.3.

TABLE 23.4. Prolo economic status

Economic score	Preoperative		Follow-up	
	No.	Percentage (%)	No.	Percentage (%)
Complete invalid	2	11	—	—
No gainful occupation (capable of independent locomotion and self-care, but unable to hold job, perform housework)	9	50	5	28
Able to work	4	22	3	17
Working with part-time or limited status	2	11	2	11
Working with no restrictions of any kind	1	5.5	8	44.5

Eighteen patients available at follow-up.

A

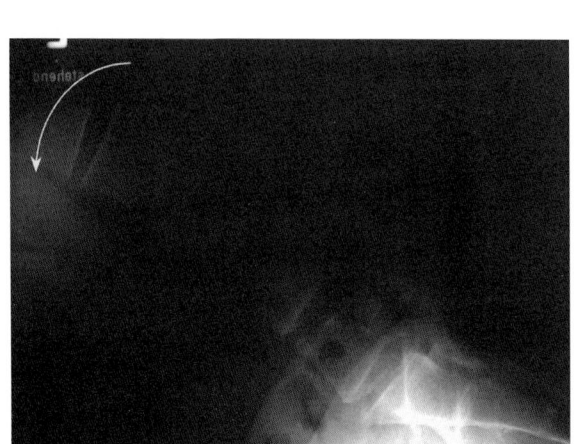
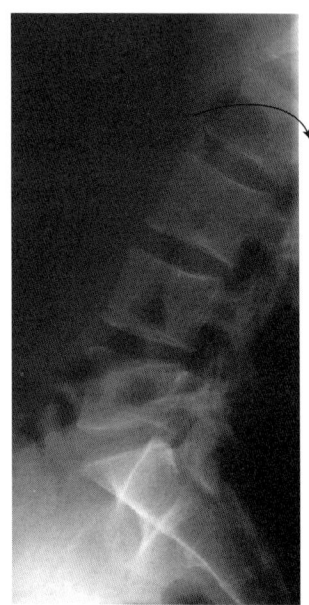

B

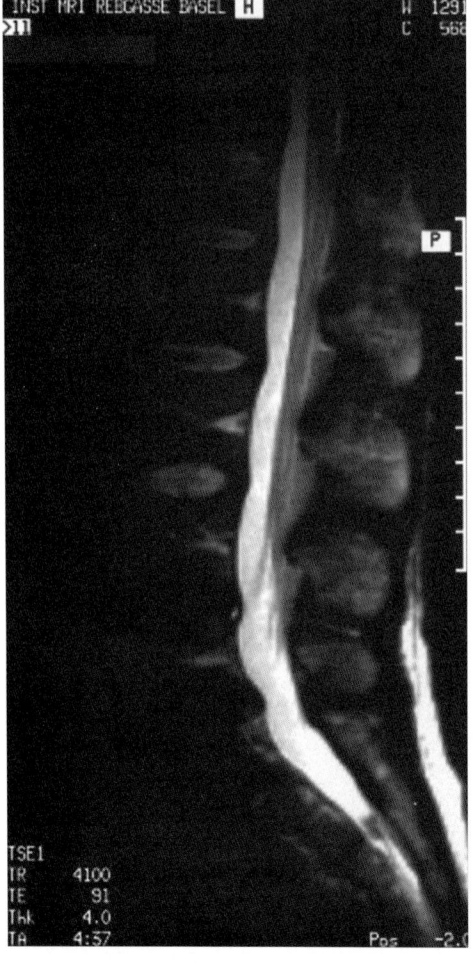
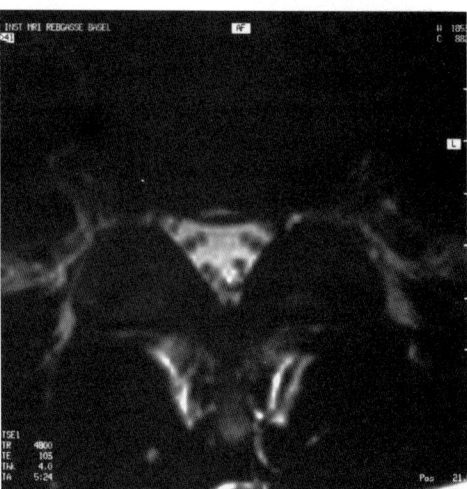
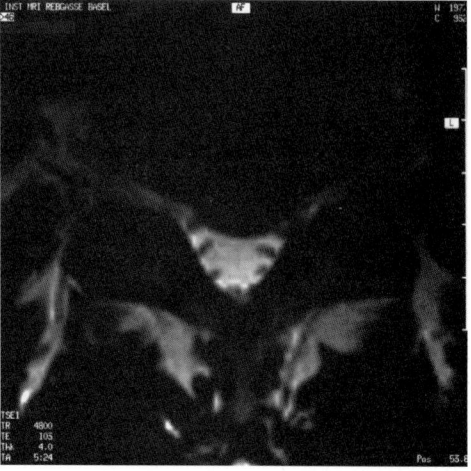

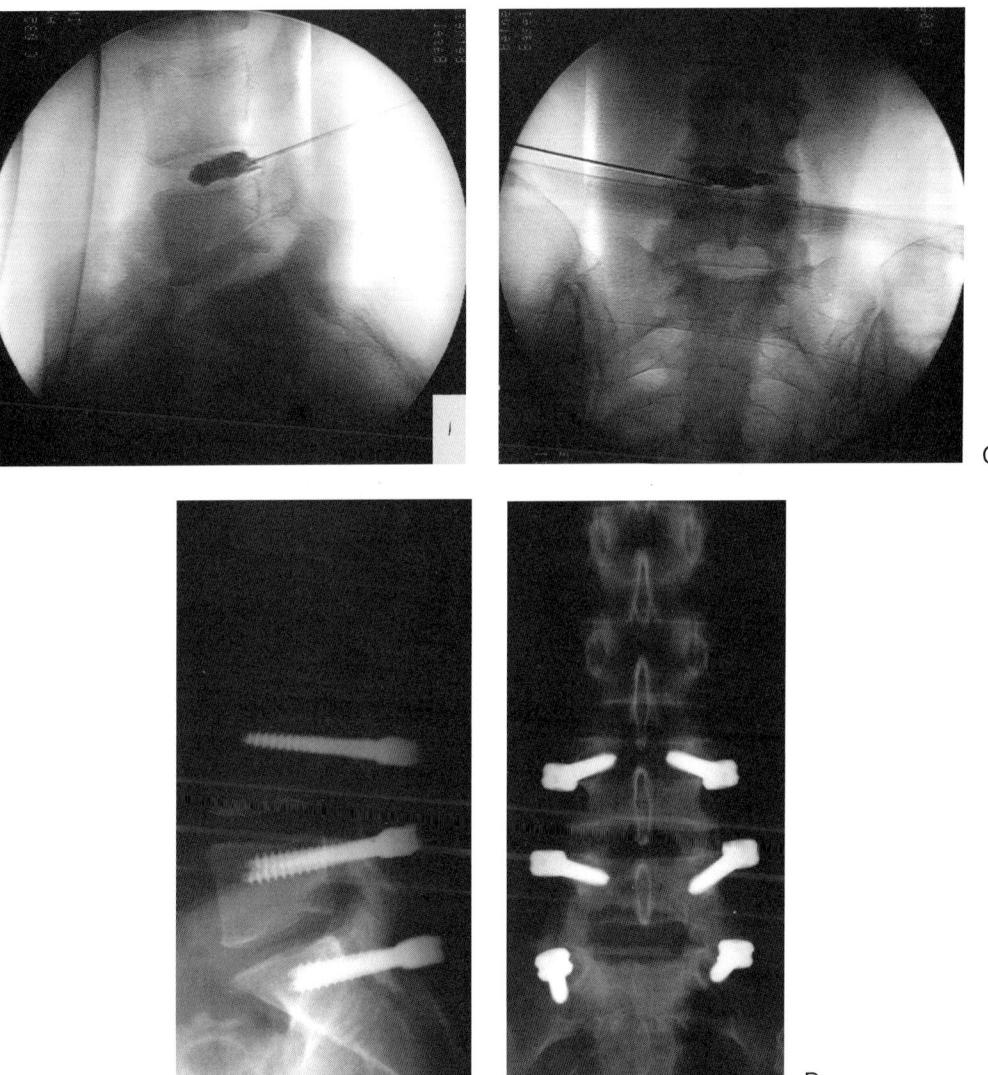

FIG. 23.2. A: Lateral bending films of a 39-year-old woman presenting with low back pain and episodes of S1 root pain demonstrate some hypermobility at L4–5 and degenerative disc disease at L4–5 and L5–S1. **B:** A magnetic resonance image demonstrates L4–5 with annular tear and L5–S1 with medial herniation. **C:** Provocative discography produced pain in both discs. **D:** Radiographs of the same patient as in **A**, **B**, and **C** following L5–S1 nucleotomy and instrumentation with a dynamic neutralization system (DYNESYS) at L4–S1.

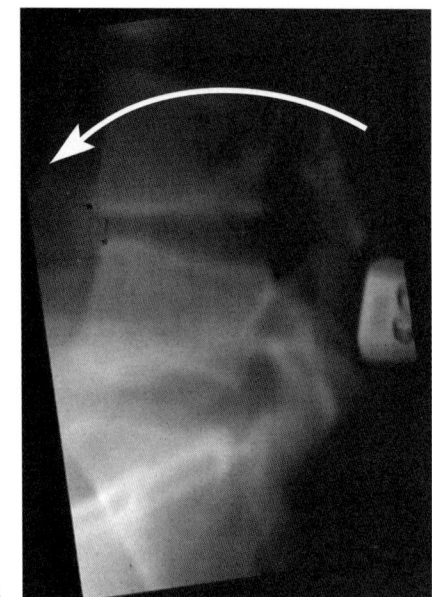
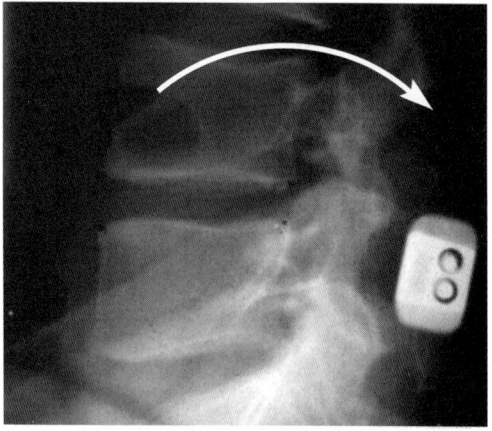
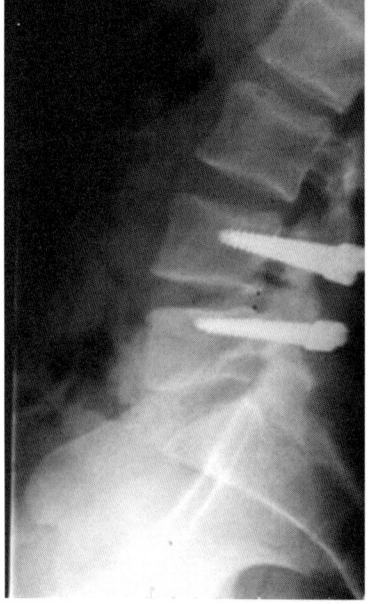
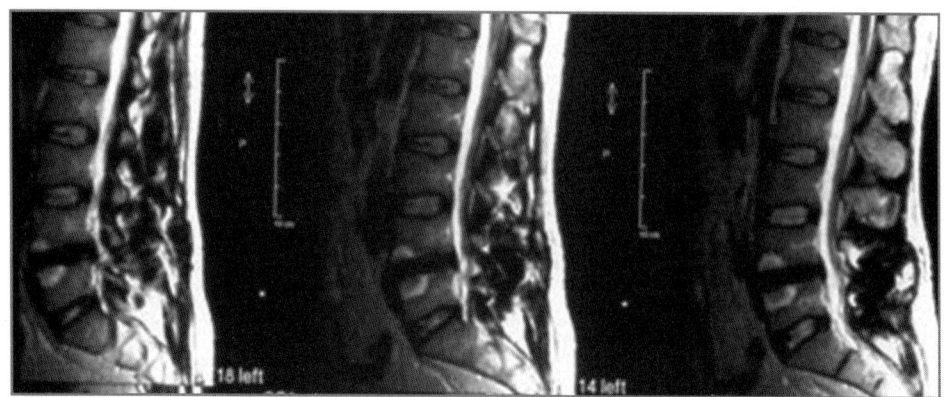

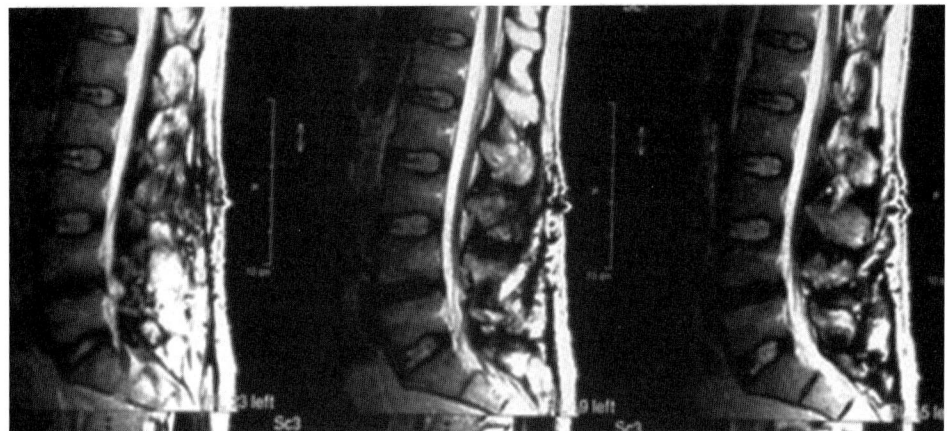

FIG. 23.3. A: Lateral bending films of a 47-year-old man, who previously had undergone decompression and interspinous stabilization of the L4—5 level, presenting with discopathy and hypermobility at L4–5. **B:** Lateral standing view of the same patient as in **A** at follow-up. **C:** Preoperative magnetic resonance image from the same patient in the T2-weighted mode demonstrating Modic type I changes at the L4–5 level, which disappeared almost completely 5 months postoperatively **(D)**.

DISCUSSION

These results are comparable with those achieved by current surgical procedures used to treat LBP, although comparisons of series are always problematic (12). Randomized controlled studies are a better alternative, but they are very rarely performed. The first difficulty encountered in comparisons is the patient populations, which vary in pathology and indications. The final difficulty is the frequent absence of a comparable presentation of results. Assessment tools that investigators agree on, such as a pain score, be it a visual analog scale (VAS) or a defined numeric pain scale system (15), and a functional assessment are often not presented. Even the validated and widely accepted ODI scores (7) are in many cases not correctly presented and are scarcely comparable. The ODI includes a statement of the patient's perception of the result and is one of the most reliable instruments for comparing the outcomes of different studies. This is less true of a pain score, be it a VAS score or a numeric score, because the results vary with instructions to the patients.

In this series, both the ODI score and the pain score at follow-up compared favorably with those in similar series. It must be emphasized that 45% of the patients had previously undergone lumbar surgery. The mean preoperative ODI score of 59.2% (12% to 92%) improved to a mean of 24.2% (0% to 62%) at follow-up, and the LBP score (1 to 10) improved from a mean of 7.7 to a mean of 3.1. These results compare favorably with those of the following studies. In a carefully designed prospective randomized study of the treatment of chronic LBP, Fritzell et al. (9) in a fusion group reported a 33% reduction in the VAS score (64 preoperatively to 43 at follow-up) and a 25% reduction in the ODI score (47% preoperatively to 36% at follow-up) at 2-year follow-up. In a prospective randomized comparison of anterior lumbar interbody fusion (ALIF) plus trans-pedicular instrumentation plus posterolateral fusion (group 1) with ALIF plus trans-pedicular instrumentation without posterolateral fusion (group 2) for comparable pathology, Schofferman et al. (31) reported an improvement in the numeric rating scale for pain (0 to 10) from a mean of 7.8 preoperatively to 4.3 at follow-up for group 1 and from 7.2 preoperatively to 4.7 at follow-up for group 2 after a mean follow-up of 34.5 months (24 to 45 months). The respective ODI scores improved from 57.5 to 38.2 in group 1 and from 61.2 to 40.5 in group 2. The mean operative times in that series were 388 minutes (group 1) and 324 minutes (group 2); in our series, it was 121 minutes. In the study of Madan and Boeree (20) of a series of 27 patients who underwent ALIF for discogenic pain, the VAS score for back pain (0 to 10) improved from a mean of 9.33 to a mean of 6.4, and the ODI score from a mean of 60.2 to a mean of 33.9 at a mean follow-up of 2.9 years (2.1 to 4.4 years). One patient required a revision at 2 weeks. In a series of 53 patients operated on for LBP with instrumented posterior lumbar interbody fusion (PLIF), Tandon et al. (34) reported a disappointing improvement in the ODI score from 51.2 to 39.1 at a mean follow-up of 2.7 years (2 to 4.7 years).

Dynamic neutralization is less invasive than most fusion procedures (6,22,23,25). This is definitely so in a combined procedure such as PLIF, transforaminal lumbar interbody fusion (TLIF), or ALIF with posterior pedicle or translaminar instrumentation. Instrumented and even uninstrumented posterolateral fusion procedures require more extensive tissue exposure and the decortication and preparation of facet joints and transverse processes. Bone harvesting causes further morbidity. Stand-alone ALIF is probably comparable in respect to overall invasiveness, but it has its own disadvantages, such as a decreased fusion rate and the inability to add posterior neurodecompressive procedures. This is also true of disc arthroplasty, which is essentially restricted to the L4–5 and L5–S1 levels and is associated with an increased risk for severe vascular complications. Furthermore, it may not sufficiently address posterior pain components. Mobile stabilization should minimize the risk for accelerated degeneration of the adjacent segment (18,30). Graf (13) introduced a trans-pedicular ligament replacement system for the treatment of painful DDD, raising many expectations (1,21) that ultimately could not be met (11,14,28). The proposed action of this pedicle screw system was based on interlocking the facet joints in maximal extension. Distraction and unloading of the disc are not possible with this system. DYNESYS provides mobile stabilization that controls motion in any plane; both compression and distraction with unloading of the disc are possible.

Because DYNESYS is a prosthetic device that in theory should serve the patient for life, screw loosening warrants special analysis. In this subgroup, screw loosening was not detected. Implant loads in a segmental lumbar setting are highly complex (29). It is hypothesized that because of its lesser degree of stiffness, DYNESYS, and therefore the screw–bone interface, may be subjected to less load than conventional internal fixator systems. However, load transfer is substantially different because the screws are not rigidly linked by a rod.

Reoperations were necessary in two cases for persistent pain in an adjacent segment. Because this occurred quite early in the postoperative course, the reason for the failure may have been a diagnostic error rather than progression of the natural history of degeneration or the transferred overload. It may also express a learning curve with respect to use of the system.

Shortcomings of this study were the small number of patients in the subgroup and the limited minimum follow-up time of 1 year rather than 2 years.

CONCLUSIONS

Dynamic neutralization has proved to be a safe and effective alternative in the surgical treatment of DDD, and its functional results compare favorably with those of other surgical procedures. It is less invasive than most fusion procedures and allows the addition of posterior nerve decompression procedures. However, this report must be considered preliminary because of the small number of patients included and the minimum follow-up time of 12 months.

ACKNOWLEDGMENTS

We are grateful to Ms. Elke Rometsch, Centerpulse Orthopedics, Ltd., for excellent preparation of the database and extensive statistical analysis. We thank Mark Myers, M.D., of Minneapolis, MN, U.S.A., for radiologic evaluation at follow-up.

REFERENCES

1. Brechbühler D, Markwalder TM, Braun M. Surgical results after soft system stabilization of the lumbar spine in degenerative disc disease—long term results. *Acta Neurochir* 1998;140:521–525.
2. Brown MF, Hukkanen MV, McCarthy ID, et al. Sensory and sympathetic innervation of the vertebral endplate in patients with degenerative disc disease. *J Bone Joint Surg Br* 1997;79:147–153.
3. Büttner-Janz K, Schellnack K, Zippel H. Biomechanics of the SB Charité lumbar intervertebral disc endoprosthesis. *Int Orthop* 1989;13:173–176.
4. Dubois G, De Germay B, Schaerer NS, et al. Dynamic neutralization: a new concept for restabilization of the spine. In: Szpalski M, Gunzburg R, Pope MH, eds. *Lumbar segmental instability*. Philadelphia: Lippincott Williams & Wilkins, 1999:233–240.
5. Dubois DD, De Germay B, Prere J, et al. Dynamic neutralisation: treatment of mobile vertebral instability. In: Kaech DL, Jinkins JR, eds. *Spinal restabilization procedures*. Amsterdam: Elsevier Science, 2002:345–354.
6. Esses SI, Sachs BL, Dreyzin V. Complications associated with the technique of pedicle screw fixation. *Spine* 1993;18:2231–2239.
7. Fairbank J, Couper J, Davies J, et al. The Oswestry Low Back Pain Questionnaire. *Physiotherapy* 1980;66:271–273.
8. Freudiger S, Dubois G, Lorrain M. Dynamic neutralisation of the lumbar spine confirmed on a new lumbar spine simulator in vitro. *Arch Orthop Trauma Surg* 1999;119:127–132.
9. Fritzell P, Hagg O, Wessberg P, et al. 2001 Volvo Award in Clinical Studies. Lumbar fusion versus nonsurgical treatment for chronic low back pain: a multicenter randomized controlled trial from the Swedish Lumbar Spine Study Group. *Spine* 2001;26:2521–2532; discussion 2532–2534.
10. Fujiwara A, Lim TH, An HS, et al. The effect of disc degeneration and facet joint osteoarthritis on the segmental flexibility of the lumbar spine. *Spine* 2000;25:3036–3044.
11. Gardner AD, Pande KC, Hassaan AM, et al. Graf stabilization of intractable lumbar instability syndrome. In: Szpalski M, Gunzburg R, Pope MH, eds. *Lumbar segmental instability*. Philadelphia: Lippincott Williams & Wilkins, 1999:175–190.
12. Gibson JNA, Grant IC, Waddell G. The Cochrane review of surgery for lumbar disc prolapse and degenerative lumbar spondylosis. *Spine* 1999;24:1820.
13. Graf H. Lumbar instability: surgical treatment without fusion. *Rachis* 1992;412:123–137.
14. Hadlow SV, Fagan AB, Hillier TM, et al. The Graf ligamentoplasty procedure—comparison with posterolateral fusion in the management of low back pain. *Spine* 1998;23:1172–1179.
15. Huskisson EC. Measurement of pain. *Lancet* 1974;2:1127–1131.
16. Husson JL, Poncer R, Polard JL. Dérangement intervertebral acquis (D.I.V.A.). In: Husson JL, Le Huec JC, eds. *Restabilisation intersomatique du rachis lombaire*. Montpellier: Sauramps Medical, 1996:13–21.
17. Kirkaldy-Willis WH, Farfan HF. Instability of the lumbar spine. *Clin Orthop* 1982;165:110–123.
18. Kumar MN, Jacquot F, Hall H. Long-term follow-up of functional outcomes and radiographic changes at adjacent levels following lumbar spine fusion for degenerative disc disease. *Eur Spine J* 2001;10:309–313.
19. Kuslich SD, Ulstrom CL, Michael CJ. The tissue origin of low back pain and sciatica. *Orthop Clin North Am* 1991;22:181–182.
20. Madan S, Boeree NR. Containment and stabilization of bone graft in anterior lumbar interbody fusion: the role of the Hartshill horseshoe cage. *J Spinal Disord* 2001;14:104–108.
21. Markwalder TM, Dubach R, Braun M. Soft system stabilization of the lumbar spine as an alternative surgical modality to lumbar arthrodesis in facet syndrome. Preliminary results. *Acta Neurochir* 1995;134:1–4.
22. Ohlin A, Karlsson M, Düppe H, et al. Complications after transpedicular stabilization of the spine. *Spine* 1994;19:2774–2779.
23. Okuyama K, Abe E, Suzuki T, et al. Posterior lumbar interbody fusion. *Acta Orthop Scand* 1999;70:329–334.
24. Panjabi MM. The stabilizing system of the spine. Part II. Neutral zone and instability hypothesis. *J Spinal Disord* 1992;5:390–397.

25. Pihlajamäki H, Myllynen P, Böstman O. Complications of transpedicular lumbosacral fixation for nontraumatic disorders. *J Bone Joint Surg Br* 1997;79:183–189.
26. Prolo DJ, Oklund SA, Butcher M. Toward uniformity in evaluating results of lumbar spine operations. A paradigm applied to posterior lumbar interbody fusions. *Spine* 1986;11:601–606.
27. Ray CD, Sachs BL, Norton BK, et al. Prosthetic disc nucleus implants: an update. In: Szpalski M, Gunzburg R, eds. *Herniation in the third millennium*. Philadelphia: Lippincott William & Wilkins, 2001;222–233.
28. Rigby MC, Selmon GPF, Foy MA, et al. Graf ligament stabilisation: mid- to long-term follow-up. *Eur Spine J* 2001;10:234–236.
29. Rohlmann A, Graichen F, Weber U, et al. 2000 Volvo Award in Biomechanical Studies. Monitoring in vivo implant loads with a telemeterized internal spinal fixation device. *Spine* 2000;25:2981–2986.
30. Schlegel JD, Smith JA, Schleusener RL. Lumbar motion segment pathology adjacent to thoracolumbar, lumbar and lumbosacral fusions. *Spine* 1996;21:970–981.
31. Schofferman J, Slosar P, Reynolds J, et al. A prospective randomized comparison of 270-degree fusions to 360-degree fusions (circumferential fusions). *Spine* 2001;26:E207–E212.
32. Senegas J, Etchevers JP, Vital JM, et al. Widening of the lumbar vertebral canal as an alternative to laminectomy in the treatment of lumbar stenosis. *J Fr Chir Orthop* 1988;1:93–99.
33. Stoll TM, Dubois G, Schwarzenbach O. The dynamic neutralization system for the spine: a multicenter study of a novel nonfusion system. *Eur Spine J* 2002;11[Suppl 2]:S170–S178.
34. Tandon V, Campbell F, Ross ER. Posterior lumbar interbody fusion. Association between disability and psychological disturbance in noncompensation patients. *Spine* 1999;24:1833–1838.
35. Thompson RE, Pearcy MJ, Downing KJW, et al. Disc lesions and the mechanics of the intervertebral joint complex. *Spine* 2000;25:3026–3035.
36. Wiltse LL, Spencer CW. New uses and refinements of the paraspinal approach to the lumbar spine. *Spine* 1998;13:1008–1012.

24

Cervical Interbody Fusion with a New Composite in Degenerative Disc Disease: A Preliminary Experience

*Richard Assaker, *Véronique Tonelle, †‡Stéphane Aunoble, and †‡Jean-Charles Le Huec

*Department of Neurosurgery, Salengro University Hospital, Lille, France;
†Department of Orthopedic Surgery and
‡ Spine Unit, Centre Hospitalier Universitaire Pellegrin, Bordeaux, France

Surgical intervention is generally considered for patients who have persistent pain or a neurologic deficit associated with a documented degenerate cervical disc when a minimum of 6 months of nonsurgical treatment has not been sufficiently effective. Anterior cervical interbody fusion is considered to be the standard of care in the surgical management of cervical spondylosis or degenerative disc disease (DDD). After the degenerate disc has been removed, an autograft or allograft strut is generally used to salvage the cervical anatomy and promote interbody fusion. Radiographic fusion and good to excellent results were obtained in 80% to 96% of patients (2–9).

However, the use of autograft is associated with significant morbidity at the graft harvest site, and the use of allograft is reported to decrease fusion rates and may transmit disease. Graft collapse is a concern with both types of graft materials (4,6,9).

These complications and concerns can be reduced by using interbody fusion cages made of metal or carbon fiber (4,6), as has been demonstrated in prospective studies.

Rhakoss-C (Orthovita, Inc., Malvern, PA, U.S.A.) is a new cervical interbody fusion device. Unlike existing interbody fusion cages, it has a radiolucency comparable with that of cortical bone, which enables visualization without distorting the radiographic signal. In addition, this composite has unique bone-bonding characteristics (1).

PATIENTS AND METHODS

This chapter reports the pilot phase of a prospective, observational cohort study in which 12 patients underwent surgery and were followed for 1 month at our two institutions. The objective of the pilot phase was to assess the following: the feasibility of using the cage and its instrumentation in patients, its radiographic appearance in humans, and its initial safety and efficacy. Patients 18 to 75 years of age were included if they had radiographic evidence of single-level disc degeneration with persistent pain refractory to 6 months of nonsurgical therapy and if they provided written informed consent to participate. Patients with multiple affected levels, a prior cervical fusion procedure, vertebral fracture or gross traumatic instability, infection, metabolic disease, or malignancy were excluded.

TABLE 24.1. *Preoperative and one-month data*

	Mean score (range)	
	Preoperative visit	One-month visit
Mean neck pain (100-mm VAS)	53.9 (12–93)	34.3 (2–84)
Mean right arm pain (100-mm VAS)	58.6 (0–100)	9.3 (0–34)
Mean left arm pain (100-mm VAS)	30.4 (0–100)	2.6 (0–20)
Mean VAS per patient (100-mm VAS)	47.6 (11.7–84)	15.4 (1.7–28)
Mean NDI score	18.5 (0–34)	15.7 (0–32)

NDI, Neck Disability Index; VAS, visual analogue scale.

Rhakoss-C was available in six different sizes (6, 7, and 8 mm in height and 13.5, 15.5, and 18 mm in width), each of these being 7 degrees lordotic. The cage was filled with β-tricalcium phosphate (Vitoss synthetic bone void filler; Orthovita, Inc.).

The Smith–Robinson approach was used to perform the surgery. Decompression of the nerve foramen was confirmed after careful removal of the disc material. Endplate preparation and hemostasis were performed after careful removal of all cartilaginous material. After placement of the cage, the construct was completed with an anterior plate (Zephyr; Medtronic, Minneapolis, MN, U.S.A.).

A 100-mm visual analog scale (VAS) was used to assess pain in the neck, right arm, and left arm separately, and the Neck Disability Index (NDI) was used to score disability. This evaluation was carried out before and 1 month after surgery, together with a detailed clinical examination. Any complication or adverse event occurring during surgery and the 1-month postoperative period was recorded. In addition, the surgeon's evaluation of the ease of using this cage and its instrumentation also was recorded.

Finally, the intervertebral disc space and sagittal alignment were measured on standard radiographs (anteroposterior and medial–lateral) obtained before and after surgery.

RESULTS

Twelve patients (eight men and four women) ages 34 to 64 years (mean, 46.1 years) were recruited and followed for 1 month during the pilot phase. All patients had radiculopathy, and one also had myelopathy. The most common surgical level was C5–6 (nine

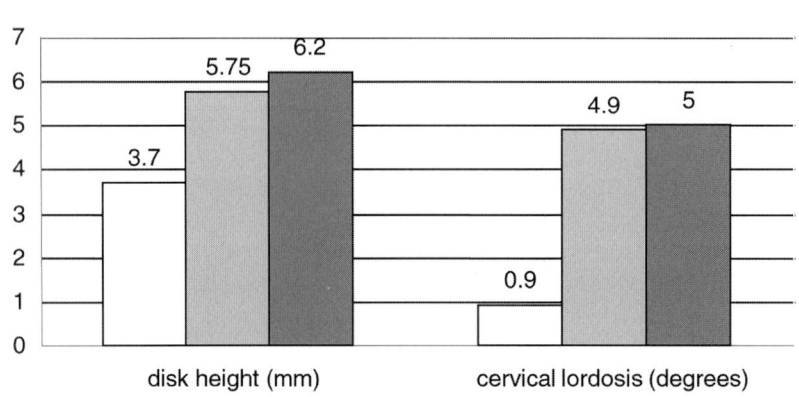

FIG. 24.1. Patient data for disc height and cervical lordosis.

cases), followed by C6–7 (two cases) and C7–T1 (one case). The 13.5-mm-wide implant was used seven times, the 15.5-mm-wide implant four times, and the 18-mm-wide implant once. The 7-mm-high implant was used most frequently (six cases), followed by the 6-mm-high implant (four cases) and the 8-mm implant (two cases).

Improvement was noted in all patients at the 1-month follow-up visit. Pain scores were reduced significantly (Table 24.1), and the height of the intervertebral disc space and lordosis were restored (Figs. 24.1, 24.2). The mean of the three pain scores on the VAS

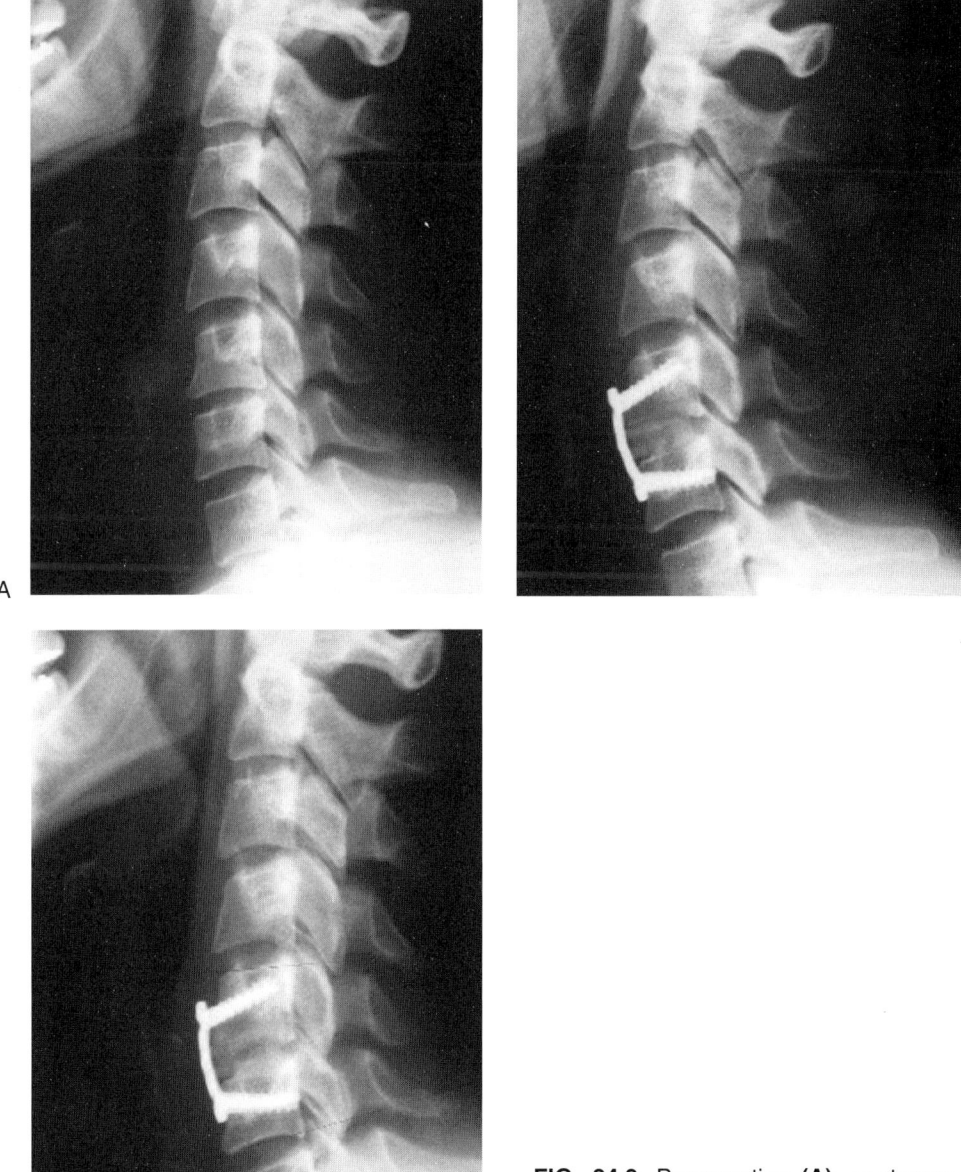

FIG. 24.2. Preoperative **(A)**, postoperative **(B)**, and 3-month **(C)** standard lateral radiographs.

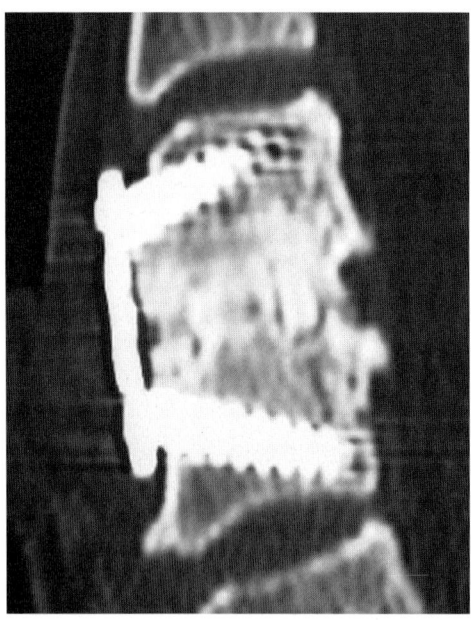

FIG. 24.3. Lateral computed tomographic scan at 6 months.

decreased from 47 mm before surgery to 15 mm at the 1-month postoperative visit, and the NDI score decreased from 18.5 to 15.7. The neurologic status was found to have improved or normalized in all patients.

Surgery with the new cage was considered by all surgeons to be very easy. No complications or adverse events occurred, except for throat irritation in one case and dysphagia in one case. These were temporary and not considered to be related to the use of Rhakoss-C or its instrumentation.

The radiographic appearance of the new composite on x-ray films (Figs. 24.2, 24.3) shows that its radiopacity is indeed comparable with that of human cortical bone and allows assessment of its position in relation to the spine and surrounding tissues. Furthermore, postoperative imaging did not reveal radiolucencies at the bone–implant interface.

DISCUSSION

This initial experience with Rhakoss-C and its instrumentation in 12 patients undergoing anterior cervical arthrodesis can be considered successful. The collection of additional data to assess its mid- and long-term effectiveness and safety in a larger number of patients is warranted.

All patients appeared to benefit from the surgery, and no device-related adverse event or complication occurred. The fact that the initial NDI scores were not very high and did not improve very much after surgery, in contrast to the VAS pain scores, suggests that the NDI may not be an appropriate tool for measuring dysfunction in the patient population studied. Although dysfunction related to DDD requiring surgery is associated mainly with symptoms of radiculopathy (10), the NDI questionnaire does not pick up these dysfunctional signs or symptoms because it focuses primarily on disability resulting from pain in the neck. This may be a consequence of the fact that it was initially constructed (at least in part) based on data from patients with whiplash injuries (10).

Finally, the visibility of the new composite is adequate, and its construct also allows good visualization of the grafted material and fusion inside the cagelike structure, as seen in the 6-month computed tomographic scan in Figure 24.3, which shows solid bony fusion inside the cage.

These data suggest that Rhakoss-C, a new synthetic cervical interbody fusion device, holds promise for the treatment of patients with significant DDD. It was able to withstand the mechanical requirements of the cervical spine, allows for good radiologic assessment of fusion, and appears to become well integrated into vertebral bone.

REFERENCES

1. *Investigator's brochure Rhakoss-C.* Malvern, PA: Orthovita, Inc., 2001.
2. Cauthen JC, Kinard RE, Vogler JB, et al. Outcome analysis of noninstrumented anterior cervical discectomy and interbody fusion in 348 patients. *Spine* 1998;23:188–192.
3. Cloward RB. The anterior approach for removal of ruptured discs. *J Neurosurg* 1958;15:602–617.
4. Debois V. Anterior cervical discectomy and vertebral interbody fusion using a carbon fiber cage with allograft bone versus an iliac crest bone graft. In: Szpalski M, Gunzburg R, eds. *The degenerative cervical spine*. Philadelphia: Lippincott Williams & Wilkins, 2001:259–264.
5. Dereymaeker A, Mulier J. La fusion vertbrale par voie ventrale dans la discopathie cervicale. *Rev Neurol (Paris)* 1958;99:99–103.
6. Matgé G. Anterior decompression and fusion with the BAK-C cage in the management of cervical spondylosis. In: Szpalski M, Gunzburg R, eds. *The degenerative cervical spine*. Philadelphia: Lippincott Williams & Wilkins, 2001:235–242.
7. Palit M, Schofferman J, Goldthwaite N, et al. Anterior discectomy and fusion for the management of neck pain. *Spine* 1999;24:2224–2228.
8. Robinson RA, Smith GW. Anterolateral cervical disc removal and interbody fusion for cervical disc syndrome. *Bull Johns Hopkins Hosp* 1955;96:223–224.
9. Sidhu KS, Herkowitz HN. Surgical management of cervical disk disease: surgical management of cervical radiculopathy, the anterior approach. In: Rothman-Simeone, ed. *The spine*, 4th ed. Philadelphia: WB Saunders, 1999:497–511.
10. Vernon H, Mior S. The Neck Disability Index: a study of reliability and validity. *J Manipulative Physiol Ther* 1991;14:409–415.

25

Ten Years On

*‡E. Raymond S. Ross, ‡Zahid Asker, and †§David G. Hughes

*Departments of *Orthopedics and †Radiology, University of Manchester, Manchester, United Kingdom; and Departments of ‡Spinal Surgery and §Neuroradiology, Hope Hospital, Salford, United Kingdom*

In many developed countries, low back pain is a prevalent problem. The cost in terms of treatment and hours lost from work can easily run into billions of dollars. Almost 75% of the U.S. population have at one time experienced back pain, and approximately 4% of the population require surgical intervention. In the United Kingdom, during any 12-month period, 7% of the adult population consult a health care practitioner with this problem (4), which will certainly grow as the population ages.

The fusion of painful segments (spinal arthrodesis) is the most common form of surgical treatment for low back pain that fails to respond to conservative means of treatment. The aim of fusion is to re-create the load-bearing path across a painful segment. In so doing, it eliminates motion. Hence, there is always a danger that fusion may induce degenerative changes in neighboring segments, which often necessitate additional fusion surgery (2).

To avoid this complication, one approach is to mimic the normal disc function of load transmission and motion through artificial mechanical means. By this means, it is hoped to circumvent the biomechanical changes normally attributed to rigid instrumentation and fusion. Several artificial disc designs have been proposed. Their aim is to reinstate stabilized physiologic motion in the lumbar spine and manage chronic low back pain syndromes that would otherwise be treated by spinal fusion.

The most widely used form of intervertebral disc replacement is the SB Charité III (Waldemar Link, Hamburg, Germany) (1). It has been in use since 1988. We present the long-term clinical and radiologic results of our series of SB Charité disc replacement.

SELECTION OF PATIENTS

The first 10 consecutive patients who underwent an SB Charité Disc III replacement were included in the study, along with two others who were later cases but of interest for reasons that will be explained. All patients initially underwent an intensive course of spinal rehabilitation and physiotherapy for at least 6 months. If they failed to respond, magnetic resonance imaging (MRI) and discography were performed. The objective was to show disc degeneration and possible painful segments. The Oswestry Disability Index (ODI) was applied preoperatively and postoperatively so that a measure of outcome could be obtained. Preoperatively, the psychologic status of the patients was also assessed with the Depression and Risk Assessment Method (DRAM) [modified Zung score and Modified Sensory Perception Questionnaire (MSPQ)]. Their clinical records were reviewed to look for any perioperative and postoperative complications. The postoperative clinical assess-

TABLE 25.1. *Postoperative assessment*

	Interobserver		Intraobserver	
	Kendall coefficient	P value	Kappa score	P value
Position of the disc	0.76	0.029	0.88	0.022
New bone formation	0.87	0.031	0.88	0.025
Osteolysis	0.75	0.021	0.83	0.012
Facet joint arthritis	0.78	0.023	0.81	0.014

ment was by postal questionnaires. At the same time, helical computed tomography (CT) with sagittal reconstruction was performed. The position of the disc, any new bone formation, and the presence and extent of any osteolysis and facet joint arthritis were noted (Table 25.1). The position of the artificial disc was graded as central, left, right, anterior, and posterior. New bone formation was classified as none or minimal, moderate but no bridging bone, and bridging bone or fused. The CT scan was assessed by three observers independently and blindly. One of the observers repeated the assessment 1 month after the first set of observations to measure intraobserver variability. Interobserver variability was measured with a nonparametric test (Kendall W test). Intraobserver agreement was measured with the weighted Cohen kappa statistic. The scores were classified into six categories by Landis and Koch: 0.81 to 1.00, almost perfect; 0.61 to 0.80, substantial; 0.41 to 0.60, moderate; 0.21 to 0.40, fair; 0.00 to 0.20, slight; and less than 0.00, poor. A two-tailed test was used to determine the statistical significance of the findings ($P = 0.05$). The clinical outcome was assessed with a nonparametric Wilcoxon two-tailed signed rank test for statistical significance ($P = 0.05$). The Spearman correlation coefficient was used to correlate the presence or absence of facet joint osteoarthritis with the postoperative clinical result.

RESULTS

The clinical details of the patients are listed in Table 25.2. The details of the spinal levels are presented in Table 25.3. Only one patient smoked at the time of surgery; however, she quit 3 years after surgery. Two patients had previously undergone discectomy before the disc replacement. No perioperative complications occurred. In one patient, a deep venous thrombosis developed that settled with conservative management. None of the patients was involved in ongoing litigation or receiving any compensation before the surgery or during the follow-up. None of them was at risk or distressed by using the DRAM score. Preoperatively, nine patients had severe disability according to the ODI score, whereas postoperatively, six patients had the same. The mean ODI score was 54 (26 to 27) preoperatively and 38 (0 to 76) postoperatively. The difference was not statistically significant ($P = 0.400$). No instances of disc dislocation or vascular or visceral injury occurred. Seventy percent of the patients had facet joint arthrosis on the CT scan.

TABLE 25.2. *Clinical details of patients*

Male-to-female ratio	2:10
Mean age (SD)	44.56 y (5.95)
Range	38.84–54.12 y
Mean follow-up (SD)	9.74 y (1.31)
Range	8.08–11.44 y

SD, standard deviation.

TABLE 25.3. Details of levels

Number of levels	No.	Level	No.
One level	5	L3–4	3
Two levels	6	L4–5	9
		L5–S1	5
Three levels	1	L5–S1, L4–5, L3–4	3
Total	12	Total	20

However, no correlation was found between the clinical result and the presence of facet joint arthrosis ($r = 0.229$, $P = 0.525$). The same was true of the relationship between the clinical results and the number of levels operated on ($r = 0.285$, $P = 0.425$). No radiologic evidence of disc loosening or bridging bone formation was detected. In one patient who underwent disc replacement at L4–5 and L5–S1, the L5–S1 replacement was converted to an anterior fusion. The radiologic marker wire broke and migrated, raising concern that it might cause neurologic damage. The three-level case was included to determine whether even within a shorter period the inclusion of three levels led to more creep or wear.

DISCUSSION

Prosthetic disc replacement has been found to be a good treatment modality for patients with degenerative disc disease (1). The intervertebral disc is a complex anatomic and functional unit. Our knowledge of the kinematics of normal discs is based on relatively little *in vivo* experimental evidence. This makes the development of an efficient and reliable artificial disc a difficult challenge. Moreover, disc function and movements are difficult to reproduce (5). Lemaire et al. (3), in their survey of various disc replacements, concluded that at this time the SB Charité is the best disc replacement compromise and can be the basis for the future development and evolution of disc replacement. However, they concluded that posterior facet arthritis, osteoporosis, structural deformities, and secondary facet pain can lead to failure.

Our study is one of the longest follow-ups of SB Charité III disc replacements. Seven patients were still experiencing significant symptoms after a mean follow-up of 9.74 years. No statistical difference was found between the preoperative and postoperative ODI scores. This is disappointing. We could not find any correlation between the clinical result and the presence of facet joint arthritis. If degenerative disc disease correlates with symptoms, then it is highly probable that the process that affects, let us say, a single level at one point in time is likely to affect other discs in the same spine over time, perhaps causing further symptoms. This makes the choice of patients for disc replacement more uncertain in our view. It also has implications for the assessment of outcome over long periods of time, such as 10 years. The lack of correlation between symptoms and facet arthritis, despite the high level of correlation between observers in detecting its presence, again begs the question of the part these joints play in symptom production.

The low level of surgical complications in this small series is encouraging for anterior approach surgery, but care must be taken, and a much larger series will be presented for comparison with the complication rates in other series.

None of the prostheses was loose on the spiral CT scan. Features that we would normally expect to find around hip or knee prostheses suggestive of high-density polyethylene wear are osteolysis and migration of the implant. In not a single level was either of these present. This is highly significant because the discs were all implanted before the development of hydroxyapatite coating. Two prostheses showed a significant loss of height. In the absence of osteolysis, this implies that creep has occurred, which is predictable theoretically, even without wear and particle formation. In the case of the retrieved prosthesis, the soft tissues were subjected to pathologic analysis, and no wear debris was noted. This finding supports the view that wear is either minimal or does not produce a detrimental particle size.

In summary, a small series of disc replacements has been reviewed. The results are optimistic in terms of wear and creep. They are less optimistic in terms of clinical outcome.

REFERENCES

1. Griffith SL, Shelekov AP, Buttner-Janz K, et al. A multicentre retrospective study of the clinical results of the Link SB Charit intervertebral prosthesis: the initial European experience. *Spine* 1994;2:1342–1349.
2. Lee CK, Lagrana NA, Parsons JR, et al. Development of a prosthetic intervertebral disc. *Spine* 1991;16[6 Suppl]:S253–S260.
3. Lemaire JP, Skalli W, Lavaste F, et al. Intervertebral disc prosthesis results and prospects for the year 2000. *Clin Orthop* 2000;337:64–76.
4. McCormick A, Fleming D, Charlton J. *Morbidity statistics from general practice. Fourth national study, 1991–1992*. London: Office of Population Censuses and Surveys, HMSO 1995 (series MB5 No 3).
5. Patwardhan A, Harvey R, Ghanayem A, et al. Load-carrying capacity of human cervical spine in compression is increased under a follower load. *Spine* 2000;25:1548–1554.

26

Total Disc Replacement for Low Back Pain of Discogenic Origin

H. Michael Mayer, Karsten Wiechert, and Andreas Korge

Spine Center, Munich, Germany

The surgical treatment of low back pain arising from the degenerating lumbar segment has always been a matter of debate. The main reason for this ongoing scientific discussion was that the only surgical option was spinal fusion, which is known to be a procedure with hardly acceptable results and a wide variety of undesired side effects and complications (5,6,7,8,10,14)

Total disc replacement was promoted after the middle of the 1980s as a potential alternative to spinal fusion in patients with severe disc degeneration, including disc space collapse, but without curvature disturbances or gross instability (3,4).

Until the end of the 1990s, total disc replacement did not gain wide acceptance for several reasons: Only one product was available on the market worldwide (3,4), the implantation required a major anterior transabdominal approach, and the indication criteria were not well defined. Because the 1990s were dominated by the development of less invasive anterior approaches to the lumbar spine, a technology without a well-defined application or predictable outcomes that required "classic" anterior access surgery appeared to have no place.

In early 2000, a new generation of implant (ProDisc; Spine Solutions, Inc., New York, NY, U.S.A.) was introduced in a multicenter clinical trial. It can be placed through a minimally invasive anterior approach and thus combines the advantages of the two technologies. This chapter outlines the implant technology, the minimally invasive access, and our preliminary results in a series of patients with a minimum follow-up of 1 year.

THE PRODISC TOTAL LUMBAR DISC

The ProDisc design is based on the physiologic form and function of the natural spinal motion segment unit. The kinematics and morphology of the implant design integrate the biomechanical and anatomic aspects of the physiologic spine.

The modular prosthesis comprises three elements: (a) an inferior cobalt–chromium–molybdenum alloy plate component, which is anchored in the endplate of the inferior vertebral body, and (b) a monoconvex ultra–high-molecular-weight polyethylene (UHMWPE) inlay securely locked in the inferior plate component, which forms a ball-and-socket joint with (c) the superior plate, which is anchored in the endplate of the superior vertebral body (Fig. 26.1). Only materials of proven biocompatibility with a successful, long-term history in joint replacement have been used.

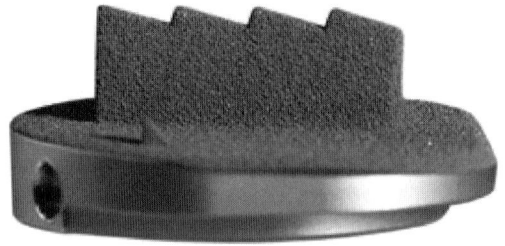
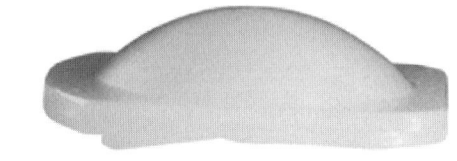
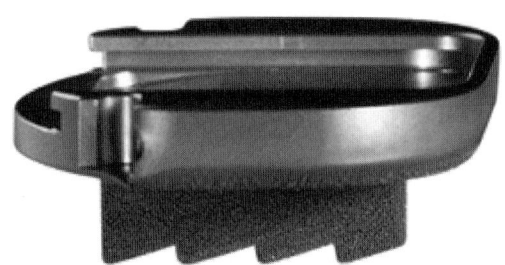

FIG. 26.1. The ProDisc modular design consists of two metal endplates and one ultra–high-molecular-weight polyethylene (UHMWPE) inlay, which is fixed in the lower endplate by a snap-lock mechanism. Modular design concept: three components. Proven implant materials: cobalt–chromium–molybdenum/ultra–high-molecular-weight polyethylene inlay/titanium. Physiologic range of motion: ball and socket joint. Modular polyethylene insertion and locking allow minimal distraction. Primary stabilization: keel/spikes/Plasmapore (Aesculap, Tuttlingen, Germany). Secondary stabilization: Plasmapore coating and osseous integration.

The superior and inferior plate components are made of a cobalt–chromium–molybdenum alloy according to International Standardization Organization (ISO) 5832-12. In both metal endplates, an osteoconductive, rough, plasma-sprayed titanium coating on the surface promotes osseous integration.

The inlay is made of UHMWPE according to ISO 5834-2. All materials in the instrumentation that come in contact with tissue are manufactured from stainless steel conforming to ISO 7153-1 ("surgical instruments, metallic materials, stainless steel").

The proper implant fit can be achieved by selecting from two sizes, three heights, and two lordosis angles. The anatomic shape of the implant provides maximum support for the endplates, which prevents migration and subsidence into the vertebral endplates. The implant is available in two angles of lordosis, 6 and 11 degrees. Disc heights of 10, 12, and 14 mm are available.

Because the design of the implant is modular, it can be inserted stepwise. The endplates are implanted without distracting the disc space. Specially designed instruments are then used to apply distraction, and the UHMWPE inlay is inserted. With this technique, "overdistraction" in the area of the spinal cord and the nerve roots can be avoided (Fig. 26.2).

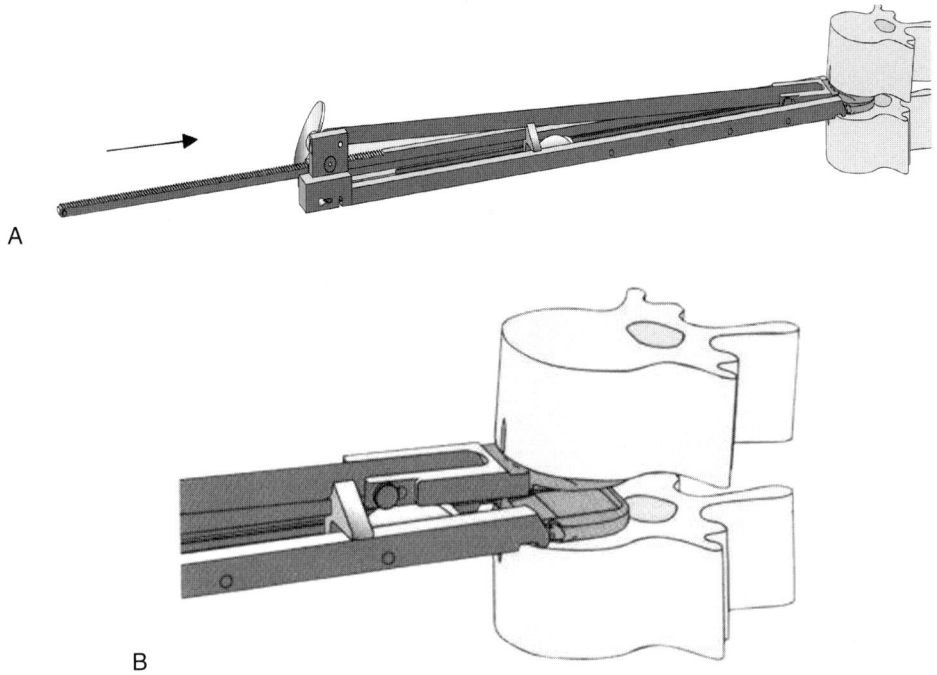

FIG. 26.2. A: Implantation of the endplates without distraction. **B:** Distraction and introduction of the polyethylene inlay.

SURGICAL TECHNIQUE

The implantation technique has been described in detail (12). The surgical access is in the midline for all levels from L2–3 down to L5–S1.

The patient is placed in a supine "Da Vinci" position (hips abducted, arms abducted 90 degrees, head of the operating table tilted down) (Fig. 26.3). The level of the disc space is localized under lateral and anteroposterior fluoroscopy (9,12). The skin incision is centered over the disc space and placed transversely in the midline for L5–S1 or slightly paramedian and to the right for L4–5 to L2–3. A mini-open laparotomy is performed, and the anterior circumference of the disc space is exposed through a retroperitoneal or transperitoneal approach. Dissection of the retroperitoneal blood vessels requires special attention and preoperative planning (12). For surgeons who are not experienced with anterior approaches, the assistance of a vascular surgeon is recommended. Once the anterior circumference of the disc space has been exposed, the midline is marked under fluoroscopic control. The disc is then removed and the segment released. Release can be difficult in cases with collapsed disc spaces, in which a resection of the posterior annulus fibrosus may be necessary. Once the disc space has been released, a probe implant is inserted to determine the size, height, and lordosis angle of the implant (Fig. 26.4). The probe implant serves as a guide for a special chisel, which creates two grooves in the superior and inferior endplates (Fig.

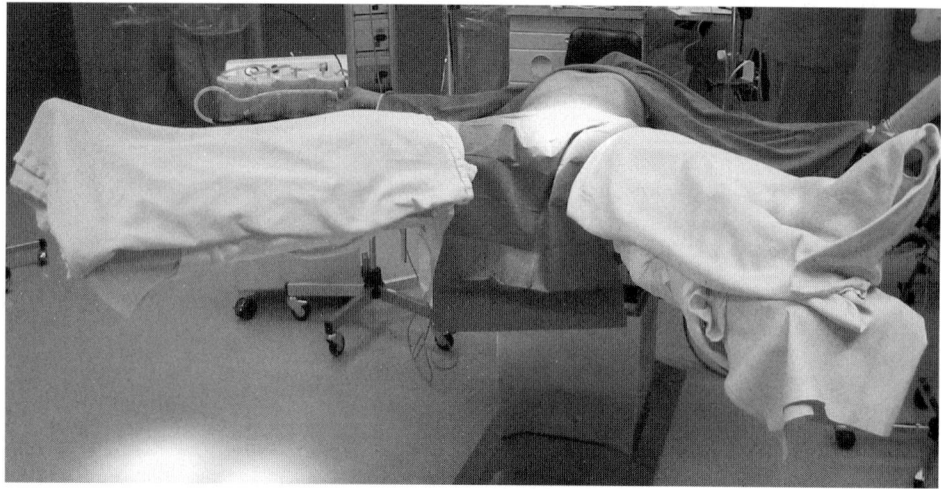

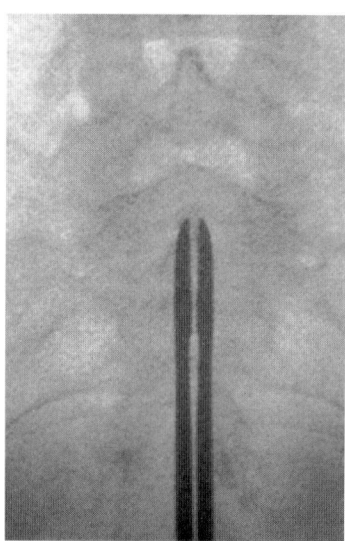

FIG. 26.3. **A:** "Da Vinci" positioning of the patient (hips abducted, arms abducted 90 degrees). **B:** Intraoperative anteroposterior roentgenogram of the lumbar spine. Marking of the midline projection.

26.5). The implant is then mounted on the application instrument and pressed with a surgical mallet into its final position. The UHMWPE inlay, which slides along two rails within the applicator, is then pushed forward, and at the same time, the disc space is distracted. After lateral roentgenographic confirmation of the correct implant position, the inlay is pushed into the lower endplate, where it snaps in firmly. After release of the distraction and removal of the applicator, the implant position is confirmed visually and with biplanar roentgenography (Fig. 26.6 A–C).

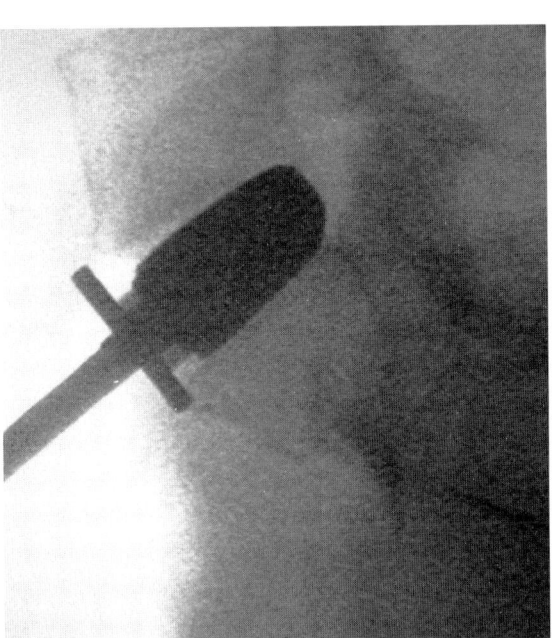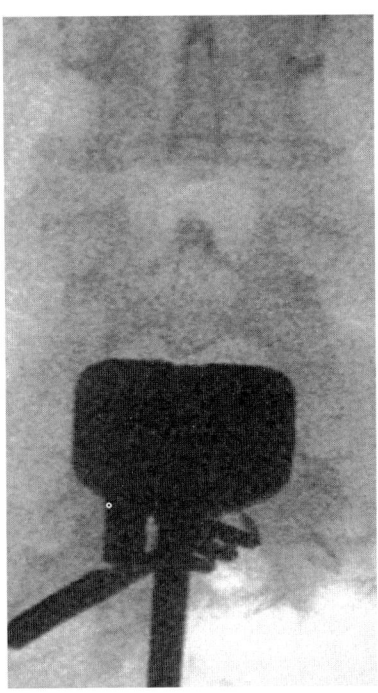

FIG. 26.4. Probe implant in place. **A:** Anteroposterior roentgenogram. **B:** Lateral view.

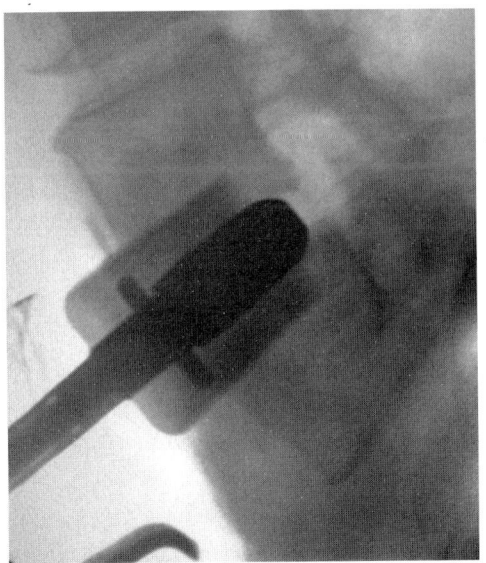

FIG. 26.5. Chiseling of the grooves in the superior and inferior endplate. Lateral roentgenogram.

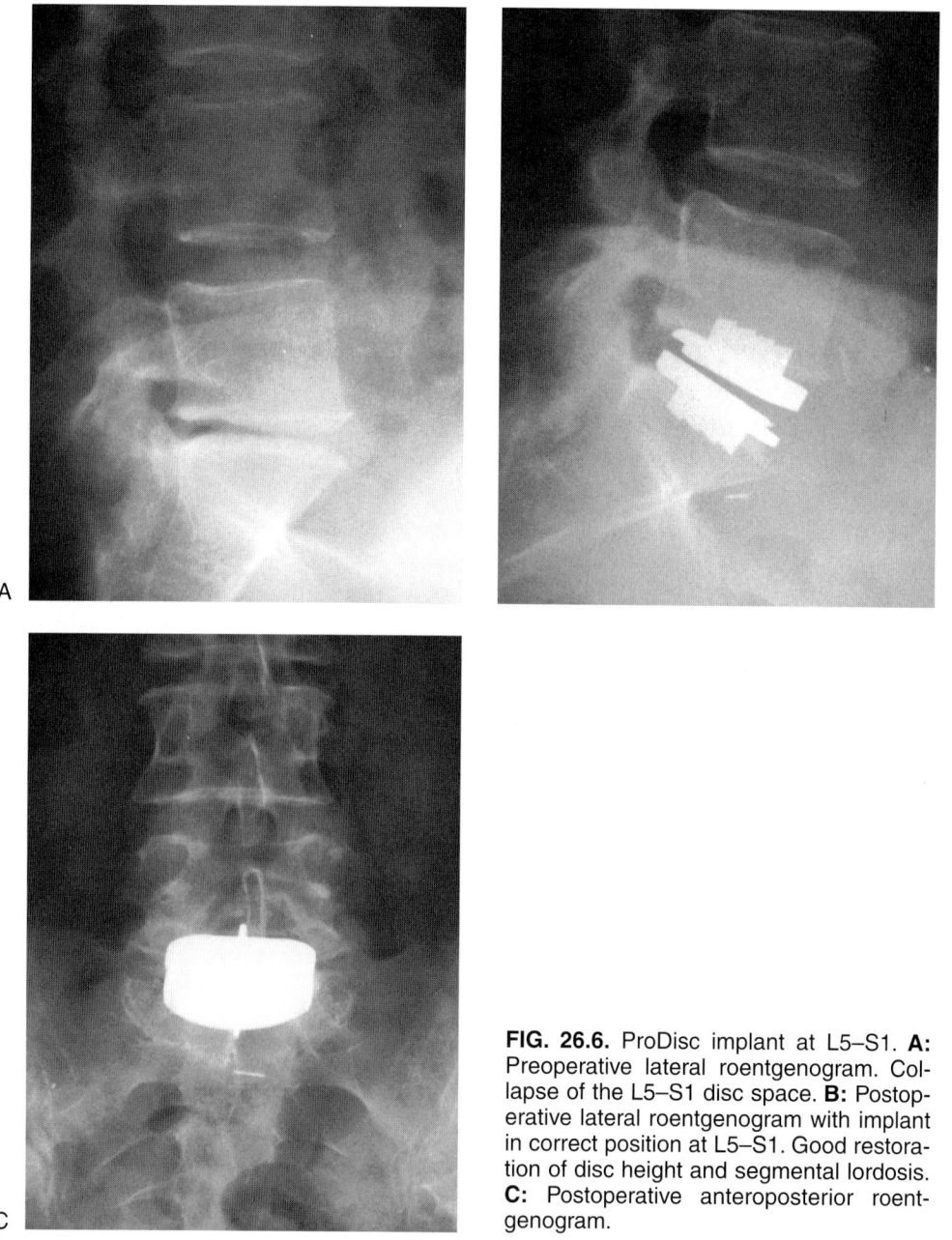

FIG. 26.6. ProDisc implant at L5–S1. **A:** Preoperative lateral roentgenogram. Collapse of the L5–S1 disc space. **B:** Postoperative lateral roentgenogram with implant in correct position at L5–S1. Good restoration of disc height and segmental lordosis. **C:** Postoperative anteroposterior roentgenogram.

PATIENTS

Between July 2000 and January 2002, 23 patients (17 women, six men) underwent surgical implantation of the ProDisc device in a prospective clinical trial. The indications were degenerative disc disease, a decompensated level adjacent to a previous fusion, and primary or postoperative degenerative disc disease without translational instability. All patients were evaluated preoperatively and postoperatively according to a standardized protocol with roentgenography, a visual analog scale (VAS) and Oswestry Questionnaire, and clinical assessment.

RESULTS

The mean follow-up was 14.7 months (range, 12 to 18 months). The average age of the patients was 43.3 years. Surgery was performed most frequently at the L5–S1 level (73.9%), followed by the L4–5 and L4–5–S1 levels (8.7% each). The average time for surgery was 128 minutes, including the double-level cases. Blood loss was 110 mL (range, 30 to 300 mL). No intraoperative complications occurred. At the time of follow-up, the mean Oswestry score was reduced by an average of 18.3% from 37.2% preoperatively. The VAS score was reduced by an average of 3.6 from 6.3 preoperatively. Of all the patients, 73.9% were completely satisfied or satisfied with the overall clinical result. One postoperative dislocation of the UHMWPE inlay resulted from poor surgical technique during the implantation. (Inlay obviously had not completely snap-locked in the lower endplate.) This young female patient had to undergo revision surgery 8 weeks after the first implantation, during which the implant was removed and a new implant inserted.

DISCUSSION

Fusion of the lumbar spine is associated with a variety of undesired side effects and complications that can be attributed to the surgical approach, type of fusion, type of implant, surgery at the donor site, or general conditions (1,6,11). The rates of specific, general, early, and late complications can reach 40% (5,11,14), which is why debate continues about whether fusion is justified at all in patients with degenerative disorders of the lumbar spine (5). A variety of "dynamic" and reconstructive techniques for the treatment of degenerative spinal disorders have now been published and are summarized under the term *spine arthroplasty* (13). The most advanced technique, however, is total disc replacement (2–4,12). Although our results must still be viewed as preliminary, total disc replacement through a limited, minimally invasive surgical access appears to be a valuable surgical alternative to spinal fusion. The complication rate in our first small series was low, and the minimally invasive surgical access is feasible and safe. The clinical results are favorable, and the range of indications is expected to increase in the future. A considerable number of patients still present with degenerative curvature disturbances, such as degenerative lumbar scoliosis and degenerative spondylolisthesis. There is no doubt that lumbar fusion is the treatment option in such cases when they do not respond to conservative therapy. Although the indications for total disc replacement are primarily restricted to one- or two-segment degenerative disc disease, we believe that this technology can be applied in new areas—for example, in combination with fusion techniques or in the dynamic restoration of a decompensated segment adjacent to a fusion.

REFERENCES

1. Baker JK, Reardon PR, Reardon MJ. Vascular injury in anterior lumbar surgery. *Spine* 1993;18:2227–2230.
2. Bertganoli R, Kumar S. Indications for full prosthetic disc arthroplasty: a correlation to clinical outcome against a variety of indications. *Eur Spine J* 2002;11:131–136.
3. Büttner-Janz K. *The development of the artificial disc: SB Charité*. Dallas: Hundley & Associates, 1992.
4. David T. Lumbar disc prosthesis—surgical technique, indications and clinical results in 22 patients with a minimum of 12 months' follow-up. *Eur Spine J* 1993;1:254–259.
5. Deyo RA. Low-back pain. *Sci Am* 1998;279:28–33.

6. Faciszewski T, Winter RB, Lonstein JE, et al. The surgical and medical perioperative complications of anterior spinal fusion surgery in the thoracic and lumbar spine of adults. *Spine* 1995;20:1592–1599.
7. Greenough CG, Taylor LJ, Fraser RD. Anterior lumbar fusion: results, assessment techniques and prognostic factors. *Eur Spine J* 1994;3:225–230.
8. Grob D, Scheier HJG, Dvorak J, et al. Circumferential fusion of the lumbar and lumbosacral spine. *Arch Orthop Trauma Surg* 1991;111:20–25.
9. Mayer HM. Microsurgical approaches for anterior interbody fusion of the lumbar spine: In: McCulloch JA, Young PA, eds. *Essentials of spinal microsurgery*. Philadelphia: Lippincott–Raven Publishers, 1998:633–649
10. Mayer HM. Microsurgical decompression of acquired (degenerative) central and lateral spinal canal stenosis. In: Mayer HM, ed. *Minimally invasive spine surgery*. New York: Springer-Verlag, 2000:105–116.
11. Mayer HM, Korge A. Nonfusion technology in degenerative lumbar spinal disorders: facts, questions, challenges. *Eur Spine J* 2002;11[Suppl 2]:85–91.
12. Mayer HM, Wiechert K, Korge A, et al. Minimally invasive total disc replacement: surgical technique and preliminary clinical results. *Eur Spine J* 2002;11[Suppl 2]:124–130.
13. Szpalski M, Gunzburg R, Mayer HM. Spine arthroplasty: a historical review. *Eur Spine J* 2002;11[Suppl 2]:65–84.
14. Turner JA, Herron, L, Deyo RA. Metaanalysis of the results of lumbar spine fusion. *Acta Orthop Scand* 1993;64:120–122.

27

The PDN Prosthetic Disc Nucleus Device: Product Design and Clinical Results

*Sinéad A. Kavanagh, and †‡§Charles D. Ray

*Department of Mechanical Engineering, National University of Ireland, Galway, Galway, Ireland; †American College of Spine Surgery, Jacksonville, Florida; ‡International Spine Arthroplasty Society, West Palm Beach, Florida; §North American Spine Society, La Grange, Illinois

Many people experience back pain during their lifetime (3,7). The causes of low back pain vary but, in most cases, some degree of intervertebral disc degeneration is involved (5). Degenerative disc disease is often characterized by a measurable decrease in disc height accompanied by a reduction in vertebral stability and the onset of sustained low back pain. These symptoms have traditionally been treated with spinal fusion, which can be effective and relieve pain; however, fusion has the disadvantages of being highly invasive and eliminating mobility in the affected vertebral segments. In addition, spinal fusion can begin a degenerative cascade in the lumbar region as the adjacent levels overcompensate for lack of motion at the fused segments (1). As an alternative to fusion, the PDN prosthetic disc nucleus device (Raymedica, Inc., Minneapolis, MN, U.S.A.) has been developed to work in a manner similar to that of a healthy disc nucleus. The device aims to reduce or eliminate the low back pain associated with degenerative disc disease by maintaining/restoring disc height while also retaining the biomechanical behavior and range of motion of the implanted level. The PDN device is designed to maintain segmental mobility by allowing the vertebral bodies to move in relation to each other in compression, rotation, and lateral bending (8).

MATERIALS AND METHODS

Device Construction

The PDN device consists of a hydrogel core encased in a polyethylene jacket (Fig. 27.1). Platinum–iridium markers are embedded in each device for radiographic visualization during and after implantation (Fig 27.2). The hydrogel core is a copolymer of polyacrylonitrile (nonhydrophilic) and polyacrylamide (hydrophilic). These polymers are combined in a ratio that allows the PDN device to absorb 80% of its weight in water, which helps to restore disc height and support the loads exerted on the lumbar spine. The hydrogel core is molded into various pellet shapes and sizes to accommodate each patient's unique endplate and disc morphology.

A tightly woven but porous jacket of high-molecular-weight polyethylene encases each hydrogel pellet, allowing it to absorb surrounding intradiscal fluid. The process by which the jacket is manufactured produces fibers with a high degree of tensile strength. The

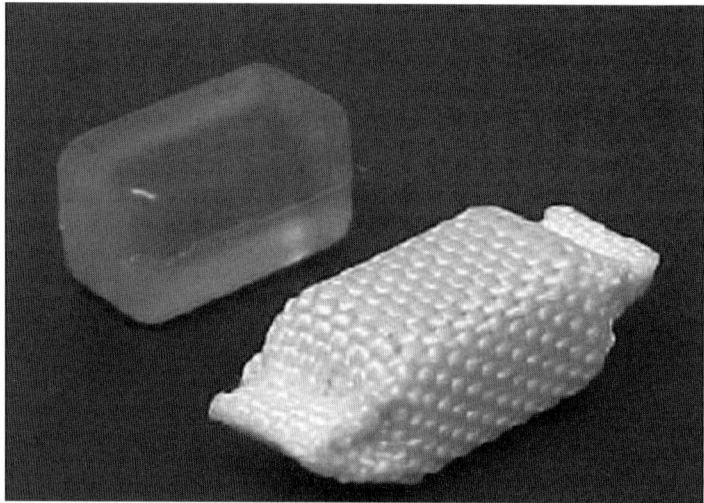

FIG. 27.1. PDN hydrogel pellet shown with and without a polyethylene jacket.

strength of the fibers is key in constraining the expansion of the hydrogel core to a predetermined dimension as it absorbs fluid; without the jacket, the hydrogel alone would not be able to support the loads exerted on the spine. The polyethylene used in the PDN device jacket is structurally different from the ultra–high-molecular-weight polyethylene (UHMWPE) used for artificial joint replacements. One of the concerns about the use of UHMWPE for artificial joints is that debris can be produced over time as a consequence of wear. Extensive testing of the PDN device and its materials have shown that the polyethylene used in the jacket does not generate biologically significant polyethylene particles with wear, even after 50 million cycles of fatigue testing (6).

Like the intervertebral disc, the PDN device exhibits viscoelastic properties. The term *viscoelastic* describes a material that behaves as both a fluid and a solid; the viscous component deforms permanently under a load, whereas the solid component supports the load

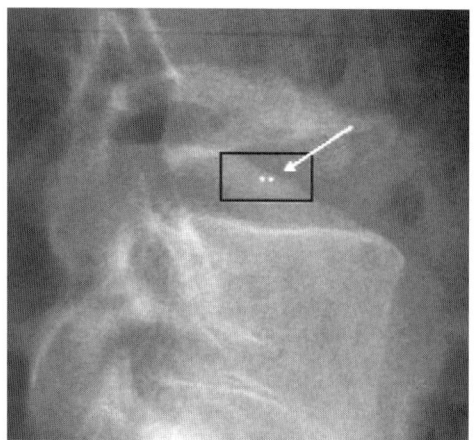 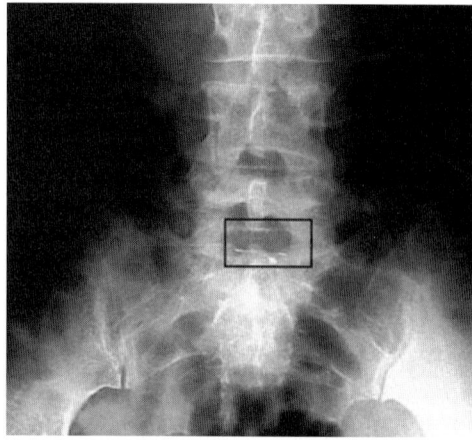

FIG. 27.2. Platinum–iridium markers are shown in the implanted PDN device on x-ray film. **A:** Lateral view of implanted disc. **B:** Anteroposterior view of implanted disc.

but returns to its original shape once the load is reduced. In a cadaver experiment, the viscoelastic behavior of the PDN device was quantified and compared with that of an intact cadaver specimen (4). A three-parameter model, which included two stiffness coefficients (describing the short-term and long-term stiffness of the material) and one viscous coefficient, was used to analyze the behavior of the devices and the cadaver specimen. The coefficient results for the devices were comparable with the values calculated for the intact intervertebral disc and other values obtained from the literature. Hence, it was concluded that the viscoelastic and material properties of the device are similar to those of a normal disc.

The PDN device with its disclike viscoelastic properties must be able to function for a long time. To evaluate the long-term performance of the device, the biomechanical properties of a cadaver motion segment were tested before and after implantation with PDN devices that were fatigued to 20 million cycles (2). The results showed that implantation of the fatigued devices restored disc height and enabled the specimen to resist compressive loading to a degree comparable with that of the intact disc.

Surgical Approach

The PDN device can be implanted through a traditional posterior hemilaminotomy technique or via the anterolateral transpsoatic approach, in which the disc is accessed from the side. In either case, the PDN device is implanted in the enucleated disc space and transversely positioned in the center of the disc (Fig. 27.3). The hydrogel core of the device is compressed and dehydrated during the manufacturing process to minimize its size, so that trauma at implantation is reduced. PDN devices can be implanted either in pairs or singly (PDN SOLO device), depending on the patient's disc size and endplate morphology.

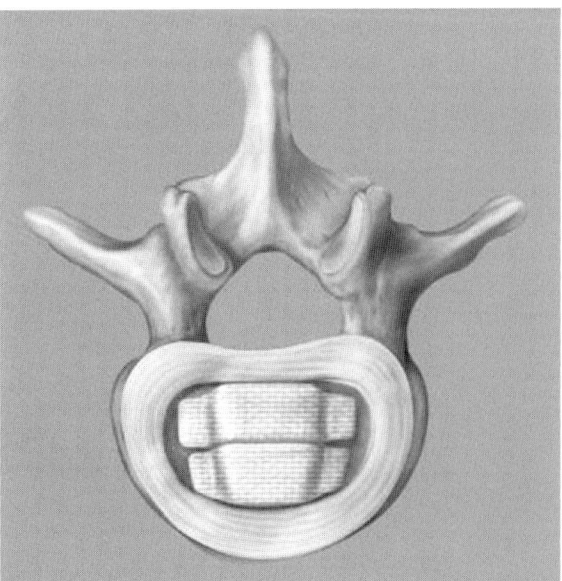

FIG. 27.3. Illustration of two PDN devices within an intervertebral disc. The nucleus pulposus is surgically removed from the disc, and the PDN devices are positioned transverse to the sagittal plane. Different device sizes and shapes are available to match the patient's endplate morphology.

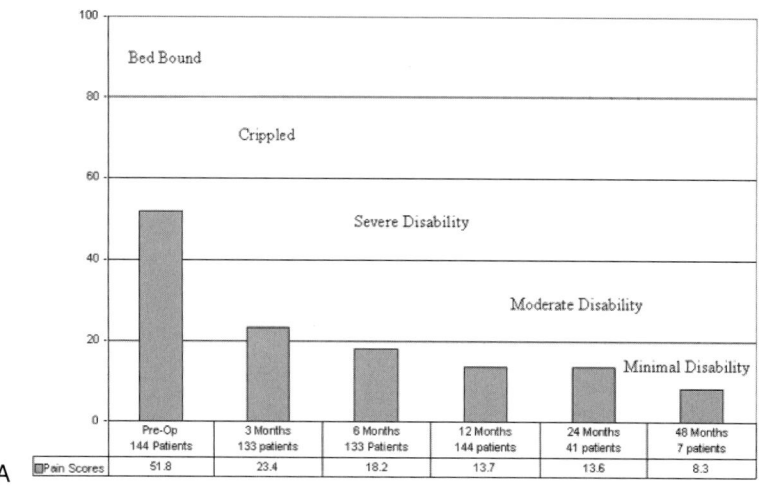
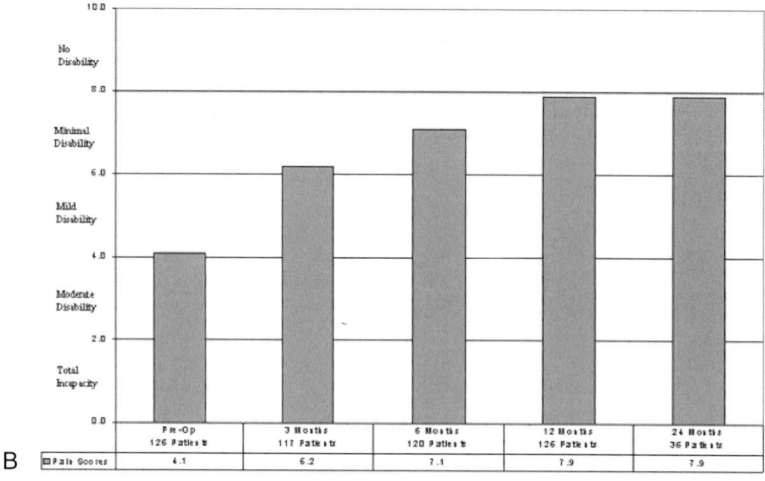
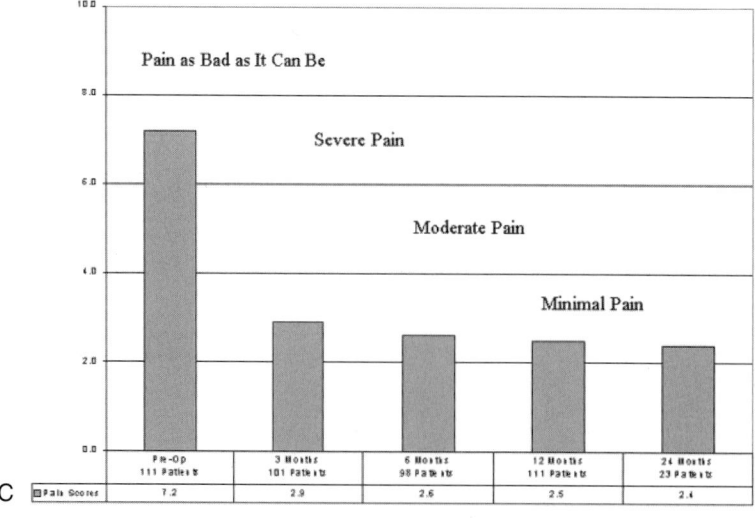

FIG. 27.4. Oswestry low back pain disability scores (%) **(A)**, Prolo functional and economic index **(B)**, and visual analog pain scale index **(C)** scores for patients with an implanted PDN device (24-month follow-up continuing to 48 months).

RESULTS

Initial clinical trials for PDN devices were conducted from 1996 through 1998. Sixty-five patients underwent implantation in this first series, with a surgical success of rate of 77% (15 of the 65 patients required either revision or explant surgery). To increase the success rate for the PDN device, a number of modifications were made: (a) The water content in the hydrogel was increased to soften the consistency of the device; (b) the PDN device models that were found to be most likely to migrate were discontinued; (c) new surgical instruments were developed to facilitate implantation; (d) fluoroscopic imaging during the implant procedure was used more often to ensure proper positioning of the device; and (e) a more restrictive postoperative patient protocol was developed and implemented.

Since these changes were incorporated, the surgical success rate for the device has improved. To date, over 1,200 PDN devices have been implanted worldwide with a success rate of over 90% in each of the past 3 years. Clinical results also are very satisfying. For a group of patients with continuous 12-month followup data, Oswestry pain scores have declined from a mean of 51.8% to a mean of 13.7% (n = 144). Prolo scores have improved from a preoperative mean of 4.1 to a postoperative mean of 7.9 (n = 126). Likewise, VAS scores (Visual Analog Scale for pain) have decreased from 7.2 to 2.5 (n = 111). Patients with 24- and 48-month followup also show the same pattern of improvement (Fig. 27.4).

DISCUSSION

A new PDN device model has been developed to satisfy further the varying needs of the patient population (Fig. 27.5). The PDN-SOLO device, as its name implies, is designed to be implanted alone, unlike the traditional devices, which have typically been implanted in pairs. The device was developed based on an analysis of 4-year follow-up clinical data, which indicated that migration was more likely to occur in patients with an anteroposterior total disc dimension of 37 mm or less when two devices were implanted. The PDN-SOLO device has been designed for patients with smaller discs (overall disc size, 37 mm or less) and for patients whose endplate configuration cannot accommodate two devices. Apart from its usefulness in smaller disc spaces, the PDN-SOLO is easier to implant than the traditional paired PDN devices.

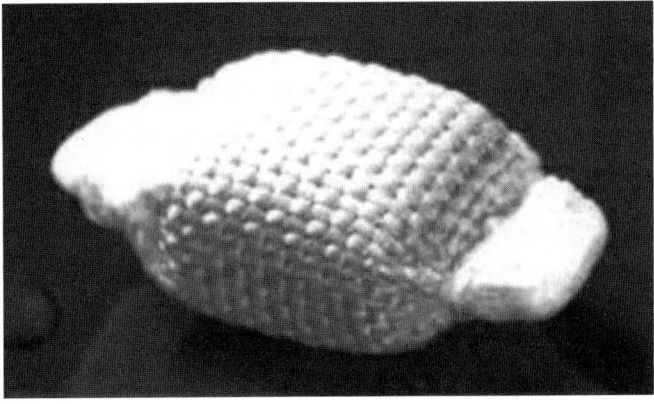

FIG. 27.5. Hydrated PDN-SOLO device.

The PDN-SOLO device is available in 5-, 7-, and 9-mm sizes to accommodate various disc heights. The materials used to manufacture the PDN-SOLO device are the same as those used to manufacture the standard PDN device models; the main difference between the devices is dimensional. The profile of the dehydrated PDN-SOLO device is essentially the same as that of standard models. However, upon implantation and hydration within the disc space, the device expands to a size 25% greater than that of a single standard device. Another feature of the new device is that the corners have been rounded and the hydrogel pellet has been molded to become more oval after hydration. The larger "footprint" and more rounded shape of the PDN-SOLO device allow it to conform to the shape of the vertebral endplates and distribute loads more evenly.

CONCLUSIONS

The PDN device is designed to reduce or eliminate the pain associated with degenerative disc disease while maintaining mobility and disc height. PDN devices come in different shapes and sizes to match the patient's disc space. The new PDN-SOLO device addresses the patient with a smaller disc space or endplate morphology that cannot accommodate paired devices.

To date, PDN devices have been implanted in more than 1,200 patients worldwide, and the clinical results, measured by Oswestry, VAS, and Prolo scores, are very encouraging. The surgical success rate for the device is also very good, with only a small percentage of patients requiring revision surgery. The device is currently available for commercial sale in Europe, South and Central America, the Middle East, Asia, and Australia. Clinical trials are ongoing in Canada and will soon begin in the United States.

REFERENCES

1. Aota Y, Kumano K, Hirabayashi S. Postfusion instability at the adjacent segments after rigid pedicle screw fixation for degenerated lumbar spinal disorders. *J Spinal Disord* 1995;8:464–473.
2. Bain AC, et al. *A biomechanical evaluation of a prosthetic disc nucleus device*. Presented at the 15th annual meeting of the North American Spine Society, New Orleans, 2000.
3. Borenstein DG. Epidemiology, etiology, diagnostic evaluation, and treatment of low back pain. *Curr Opin Rheumatol* 1999;11:151–157.
4. Kavanagh S, Bain A, Sherman T, et al. *Biomechanical evaluation of a fatigued prosthetic disc nucleus*. Poster presentation at the EuroSpine Conference, Gothenburg, Sweden, September 2001.
5. Luoma K, Riihimaki H, Luukkonen R, et al. Low back pain in relation to lumbar disc degeneration. *Spine* 2000;25:487–492.
6. Norton BK. *Polyethylene wear debris: is it relevant to the PDN prosthetic disc nucleus?* [Internal Research Publication]. Minneapolis, MN: Raymedica, Inc., 1998.
7. Reigo T, Timpka T, Tropp H. The epidemiology of back pain in vocational age groups. *Scand J Prim Health Care* 1999;17:17–21.
8. Wilke HJ, Kavanagh S, Neller S, et al. Effect of a prosthetic disc nucleus on the mobility and disc height of the L4–L5 intervertebral disc postnucleotomy. *J Neurosurg (Spine 2)* 2001;95:208–214.

28

The Evidence Base for the Treatment of—Not Degenerative Disc Disease—but Back Pain

Alf Nachemson

Department of Orthopedics, Göteborg University; Sahlgrenska University Hospital, Göteborg, Sweden; and Department of Orthopedics, Georgetown University, Washington, DC

With our proven difficulties in precisely diagnosing the cause of pain in patients with both acute and chronic back pain, it is my strong view that the term *degenerative disc disease* is a misnomer. Thus far, back pain is a symptom of unknown etiology, just like fewer. In about 90% of persons with back pain, the exact diagnosis eludes us, although this does not exclude the intervertebral disc as a possible generator of pain. In particular, pain occurs when a disc hernia causes radiculopathy. However, these cases constitute a minority of our difficult patients, about 5% to 10%. The effect of ordinary surgical removal of a disc hernia has been proved (8), whereas the removal of a degenerate/aging disc with or without fusion yields an unpredictable and rather modest clinical benefit (7,9).

An evidence base for the general treatment of low back pain (LBP) does exist, however, and I am happy to delineate such effective treatment after 50 years of studying back pain, including the last 10 years as chairperson of the Cochrane Collaboration Back Review Group, the output of which can be found at *http://cochrane.iwh.on.ca/review.htm* (2). This evidence base is also clearly described in my book (6). Thus, there is reason for optimism regarding at least a partial solution for the great majority of our patients with back pain, although it should be emphasized that the global problem is not only medical but also social and political (4,11). A final substantial reduction of this problem afflicting both patients and society will entail multifaceted collaboration.

In an overview of the results of the various treatment methods, agreement has been reached regarding levels of evidence:

Level A. *Strong evidence*—findings concur in several randomized controlled trials of high quality.

Level B. *Moderate evidence*—findings concur in one randomized controlled trial of high quality and one or more randomized controlled trials of low quality, or findings concur in several studies of low quality.

Level C. *Limited evidence*—based on findings of one randomized controlled trial (of high or low quality) or contradictory findings in several studies.

Level D. *No evidence*—no randomized controlled trials or other types of studies of satisfactory scientific quality.

ASSESSING PAIN IN THE NECK AND LOW BACK

Thorough, systematic anamnesis and a physical examination constitute a good foundation for diagnosing back pain according to many studies reflecting moderate evidence (B). Furthermore, many studies show that the caregiver's involvement and ability to listen to the patient's concerns—not only about pain and its localization but also about the consequences of pain and how it is dealt with—are essential to a proper diagnosis. Along with anamnesis and physical examination, listening and talking allow the patient and caregiver to reach agreement on the best treatment. They are also sufficient for identifying the few cases that must be referred for further investigation when a specific cause or serious disease may be responsible for the pain.

If pain persists for 3 to 4 weeks, further investigation should be carried out with one of the validated available questionnaires, which can identify other relevant problems (e.g., in the work environment or the psychosocial situation in general) (B).

A basic roentgenographic examination seldom provides guidance in the diagnosis, except in cases in which specific trauma or serious disease is suspected. As a rule, computed tomography (CT) and magnetic residence imaging (MRI) do not identify where pain is located, except, again, in patients with specific disease. A herniated disc pressing on a nerve root can cause severe sciatica. This condition can be visualized and confirmed by CT or MRI, which are of proven value when clinical symptoms of nerve root involvement are correctly correlated with imaging findings (A).

The advantage of CT is that the procedure is noninvasive, and MRI additionally does not expose the patient to radiation. However, false-positive findings are associated with these studies. This risk is substantial, both regarding herniated discs and changes in discs resulting from aging and narrowing of the spinal and root canals, which all appear in approximately 40% to 50% of symptom-free persons.

Only limited evidence is available for many other diagnostic methods and their benefits (C). This applies to measurement of range of motion, evaluation of muscle strength and condition, facet joint or nerve root blockade, spectrometry, discography, electromyography or neurophysiology studies, and radiographic measurement of segmental movements and various spinal diameters. Actually, limited evidence (C) suggests that some of these are of no benefit at all.

Moderate evidence (B) suggests that thermography and ultrasonography do not contribute information toward establishing a diagnosis. Here, it should be noted that for a diagnostic method to be based on evidence, it must lead to a treatment method that has been proved useful scientifically.

CONSERVATIVE TREATMENT OF ACUTE AND CHRONIC LOW BACK PAIN

Conservative treatment refers basically to all nonsurgical treatment methods, including psychologic treatment, which is discussed separately later. Conservative treatment methods include drugs, acupuncture, injections of various types, back exercises, back school, manual treatment, manipulation, physical methods, traction, corsets, transcutaneous electric nerve stimulation (TENS), behavioral therapy, multidisciplinary treatment, biofeedback, rest, and activation. At the end of this chapter, the evidence regarding the effects of the various treatment methods is summarized. Here, the only conclusions presented for conservative treatment methods are those supported by strong evidence (A). It should be noted, however, that the treatment methods with level B evidence are also supported by relatively good scientific documentation.

28. EVIDENCE BASE FOR TREATMENT OF—NOT DDD—BUT BACK PAIN

For *acute* and *subacute* (0 to 3 months) LBP, strong evidence (A) indicates the following:

- Continuing with normal activities results in faster recovery and fewer chronic functional disorders.
- Antiinflammatory and muscle relaxant drugs offer effective relief of uncomplicated, acute LBP. (However, these drugs have some side effects.)
- Bed rest is *not* effective treatment for acute LBP.
- Exercises involving bending, traction, aerobics, and stretching do *not* effectively cure acute LBP.

For *chronic* (lasting longer than 3 months) LBP, strong evidence (A) indicates the following:

- Manual treatment/manipulation, back training, and multidisciplinary treatment are effective in relieving pain; multidisciplinary treatment also improves function.
- Intensive treatment at a health resort reduces pain in the short term for elderly patients (older than 60 years of age) with chronic low back problems.

CONSERVATIVE TREATMENT OF ACUTE AND CHRONIC NECK PAIN

Conventional treatment methods that are normally used to treat neck pain are largely similar to those used to treat low back problems. The treatment methods reviewed include drugs, physical training, manual treatment, massage, body exercises, muscle training, heat packs, ergonomic counseling, traction, acupuncture, TENS, electromagnetic treatment, magnet therapy, patient education, behavioral therapy, steroid injections, and treatment with neck collars, infrared light, ultrasound, lasers, cooling spray, and stretching.

Very few studies in this field are of high scientific quality. In summary, only moderate or limited evidence is available to show that any of the treatment methods are effective in relieving acute or chronic neck pain. However, strong evidence shows that acupuncture is *not* an effective method of treating *chronic* neck pain (A).

SURGICAL TREATMENT OF SCIATICA AND CHRONIC LOW BACK PAIN

Surgery for *herniated discs* in patients with sciatica, which reduces pressure on a painful nerve root and chemical irritation, is of proven efficacy (A), although the reviewers point out that the evidence is indirect (8). Numerous surgical methods, including minimally invasive surgery, are used to treat herniated discs—with or without the help of lasers or microscopes. No scientific evidence shows that these surgical methods yield better results or cause fewer serious complications than conventional surgery (C)

As mentioned in the Cochrane Review of Gibson et al. (8), including the update presented in this book, and in the landmark Swedish multicenter prospective randomized trial published by Fritzell (7) and Hägg (9), fusion for chronic LBP of more than 6 months' duration, particularly in patients without psychosocial deterrents for recovery and with a radiographic demonstration of a single involved disc at a low level (low predictive power), is somewhat better than continuing physical therapy; however, the improvement, regardless of whether an ordinary fusion, fusion with pedicle screws and plates, or 360-degree fusion is performed, is moderate indeed. Only a 30% improvement in the Oswestry score and approximately the same in the visual analog scale (VAS) score for pain reduction is achieved (level B evidence). However, the rate of complications, both acute and after 2 years, is significantly greater with metallic implants or with 360-degree fusion than with an ordinary fusion—30% versus 6%.

The randomized studies reviewed (8) showed surgery for a herniated disc to be more effective than chemonucleolysis (A), which in turn was more effective than placebo (A). Chemonucleolysis is an alternative to surgery in which the chymopapain enzyme is used to dissolve the soft nucleus of the disc chemically. The results of surgery following failed chemonucleolysis are inferior to those of primary open surgery (C).

SURGERY FOR NECK PAIN

The studies reviewed address the surgical treatment of chronic pain resulting from whiplash injuries, herniated discs, or spondylosis.

Only two randomized controlled studies of surgery for spondylosis, with or without herniated disc, were found (3,10). These reported no advantages from surgery (B). Regarding whiplash injuries, no evidence indicates that surgery is superior to conservative treatment. No studies have been performed.

PSYCHOLOGIC TREATMENT METHODS

Psychologic treatment is used to complement other treatment and is often included as part of the increasingly common multidimensional pain treatment programs. Cognitive behavioral therapy focuses on managing the problems, feelings, thoughts, and behaviors that pain and functional disabilities may cause.

Many randomized controlled studies have addressed cognitive behavioral therapy. Although it is difficult to assess the specific impact of cognitive behavioral therapy in multidimensional programs, studies show that programs including this type of treatment achieve better results than other types of treatment in patients with *chronic* back problems (A). This particularly applies to the effects of treatment on anxiety, physical function, and use of medication.

INFLUENCE OF SOCIAL FACTORS

Social factors that have been reviewed include the following (11): the role of culture and family; the influence of unemployment on the consequences of back pain, its intensity, and duration; the role of access to social welfare payments and early pension, and their monetary value; and the importance of relations with work colleagues and the degree of work satisfaction in this context. In addition, special forms of workers' compensation insurance systems appear to influence the results of treatment and disability.

Neck and back pain occur in all societies, but cultural groups differ in how they perceive symptoms and deal with them. Weak scientific evidence (C) shows that genetic factors do not play a role in the occurrence of back pain, except possibly in disc aging and herniation.

Many studies show that poor social conditions are closely associated with poor general health, including back pain. Regarding back problems as a risk factor for unemployment and early retirement, several studies show conflicting results without a clear cause-and-effect relationship. Rather, it appears that age, psychologic factors, and access to insurance are important explanatory variables in this context.

Several studies show that neck and back pain are not always isolated clinical problems; rather, they are often associated with other types of pain, other diseases, stress-related symptoms, and work-related or other social problems. Scientific evidence shows that negative psychosocial aspects of working life, such as poor work satisfaction and poor relationships with others, are associated with more frequent reports of neck and back problems. At present, no confirmed biologic mechanisms have been identified to explain how psychosocial factors would *cause* back pain, nor has any evidence been found of a direct causal relationship.

In summary, extensive but scientifically weak evidence suggests that social factors can influence the tendency to recognize back pain and attitudes toward pain, functional disabilities, absenteeism, and early retirement. Some of these factors can be quite powerful and, at least in some situations, may have a greater effect on the back or neck than physical problems.

ROLE OF PRIMARY CARE

Many earlier reviews from different countries have led to evidence-based guidelines for the care of patients with back pain. These have focused on primary care.

The scientific studies currently available show that the interventions provided within primary care are the only ones that most patients with back problems require. These studies also show that a primary care physician's most important task is not to intervene unnecessarily. Subjecting a patient to ineffective examinations and treatments carries some risk that the patient's back problem will develop into a chronic, lifelong disorder.

In primary care, the consultation itself offers a major opportunity to influence both the acute and the longer-term course of a back problem. An essential aspect of the consultation is the involvement of the caregiver and the ability to work with and listen to the patient's perception of back pain, mainly how it affects daily life. The opportunity for the physician and patient to arrive at a common understanding about the nature and course of back pain is of major importance for the prognosis and is highly dependent on a good patient–doctor relationship.

CONCLUSIONS

- Pain in the low back and neck is common. LBP affects up to 80% of all people at some time during life, and neck pain affects up to 50% of the population (5). In the overwhelming majority of cases, back pain does not signal a serious disease or indicate that one should avoid normal daily activities. On the contrary, scientific studies show that healing is promoted by staying active, returning to work, and exercising at an appropriate level and with increasing intensity.
- A thorough anamnesis and physical examination are important for relieving anxiety about the consequences of pain and sufficient for identifying those patients who should be referred to a specialist for further examination and treatment (e.g., patients with severe infection, specific rheumatic disease, suspected cancer, or other serious conditions).
- For most people with back pain, the interventions that can be offered in primary care are the only ones needed. The physician's attitude and ability to listen to and empathize with the patient are important for achieving a common understanding about which treatment strategies are likely to be effective. The physician's demeanor is also important in regard to the future course of the patient's back pain and compliance with treatment advice.
- Back pain and its consequences are not isolated physical problems; rather, they are often associated with other conditions, such as social, psychologic, and workplace-related fac-

tors. These factors (e.g., stress, worry, and anxiety), along with the patient's own perceptions of and ability to manage the problem, can have a decisive effect on the transition from acute to more chronic pain. The obvious role of psychosocial factors in this respect suggests that such factors should be considered an integral part of back pain in relation to preventive efforts, both in the initial phase of treatment and later during rehabilitation.

- Many treatment methods are currently used, but often little scientific evidence of their benefit is available. Some treatment methods are used despite scientific evidence showing that they do not benefit the patient. The appropriateness of subsidizing ineffective treatments with public funds should be investigated.
- The primary focus in a patient with back pain should be on the pain itself and the human suffering it causes. Back pain has an extensive economic effect on both individuals and society. At least in Sweden, the annual direct costs of health care and the costs of sick leave and early retirement resulting from back pain are more than three times higher than the corresponding costs for all cancer diseases. Against this background, it is remarkable that research on back pain, particularly research related to prevention, relief, and rehabilitation, is relatively limited in scope. Agencies that have a responsibility for and interest in effectively managing back problems should take initiatives to stimulate and focus research in this field and disseminate the information that is currently available; they should also promote the application of evidence-based medicine for patients with back pain.

SUMMARY OF EVIDENCE

Conservative Treatment Methods for Low Back Pain

Medication. Strong scientific evidence shows that nonsteroidal antiinflammatory drugs (NSAIDs) and muscle relaxants (e.g., benzodiazepines) relieve pain in patients with acute or subacute low back problems (i.e., problems that have lasted up to 3 weeks or up to 12 weeks) (A). However, antiinflammatory drugs can have serious side effects, particularly in elderly people, and muscle relaxants can cause tiredness and dependency, even after short-term use. Furthermore, moderate scientific evidence indicates that paracetamol effectively relieves acute LBP (B).

Limited scientific evidence suggests that these drugs are effective in treating chronic LBP (C). For example, only one study was found that compared the effect of muscle relaxants with the effects of placebo (i.e., no active treatment), but no such studies have addressed analgesics and NSAIDs in people with chronic low back problems.

No studies have assessed the effects of antidepressants in treating acute low back problems (D). However, moderate evidence suggests that these drugs do *not* have any effect on pain and mobility in patients with chronic low back disorders (B).

Only limited evidence supports the effectiveness of colchicine (medication for gout) and cortisone in tablet form (systemic steroids) in patients with acute LBP (C). Serious side effects have been reported for colchicine, but side effects of systemic steroids develop only after long-term use.

Injections. Several different types of injections are used at times to treat both acute and chronic back problems. The injections reviewed were epidural steroid injections (i.e., injections in the spinal cord canal), injections in trigger points and ligaments, and injections in facet joints.

Limited evidence suggests that epidural steroid injections are more effective than placebo for acute and chronic low back problems involving nerve root pain (C).

No studies have addressed the effects of injections on acute low back problems without nerve root pain (D). However, moderate evidence suggests that injections do *not* have any effects on chronic LBP without root symptoms (B).

No evidence is available on the effects of injections in trigger points, ligaments, or facet joints (D).

Back school. Limited evidence is available on the effects of back school on chronic and acute low back problems (C).

TENS. Limited evidence is available on the effects of TENS on acute and chronic low back problems (C).

Traction. Limited evidence suggests that traction effectively treats acute low back problems (C). However, strong evidence shows that it is *not* effective in treating chronic low back problems (A).

Acupuncture. No evidence is available on the effects of acupuncture in treating acute LBP (D), and only limited evidence (C) indicates that acupuncture is effective in treating chronic LBP.

Physical treatment methods. No evidence is available on the effects of cold, heat, shortwave diathermy, massage, or ultrasound in treating acute low back problems (D).

Low back corsets and other supportive devices. No evidence is available on the effects of different types of supportive devices in treating acute low back problems (D), and only limited evidence regarding their effects on chronic low back problems (C).

Back exercises/back training. Strong evidence shows that back training is an effective treatment for chronic LBP (A). Strong evidence also indicates that most types of specific back exercises (e.g., bending, traction, aerobic training, strength training, stretching) are *not* more effective than other interventions in treating acute LBP (A).

Manual therapy (manipulation and mobilization). Strong evidence shows that manual therapy provides short-term relief of chronic LBP (A), and moderate evidence indicates that it has corresponding effects on acute LBP (B). Moderate evidence also indicates that these methods provide better short-term relief of chronic LBP than routine care from a general practitioner, bed rest, analgesics, or massage (B). Limited evidence suggests that manipulation is more effective than physiotherapy or drugs in relieving acute LBP (C). The long-term effects of manipulation are supported only by limited evidence (C). A small but serious risk for neurologic complications is associated with manipulation therapy in patients with progressive neurologic deficit.

A Cochrane Review by Assendelft et al. (1) has demonstrated that manual therapy is superior only in comparison with treatment that has been shown to be of little benefit or ineffective. In comparison with medical practitioners' treatment, manual treatment appears to be equally effective for acute, subacute, and chronic back pain.

Behavioral therapy. The evidence is limited that behavioral therapy is effective in treating acute LBP (C), but moderate evidence is available concerning its effects on chronic LBP (B).

Multidisciplinary treatment. Strong evidence shows that multidisciplinary treatment, which includes cognitive behavioral therapy, effectively relieves pain and improves function in patients with long-term and severe chronic LBP (A).

Biofeedback. Moderate evidence suggests that electromyography-based biofeedback is *not* effective in treating chronic low back problems (B).

Health resorts. Strong evidence shows that intensive treatment at a health resort reduces short-term pain in elderly patients with chronic low back problems (A).

Bed rest. Strong scientific evidence shows that bed rest is *not* an effective way to treat acute LBP (A). The previous perception that 1 to 2 days of bed rest is effective in treating uncomplicated acute LBP has been rejected in scientific studies. Extended bed rest may cause complications such as joint stiffness, muscle atrophy, osteoporosis, pressure sores, and thromboembolism.

Continued activity. Strong scientific evidence shows that a gradual resumption of activity in patients with subacute LBP, in combination with treatment of pain behavior, helps reduce chronic functional problems and sick leave from work (A).

Conservative Treatment Methods for Neck Pain

Laser treatment. Limited evidence is available on the effects of laser treatment for acute and chronic neck pain (C).

Infrared light. Only limited evidence indicates that infrared light has any effect at all on acute neck pain (C).

Electromagnetic therapy. Only limited evidence supports the effectiveness of electromagnetic therapy in treating acute neck pain (C).

TENS. Only limited evidence is available on the effects of TENS in treating acute neck pain (C).

Steroid injections. Limited evidence suggests that steroid injections are *not* effective in treating neck pain (C).

Acupuncture. No evidence is available on the effects of acupuncture in treating acute neck pain (D). However, strong evidence shows that acupuncture is *not* an effective treatment for chronic neck pain (A).

Traction. Limited evidence suggests that traction is *not* effective in treating acute neck pain (C), and moderate evidence suggests that it is *not* effective in treating chronic neck pain (B).

Cooling spray and stretching. Only one controlled study of patients with acute neck pain addressed the effects of cooling spray combined with passive stretching—a common treatment method in sports medicine. The study is of low scientific quality and showed no differences in outcome between active treatment and placebo (C).

Neck support. Limited evidence suggests that a neck collar is *not* effective in treating acute or chronic neck pain (C).

Manual therapy. Only limited evidence is available on the effects of separate manual therapy for acute neck pain (C), but moderate positive evidence supports the effects of manual therapy applied as one of several methods in a treatment program for acute neck problems (B). Regarding chronic neck pain, strong evidence shows that manipulation is *not* more effective than physiotherapy methods (A), and moderate evidence suggests that manipulation is *not* an effective treatment for chronic neck pain (B).

Other types of physiotherapy (massage, body movements, and instruction). Strong evidence shows that these physiotherapy methods are *not* more effective than alternative forms of treatment (e.g., group exercises, manual therapy, and routine care from a general practitioner) in treating chronic neck pain (A).

Patient education. Limited evidence suggests that various types of instruction help reduce acute neck pain (C).

Behavioral therapy. Limited evidence suggests that behavioral therapy is effective in treating chronic neck pain (C).

Medication. Limited evidence is available on the effects of pain-relieving drugs in treating acute neck pain (C), and limited evidence that muscle relaxants are effective in treating chronic neck pain (C).

Physical training. Moderate evidence suggests that active training is more effective than passive methods (e.g., massage, heat therapy, and stretching) in treating acute neck pain (B).

Surgical Methods

Strong indirect evidence shows that surgical removal of a disc herniation in patients with pronounced lumbar root pain lasting several weeks is effective (more effective than chemonucleolysis, which in turn is more effective than placebo) (A). However, moderate evidence suggests that corresponding surgery is *not* effective in treating neck problems (B). Moderate evidence (B) is available concerning some positive effects of fusion surgery in treating chronic pain in the low back. Moderate evidence (B) indicates that additional fixation with implants *does not* improve clinical results in the lumbar spine.

Psychologic Treatment Methods

Strong evidence shows that cognitive behavioral therapy reduces problems in patients with chronic back pain (A). The effects are mainly on psychologic and physiologic function, pain, and medication use. Limited evidence suggests that cognitive behavioral therapy influences the patient's return to work (C). No evidence is available on the effects of cognitive behavioral therapy in treating acute back or neck problems (D).

REFERENCES

1. Assendelft WJ, Morton SC, Yu EI, et al. Spinal manipulative therapy for low back pain: a meta-analysis of effectiveness relative to other therapies. *Ann Intern Med* 2003;138:887–881 Review Summary for patients in: *Ann Intern Med* 2003;138:I33.
2. Cochrane Back Review Group. www.cochrane.org.
3. Fouyas IP, Statham PFX, Sandercook PAG, et al. *Surgery for cervical radiculomyelopathy*. Oxford: Cochrane Library, Issue 4, 2002.
4. Hoogendoorn WE, Van Poppel MNM, Bongers PM, et al. Systematic review of psychosocial factors at work and private life as risk factors for back pain. *Spine* 2000;25:2114–2125.
5. Nachemson A. Ont i ryggen—orsaker, diagnostik och behandling [in Swedish]. Stockholm: Statens Beredning für Utvärdering au medicinsk metodik, 1991.
6. Nachemson A, Jonsson E. *Neck and back pain. The scientific evidence of causes, diagnosis and treatment*. Philadelphia: Lippincott Williams & Wilkins, 2000.
7. Fritzell P. *Fusion for chronic low back pain. Treatment effects, complications and cost-effectiveness. The Swedish Lumbar Spine Study* [Thesis]. Göteborg, Sweden: Sahlgrenska Academy at Göteborg University, 2002.
8. Gibson JNA, Grant IC, Waddell G. Surgery for lumbar disc prolapse and degenerative lumbar spondylosis [Cochrane Review]. *Spine* 1999;24:1820–1832.
9. Hägg O. *Measurement and prediction of outcome. Application in fusion surgery for chronic low back pain. The Swedish Lumbar Spine Study* [Thesis]. Göteborg, Sweden: Sahlgrenska Academy at Göteborg University, 2002.
10. Kadanka Z, Mares M, Bednarik J, et al. Approaches to spondylotic cervical myelopathy. conservative versus surgical results in a 3-year follow-up study. *Spine* 2002;20:2205–2211.
11. Waddell G, Aylward M, Sawney P. *Back pain, incapacity for work and social security benefits: an international literature review and analysis*. Department for Work and Pensions. London: The Royal Society of Medicine Press, 2002.

29

The Need for Central Registration: Spine Tango

A European Spine Registry

*Christoph P. Roeder, *Amer I. EL-Kerdi, †‡Dieter Grob, and §¶Max Aebi

*Institute for Evaluative Research in Orthopaedic Surgery, and §Center for Orthopaedic Research, University of Bern, Bern, Switzerland; †Department of Orthopedic Surgery, Zurich University; ‡Department of Spine Surgery, Division of Orthopedics, Schulthess Clinic, Zurich, Switzerland; and ¶Orthopedic Department, Salem Hospital, Bern, Switzerland

All over the world, efforts have been made to set up registries on regional, state, and even national levels; consequently, the number of articles in the literature reflects the establishment and activity of all these new and young institutions (1,3,7,11,12). The Swedish Hip Registry, considered one of the oldest and best-functioning registries, has proved valuable in eliminating poorly performing materials and implants, and it was key in changing treatment practices based on evidence (4). In imitation of the Swedish model, registries have been set up in Germany (7), Canada (1), New Zealand (12), Norway (3), Finland, England, and many young Eastern European countries. Their focus has extended beyond the replacement of major joints, such as total hip and knee arthroplasty, and new registries have been set up for joint replacement procedures that are less frequently performed, such as shoulder and elbow arthroplasty (11).

All authors stress the fact that their registry questionnaires are to be considered a minimal data set, so as not to create too much extra work for surgeons and thereby lower the response rates (3,7,12). In addition, many registries try to construct their questionnaires in such a way that the collection of data becomes a team effort on the part of operating room staff, surgeons, secretaries, and residents.

Spine surgery is a challenge for all registry endeavors. Because of the variety of levels, pathologies, accesses, and surgical techniques, all attempts to invent a short yet comprehensive questionnaire have failed. Therefore, institutions that have developed questionnaires or registries have focused on some of the main aspects of spine surgery. The North American Spine Society has developed mostly patient-based questionnaires for cervical and lumbar spine problems and for scoliosis (2,9). The Swedish Spine Registry was even named the "Swedish National Register for Lumbar Spine Surgery," indicating that the focus was only on lumbar pathologies and interventions (14). In comparison with older registration and documentation initiatives in other orthopedic subspecialties (6), the outcomes movement has led to a dramatic shift toward patient-based documentation (5,15). Hence, the burden of answering long and detailed questionnaires was taken away from the busy clinician and put into the hands of the patient who has been empowered with more responsibility to participate in decision making and quality assessment. A modern, surgeon-based documentation system was described by one of the authors of the Swedish Spine Registry in three words: simplicity, simplicity, simplicity (P. Fritzell, personal communication, 2002).

SPINE TANGO—THE EUROPEAN INITIATIVE

Under the auspices of the Spine Society of Europe, a project was launched to design and implement a documentation system for spinal surgery in 2000. This effort, introduced as the "Spine Tango," was conducted in collaboration with the Institute for Evaluative Research in Orthopaedic Surgery at the University of Berne, Switzerland, formerly the Maurice E. Müller Center for Education and Documentation (MEM-CED), which has acquired profound expertise in documentation and data collection because it has arguably been hosting the oldest and most detailed hip arthroplasty registry in the world. Its earliest records date back to 1968, and currently, more than 48,000 primary interventions, 12,000 revisions, and roughly 71,000 follow-up controls are archived in the database. Data collection took place on a voluntary basis and was standardized according to the International Documentation and Evaluation System (IDES) (10). Data were collected in more than 40 hospitals in various European countries, including Austria, Belgium, Switzerland, Germany, Great Britain, France, Italy, and the Netherlands.

The Spine Tango is probably the first spine registry initiative to face the challenge of developing a comprehensive questionnaire covering all major spine pathologies and interventions and spanning all anatomic levels. To accomplish this task, a technically demanding computer application was an obvious prerequisite. The need for such an application coincided with the prototype release of an on-line tool for data collection developed by the MEM-CED. The decision to use Internet technologies to enhance centralized data collection seemed obvious to the Spine Tango team, given the cumbersome and inaccurate paper-based methods that had been used previously. Paper-based forms are traditionally filled in by clinical users, sent to a central data collection office, and then entered into a database by means of various customized local software solutions, which are sometimes optionally interfaced to optical character or mark readers. The enormous human and financial resources needed to read in paper-based data, and especially to correct and complete invalid data sheets, were the driving force behind conceptually changing these outdated methods by technologically moving data entry back to the peripheral user. All the while, new documentation features and interfaces were introduced to facilitate further the registration of data.

MEDICAL INFORMATION TECHNOLOGY INNOVATIONS

The new on-line documentation system of the MEM-CED is slowly being recognized as a powerful generic centralized documentation application. Along with its numerous simplified tools for collecting medical, implant, radiologic, and patient data, a real information technology innovation was developed. Embedded in an orthopedic portal called *Orthoglobe*, accessible at *www.orthoglobe.com*, the academic on-line joint registry application currently offers a wide array of questionnaires and on-line tools for data collection and administration. In addition to the Spine Tango, it offers the orthopedic community the European Federation of National Associations of Orthopaedics (EFORT) and IDES registries for total hip arthroplasty, the IDES total knee arthroplasty registry, and several ongoing multicenter studies for restricted user communities that deal with spine trauma, fractures in children, motion-preserving spine stabilization, and meniscus implants.

Several complementary solutions can be used to collect and extract data (Fig. 29.1). Although the most direct method of data entry is to use the on-line interface, a second alter-

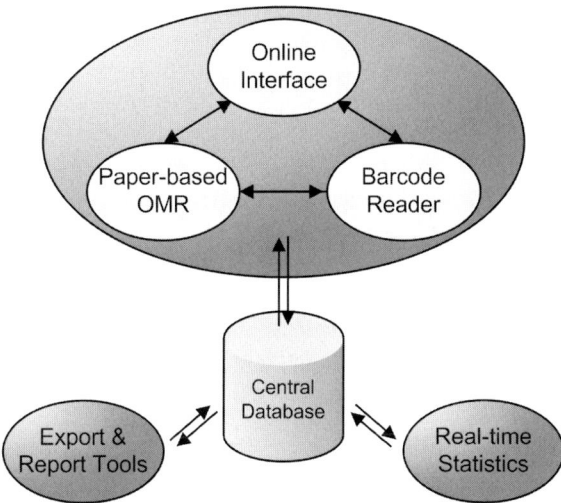

FIG. 29.1. Overview of documentation information technology solution. *OMR*, optical mark reader.

native off-line solution is to use hand-held barcode readers. A third possibility of data collection is based on an MEM-CED proprietary on-line interface to traditional paper-based data registration that uses an optical mark reader. Regardless of the method by which data are registered, all data are finally routed back to the on-line–accessible central database, where the user can verify, edit, and submit data. On-line validation rules guarantee that only medically and logically valid and complete data sets are submitted. Otherwise, the data set is rejected as users are warned to make corrections. This ensures the quality and integrity of the data stored in the database. Once data have been submitted, they cannot be altered. Various features are in place for on-line data analysis to recover time spent in documentation. Forms can be printed in a rough question-and-answer format, and soon the documented information is available within a body of text that can be edited so that user-customized reports and letters can be created with the collected data. Additionally, direct on-line–accessible real-time queries of personal user statistics and comparison with the data pool for benchmarking are possible. Moreover, data can be downloaded to the user's own computers for further customized statistical analysis. An on-line tool to upload up to six digital x-ray films per documented case is also available.

Because of the unique nature of the doctor–patient relationship and the sensitivity of health care data, exchanging and collecting information on the World Wide Web raises many concerns regarding privacy and confidentiality. Therefore, the official security policy of the MEM-CED and the Orthoglobe portal is to take every measure possible to guarantee the security and integrity of entrusted data. This is accomplished by using only International Standardization Organization (ISO)–compliant systems with a physically secure and segregated network setup protected by firewalls and antivirus filtering. In addition, all data are transferred via 128 bit–encrypted channels conforming to the highest levels of security, similar to those used in electronic business solutions.

A EUROPEAN REGISTRY—UNITY IN DIVERSITY

The biggest obstacle in establishing a European registry is the heterogeneity of interests and ideas regarding content and techniques of documentation. There is no doubt that the Internet is the best and least expensive means available for networking all those involved and gathering data sets in a central database. In addition, no costly hardware and software purchases are necessary to run or maintain the installation because system upgrades and maintenance are conducted only at the central control unit. Nevertheless, the amalgamation of different sets of questions into a single questionnaire to satisfy various European, national and regional, and even individual needs, while still ensuring the extraction only of data of interest to the respective user, remains an insurmountable obstacle in any documentation system.

In developing an on-line tool for a European mission, the MEM-CED has engineered an information technology solution that measures up to the expected complexity of several levels of content within one and the same questionnaire. After a core data set for a European register has been adopted, each participating nation can define additional questions that it would like to incorporate into its national documentation system. Therefore, participating surgeons can choose their national registry questionnaire but still meet European standards. Moreover, they are provided with an on-line tool to generate questions for their individual in-house interests. This is accomplished by introducing a new scheme of real-time retrospective and prospective documentation. In such a system, each study questionnaire is divided into subforms that best emulate the data collection work flow in hospitals (Fig. 29.2). The overwhelming advantage of such a model is that subforms can be filled out by different users independently of one other while at the same time validation rules built into the generic system ensure that data are logically and medically validated before submission.

Because data sharing is defined at the department level, all surgeons within a department can make use of the individually created sets of added-on questions, whereas users outside the department or hospital cannot see or use these extensions. To increase flexibility and application tidiness, the various sets of additionally created questions are provided in the form of a menu of optional packages that can be actively selected and linked to the European and national questions, thereby enabling the concept of a multilevel documentation. The European core data are anonymously pooled at the central data collection unit, and benchmarks are created. Hospitals are given the opportunity to compare their core parameters with the European or national averages by performing on-line live queries of the database. The national data sets belong to the society under whose auspices the registry was established. Only the surgeon who entered the data is able to retrieve the complete set of parameters, including patient-based information.

Far more difficult than constructing complicated information technology architecture is defining a core data set for the various orthopedic subspecialties. Regarding a core

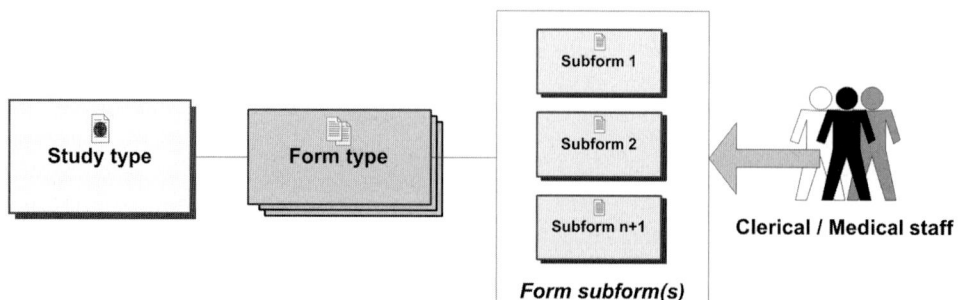

FIG. 29.2. Breakdown of study forms into sizable subforms.

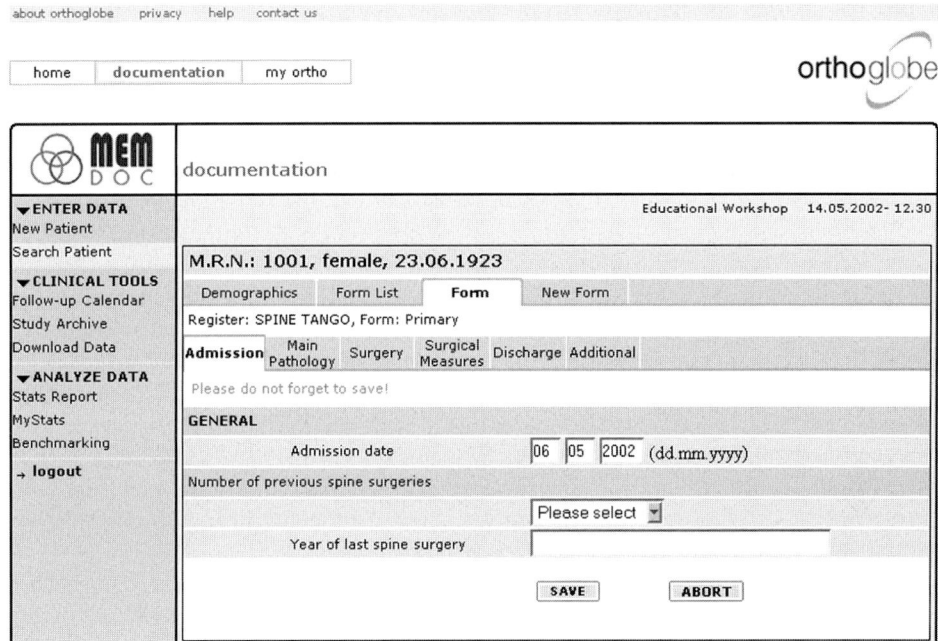

FIG. 29.3. Spine Tango primary intervention questionnaire.

questionnaire for the Spine Tango, an initiative was undertaken in cooperation with the Spine Department at the Schulthess Clinic, Zurich, Switzerland, to develop a set of questions suitable for a European Spine Registry. For reasons of data validation, the possibility of real-time documentation, and sharing of the documentation workload, the core questions are subdivided into five subforms: admission, main pathology, surgery, surgical measures, and discharge (Fig. 29.3). Under the "additional" menu, several optional modules are also available: social, clinical assessment cervicothoracic, clinical assessment lumbar, imaging, functional tests and invasive imaging, and the Oswestry score. Moreover, a second intervention surgery and surgical measures subform for combined access or two-step intervention can be activated for a precise documentation of cases with two accesses or even two interventions within one hospital stay. The intent is to provide interested users with an opportunity to document information beyond the core data set with standard add-on modules.

IMPLANT DOCUMENTATION—HIGH TECH FOR PRECISION AND TIME SAVING

One of the main reasons for setting up joint replacement and implant registries is that many implants are put on the market after laboratory testing only. However, the real testing arenas for implants are the patients themselves, in whom all the factors affecting implant performance, such as design, choice of materials, manufacturing issues, patient characteristics, and surgical techniques, come into play (8). A minimum follow-up of 10 years is normally required to judge a joint replacement as realistically successful (13). However, many institutions that possess such data often cannot compare them with those of other institutions and authors because of the technologic and content limitations of the different methods used for data collection and analysis.

Implants are also an essential part of modern spine surgery, and the increased use of artificial materials during past years makes the postmarketing surveillance of products as necessary as in the joint replacement sector. To overcome the problem of incompatible documentation techniques and parameters of interest, and to follow new or questionable products and implant designs for extended postoperative periods, the MEM-CED has integrated a unique implant-tracking tool to complement the documentation system.

A major European implant producer has introduced a barcode-based implant-tracking system for ordering and stocking purposes. The so-called SEDICO (secure data integration concept) system is being marketed in an open partner concept because other large implant producers are already participating and using the new technology. All materials with article and lot numbers in barcode format are registered with a barcode scanner when they are unwrapped by the operating room staff and delivered to the surgeon. Via telephone modem, the article and lot numbers are sent to the producers for restocking. Hospitals, which are part of the fast-growing SEDICO user community and document with the MEM-CED on-line system, can rely on the automated background linking of article and lot numbers of implants to their documented cases.

Hence, a unique and proprietary interface is in place to ensure that a copy of all implant data sets is independently sent to the registry database and made available on-line within minutes. As a result, a single product can be evaluated precisely, and furthermore, an early warning system for poorly performing implants is established because all other implants belonging to a particular production run can be recalled by using the lot numbers. Users who do not want to or cannot install the SEDICO system are offered updated on-line product catalogs of all participating implant suppliers within the documentation system. With the search tools in place, an implant can be selected and also linked to the respective case. However, lot numbers are not registered with this implant-tracking search option.

REFERENCES

1. Bourne RB. The planning and implementation of the Canadian Joint Replacement Registry. *Bull Hosp Jt Dis* 1999;58:128–132.
2. Daltroy LH, Cats-Baril WL, Katz JN, et al. The North American Spine Society lumbar spine outcome assessment instrument: reliability and validity tests. *Spine* 1996;21:741–749.
3. Havelin LI. The Norwegian Joint Registry. *Bull Hosp Jt Dis* 1999;58:139–147.
4. Herberts P, Malchau H. How outcome studies have changed total hip arthroplasty practices in Sweden. *Clin Orthop* 1997;344:44–60.
5. Johanson NA. Outcomes assessment. In: Callaghan JJ, Rosenberg AG, Rubash HE, eds. *The adult hip*. Philadelphia: Lippincott–Raven Publishers, 1998:853–863.
6. Johnston RC, Fitzgerald RH, Harris WH, et al. Clinical and radiographic evaluation of total hip replacement. A standard system of terminology for reporting results. *J Bone Joint Surg Am* 1990;72:161–168.
7. Lang I, Willert HG. Experiences with the German Endoprosthesis Register [in German]. *Z Arztl Fortbild Qualitatssich* 2001;95:203–208.
8. Maloney WJ. National joint replacement registries: has the time come? *J Bone Joint Surg Am* 2001;83:1582–1585.
9. North American Spine Society. www.spine.org.
10. Paterson D. The International Documentation and Evaluation System (IDES). *Orthopedics* 1993;16:11–14.
11. Rahme H, Jacobsen MB, Salomonsson B. The Swedish Elbow Arthroplasty Register and the Swedish Shoulder Arthroplasty Register: two new Swedish arthroplasty registers. *Acta Orthop Scand* 2001;72:107–112.
12. Rothwell AG. Development of the New Zealand Joint Register. *Bull Hosp Jt Dis* 1999;58:148–160.
13. Sochart DH, Long AJ, Porter ML. Joint responsibility: the need for a national arthroplasty register. *BMJ* 1996;313:66–67.
14. Stromqvist B, Jonsson B, Fritzell P, et al. The Swedish National Register for Lumbar Spine Surgery: Swedish Society for Spinal Surgery. *Acta Orthop Scand* 2001;72:99–106.
15. Weinstein JN, Deyo RA. Clinical research: issues in data collection. *Spine* 2000;25:3104–3109.

30

Assessment of Health-Related Quality of Life

Christian Mélot

Faculty of Medicine, Free University of Brussels; and Department of Intensive Care, Erasme University Hospital, Brussels, Belgium

The term *health-related quality of life (HRQL)* is often used because some aspects of the quality of life are not generally considered as part of "health" (e.g., income, freedom, quality of the environment).

HRQL is important for measuring the impact of chronic disease on daily life. Physiologic measures provide information to clinicians but are of limited interest to patients. They correlate poorly with functional capacity and well-being, the areas of greatest concern to patients and with which they are most familiar.

Moreover, the number of clinical trials incorporating measurements of HRQL has increased in recent years. Patients, clinicians, pharmaceutical companies, and regulatory authorities acknowledge the need to assess the impact of treatments on patients' quality of life—essentially in regard to chronic diseases, for the licensing of new medications, and in health care policy decisions for allocating available resources.

Most commonly, questionnaires comprising a number of items or questions are used to measure HRQL. These items are added up in a number of domains, also called *dimensions*. A domain or dimension is an area of behavior or experience that we are trying to measure. Two basic approaches to HRQL measurement are available: generic instruments, which provide a summary of HRQL, and specific instruments, which focus on problems associated with single disease states, patients groups, or areas of function. The two approaches are not mutually exclusive.

Combining HRQL measures with life expectancy allows the computation of health-adjusted life-years (HALYs) as summary measures of population health; these make it possible to consider the combined impact of death and morbidity simultaneously. Health-adjusted life expectancy (HALE) estimates the average time in years that a person at a given age can expect to live in the equivalent full health by combining life tables with cross-sectional age-specific HRQL data. In HALE, the contribution of any specific disease or condition to decrements in health is not presented. Rather, HALE seeks to provide an overview of the morbidity and mortality burden of a population.

DESCRIBING HEALTH: THE HIERARCHY OF PATIENT OUTCOMES

The meanings of the terms *quality of life*, *health status*, and *patient outcome*, as generally used, overlap. Patient outcome usually refers to a final health status measurement after the passage of time and the application of treatment. In the future, patient outcome will be increasingly described by a cumulative series of health status measurements.

It is highly desirable to represent any of these terms by a single number. Unfortunately, the calculation of a single index number that can serve as a primary dependent variable in clinical studies presents major obstacles. A single index number can be developed in two ways. First, it can be obtained directly. For example, one can use an analog scale question with an appropriate item asking subjects to make a mark that represents, broadly considered, their health status at the moment. Such a simplistic approach can in fact be useful for validating more sophisticated approaches, but experience with such scales has shown that they are very insensitive and fail to identify the specific positive and negative inputs that are included in the global judgment. The second approach is to calculate a single index number indirectly by combining numbers from different scales representing different facets of health status.

Dimensions of Health Outcomes

Implicit in the concept of patient outcome assessment is a shift from reliance on measures of medical processes (autoantibody titer, joint space narrowing, erosions on x-ray films) toward elements that are of direct importance to the patient (pain, discomfort, anxiety, depression). Patients want to be alive as long as possible, function normally, be free of pain and other physical, psychologic, or social symptoms, be free of iatrogenic problems resulting from the treatment regimen, and remain solvent (Fig. 30.1).

These five dimensions (death, disability, discomfort, drug side effects, and cost) define patient outcome (10,11). The dimensions must be considered mutually exclusive and collectively exhaustive. All the available questionnaires explore several of these dimensions (Fig. 30.2).

The outcome hierarchy makes dimensions and components comprehensible. A treatment that does not affect at least one major dimension positively is unlikely to be a major contribution. The need for outcome studies becomes increasingly important in health assessment.

Measurement Instruments

Instruments that measure quality of life consist of questionnaires, most often self-administered by patients. This type of evaluation has the advantage of being simple and inexpensive; however, the rate of incomplete replies is higher than when questionnaires are administered by investigators, and one cannot be sure that the questions have been perfectly understood. The advantages and disadvantages of the various modes of administration of HRQL questionnaires have been analyzed (15).

Among psychometric instruments, one can distinguish between generic and specific instruments. Generic instruments evaluate an individual person's state of health, whatever disease he or she may have, and can be used in the general population. They are particularly useful for comparing different disorders and can be used to establish health policies. Specific instruments are particularly adapted to the study of a given disease (rheumatoid arthritis, osteoporosis), syndrome [low back pain (LBP)], or population (children, the elderly). Directed to the aspects of health most affected by the disease for which they have been developed, these instruments are in principle more sensitive to change than generic measures. Whether generic or specific, these instruments contain a variable number of closed standardized items. The response mode is by the way of a visual analog

30. ASSESSMENT OF HEALTH-RELATED QUALITY OF LIFE

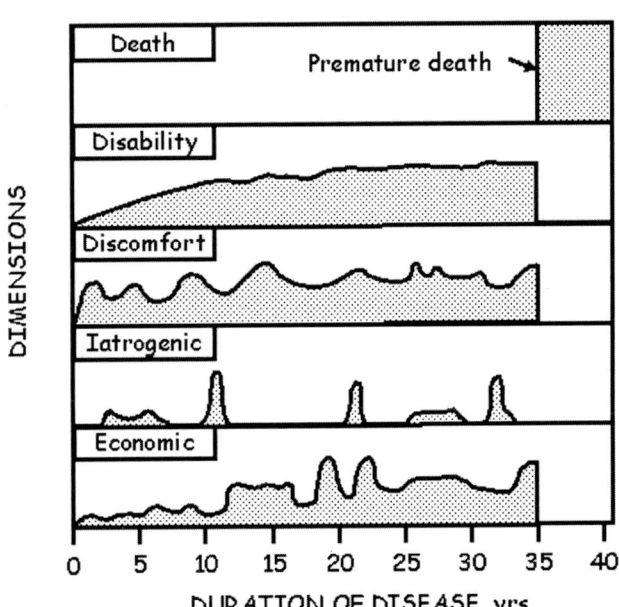

FIG. 30.1. The five primary dimensions of patient outcomes in chronic disease. The health outcomes of a patient with low back pain are represented over time. During 35 years of illness, the patient experiences economic difficulties, iatrogenic problems, and physical and psychologic discomfort; becomes progressively disabled; and dies prematurely. (Adapted from Fries JF, Spitz PW. The hierarchy of patient outcomes. In: Spilker B, ed. *Quality of life assessments in clinical trials.* New York: Raven Press, 1990:25–35.)

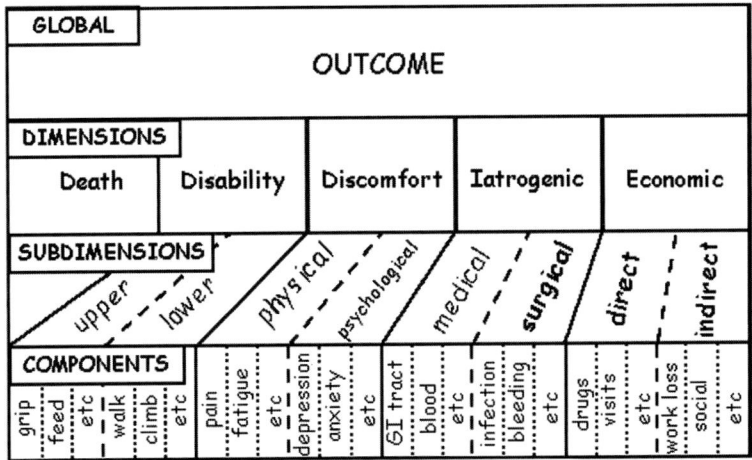

FIG. 30.2. The hierarchy of patient outcomes. Questionnaires address factors related to each of the components. (Reproduced from Fries JF, Spitz PW. The hierarchy of patient outcomes. In: Spilker B, ed. *Quality of life assessments in clinical trials.* New York: Raven Press, 1990:25–35, with permission.)

scale or, more often, a Likert ordinal scale. With most psychometric instruments, one can calculate a score for each of the dimensions making up the instrument and derive a quality-of-life profile. Summing the scores to give a single value is rarely proposed because of the resulting loss of information.

Main Generic Measures

Sickness Impact Profile

The Sickness Impact Profile (SIP) is a multidimensional measure of self-reported health status. It consists of 136 statements about limitations in 12 categories of function: ambulation, mobility, body care and movement, social interaction, alertness, emotional behavior, communication, sleep and rest, eating, work, home management, and recreation (2,3). The SIP can also be administered by an investigator or filled in by someone close to the patient. Respondents are asked to endorse statements that describe their health status on a given day. Scores are computed for the overall instrument, for each of the 12 categories, and for two major dimensions of health (physical health, which reflects limitations noted in the first three categories, and psychologic health, which reflects limitations noted in the second three categories). The overall scores can range from 0 to 100. Scores higher than 10 represent severe disability, and a difference in a score of 2 to 3

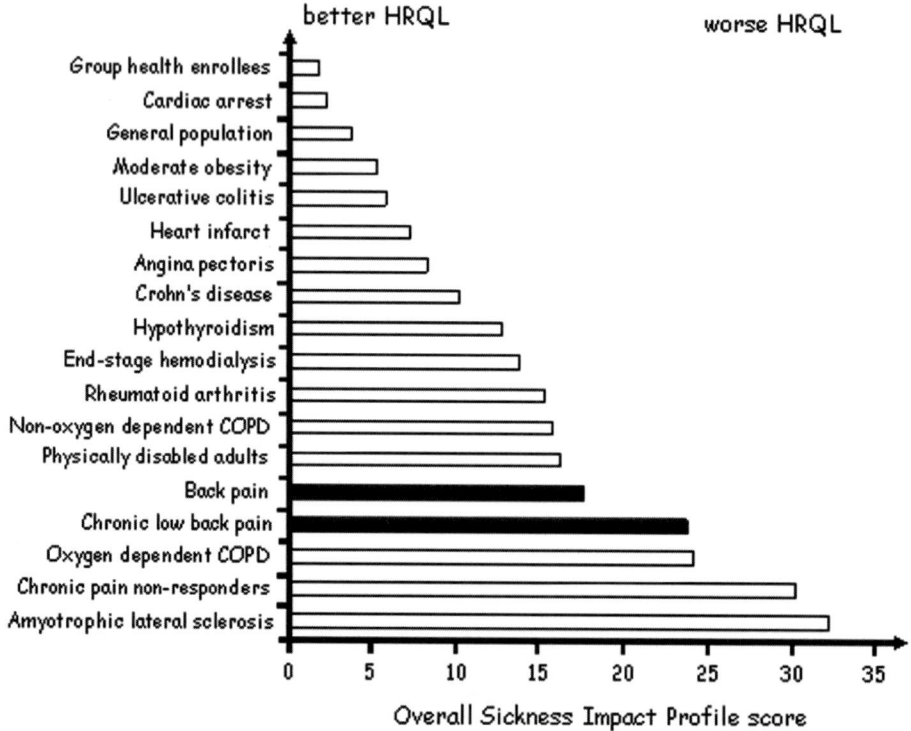

FIG. 30.3. Use of the Sickness Impact Profile score to evaluate health-related quality of life (*HRQL*) in different conditions. A score higher than 10 indicates severe disability. *COPD*, chronic obstructive pulmonary disease. (Data from Bergner M, Bobbitt RA, Pollard WE, et al. The Sickness Impact Profile: validation of a health status measure. *Med Care* 1976;14:57–67.)

points reflects a meaningful difference in function (29). Scores average between 2 and 3 for the general population and higher than 20 for patients with chronic LBP (3) (Fig. 30.3). A short version of 68 items has been proposed and validated (7).

Nottingham Health Profile

The Nottingham Health Profile is a much shorter generic questionnaire that contains only 38 questions grouped into six dimensions. A score is obtained for each of the questionnaire's six dimensions (pain, emotional reactions, physical mobility, sleep, energy, social isolation). This self-administered questionnaire is easy to use and well accepted. Replies consist of a dichotomous yes or no (18).

Medical Outcomes Study Short Form 36

Derived from the Medical Outcome Study, an observational study comprising a large number of patients (more than 20,000) who had undergone medical treatment, the Medical Outcome Study Short Form 36 (MOS SF-36) is a self-administered questionnaire that provides a quality-of-life profile with a score for each of its eight dimensions (physical functioning, role physical, bodily pain, general health, vitality, social functioning, role emotional, mental health). It contains 36 items, and the reply modes are 3- to 5-point Likert ordinal scales (34). The MOS SF-36 is a reference generic instrument.

Quality of Well-Being

The Quality of Well-Being is an index that attributes a global score of well-being to the state of health of a person during the past 6 days on a continuum ranging from death to optimal function. It uses a combination of three scales of daily functioning (mobility, physical activity, social activity) and a list of 27 symptoms or problems weighted for social preferences (1).

EuroQoL EQ-5D

The EuroQoL EQ-5D was developed by a multidisciplinary group of researchers from five European countries. It defines health status in terms of five dimensions: mobility, self-care, usual activity, pain/discomfort, and anxiety/depression (8). Three response levels are available for each question: no problem, some problems, and extreme problems. The instrument yields a total of 243 possible health states. A single overall score can also be obtained from the EuroQoL "thermometer," on which respondents mark their overall perceived state of health from "worst imaginable" to "best imaginable."

Specific Measures of Low Back Pain

Several syndrome-specific questionnaires has been developed for patients with LBP (4,21).

Oswestry Disability Index

The Oswestry Disability Index indicates the extent to which a person's functional level is restricted by pain. The 10 sections of the scale refer to activities of daily living that can be disrupted by LBP. Each section contains six statements, each describing a greater degree of difficulty in a particular activity than the preceding statement. The six statements are scored from 0 to 5 (9). The scores of all sections are added to give a highest possible score of 50. The original questionnaire was slightly modified by the Medical Research Council. The Oswestry and the revised Oswestry scores were found to be equally reliable and valid (17).

Million Visual Analog Scale

Million et al. (26) developed a 15-item checklist about degree of disability and intensity of pain to measure progress in patients with back pain. They selected a series of questions relating to various aspects of pain, such as the influence of circumstances and activities on the pain and the effects of the pain on the patient's capacity to lead a normal life. The score is integrated by adding the equally weighted scores.

Roland–Morris Disability Questionnaire

The Roland–Morris Disability Questionnaire (RMDQ), which is also called the *St. Thomas Questionnaire,* was derived from the SIP. The RMDQ was constructed by choosing 24 yes-or-no items relevant for back pain from the SIP that cover a range of aspects of daily living (31). The RMDQ is scored simply by adding the equally weighted number of positive responses. An individual patient's score can vary from 0 (no disability) to 24 (severe disability). Patrick et al. (28) developed a slightly modified version of the RMDQ that excludes five items that were relatively nonresponsive in two different studies of patients with acute and chronic LBP. It adds four new items from the SIP.

Waddell Disability Index

The Waddell Disability Index is a short yes-or-no checklist. Waddell and Main (33) defined disability as the resulting loss of function based on general activities of daily living. Loss of function is assessed according to nine basic physical activities of daily living commonly restricted by LBP. The score is integrated by adding the equally weighted positive items and can vary from 0 to 9.

Low Back Outcome Score

The Low Back Outcome Score is a 13-item questionnaire intended as a comprehensive rating system for patients with back pain. It includes weighted questions that pertain to current pain, employment, domestic and sports activities, use of drugs and medical services, rest, sex life, and daily activities (14).

Clinical Back Pain Questionnaire

The Clinical Back Pain Questionnaire, also known as the *Aberdeen Low Back Pain Scale,* was devised from questions commonly used in the clinical assessment of patients with LBP (32). The questions assess the effect of various activities on the level of pain; location and duration of pain; use of analgesics; weakness; days in bed; and interference with sleep, physical activities, work, sex life, and leisure caused by pain.

Low Back Pain Rating Scale

The Low Back Pain Rating Scale comprises three scales: pain, disability, and physical impairment (25). Impairment is measured by testing endurance and flexibility; this part is omitted if the scale is self-administered. The disability component consists of 15 questions pertaining to various specific activities, contact with people, ability to work, and expectations of future pain. The components are weighted as follows: 60 points for pain, 30 points for disability, and 40 points for physical impairment.

Quebec Back Pain Disability Scale

The Quebec Back Pain Disability Scale is a 20-item scale that measures physical disability associated with back pain (20). The items refer to specific activities: sleeping and resting, sitting, standing, ambulation, movement, bending and stooping, and handling large or heavy objects. Each activity is rated on a 6-point difficulty scale. Intensity of pain and social role and activities are not included.

Lumbar Spine Questionnaire

The Lumbar Spine Questionnaire, promoted by the North American Spine Society and American Academy of Orthopedic Surgeons, incorporates a modified version of the Oswestry Disability Index (6). In addition, the questionnaire contains a neurogenic symptoms scale, questions about satisfaction with one's current condition, and a scale of expectations met.

Resumption of Activities of Daily Living Scale

The Resumption of Activities of Daily Living Scale measures the extent to which a person with back pain has resumed his or her usual activities since the time of injury (36). The activities include sleep, sex, self-care, household chores, shopping, socializing, traveling, recreational activities, and paid employment. Each item is rated on a graphic scale ranging from 0 to 100%.

Dallas Pain Questionnaire

The Dallas Pain Questionnaire was developed to assess the extent to which chronic spinal pain affects four aspects of a patient's life: daily and work–leisure activities, anxiety–depression, and social interest. Two domains are explored by the Dallas Pain Questionnaire: functional activities and emotional capacities (22).

Minimal Clinically Important Difference

When the effects of treatment effect on chronic LBP are measured with multiple-item outcome instruments, it is necessary, both for clinical decision-making and research purposes, to understand the clinical importance of the outcome scores. Evidence suggests that a statistically significant change in a score does not necessarily indicate a change that is clinically important. The minimal clinically important difference (MCID) has been introduced in an effort to define the smallest meaningful change in score (35). Jaeschke

TABLE 30.1. *Minimal clinically important difference for low back pain evaluated with the visual analog scale, Oswestry Disability Index, Roland–Morris Disability Questionnaire, Sickness Impact Profile, and Medical Outcome Study Short Form 36*

Scale	MCID	Range of the scale
VAS	18	0–100 mm
ODI	10	0–100
RMDQ	2–3	0–24
SIP	2–3	0–100
MOS SF-36	10	0–100

MCID, minimal clinically important difference; MOS SF-36, Medical Outcome Study Short Form 36; ODI, Oswestry Disability Index; RMDQ, Roland–Morris Disability Questionnaire; SIP, Sickness Impact Profile; VAS, visual analog scale.

Data from Bombardier C, Hayden J, Beaton DE. Minimal clinically important difference. Low back pain: outcomes measures. *J Rheumatol* 2001;28: 431–438; Hägg O, Fritzell P, Nordwall A. The clinical importance of changes in outcome scores after treatment for chronic low back pain. *Eur Spine J* 2003;12:12–20.

et al. (19) defined the MCID as "the smallest difference in score in the domain of interest which patients perceive as beneficial." The MCIDs for some generic and specific instruments used to evaluate patients with LBP are presented in Table 30.1 (5,16).

Selection of Instruments

It is generally recommended that the investigators use both generic and specific measures. This review has identified several back-specific scales that can be used to assess the physical function of patients with back pain. The most widely accepted are the Roland–Morris and Oswestry questionnaires. In choosing an outcome measure, the investigator should take into account the type of patients studied and the specific objectives of the investigation. Choosing a measure optimally adapted to the study may conflict with efforts to standardize instruments. Such dilemmas can be resolved through the application of modern psychometric methods based on the Rash model and item response theory (23,30).

HEALTH-ADJUSTED LIFE-YEARS

HALYs are summary measures of population health that make it possible to consider the combined impact of death and morbidity simultaneously. This feature makes HALYs useful for comparisons across a range of illnesses, interventions, and populations. HALYs include disability-adjusted life-years (DALYs) and quality-adjusted life-years (QALYs).

The morbidity or quality of life component of HALYs is referred to HRQL and is captured on a scale of 0 to 1, representing the extremes of death and full health (12). The HRQL associated with different conditions of health and disease is multiplied by life expectancy; then, depending on the underlying methodology, it produces an estimate of DALYs or QALYs associated with different levels of health.

HALE, a related type of summary measure of population health, estimates the average time in years that a person at a given age can expect to live in the equivalent full health.

Life tables are combined with cross-sectional age-specific HRQL data. It should be noted that in HALE, the contribution of any specific disease or condition to decrements in health is not presented. Rather, HALE seeks to provide an overview of the morbidity and mortality burden of a population.

Quality-Adjusted Life-Years

QALYs were developed in the late 1960s by economists, researchers, and psychologists, primarily for use in cost–utility analysis (24). Cost–utility analyses of medical interventions have been conducted for more than 30 years. QALYs are routinely used in assessments of medical care, technology, and public health interventions. Given a specific budget constraint, QALYs are maximized by increasing the "utility" of individuals and aggregates of individuals. Utility can be understood as the value, or preference, that people have for health outcomes along a continuum anchored with death (= 0) and perfect health (= 1).

Disability-Adjusted Life-Years

In 1993, a World Bank and World Health Organization collaboration resulted in the publication of a volume that sought to quantify the global burden of premature death, disease, and injury and to make recommendations that would improve health. DALYs were developed on that occasion to quantify the burden of disease and disability in populations and to set priorities for resource allocation. DALYs measure the gap between the health of a population and a hypothetical ideal for health achievement.

Calculating Quality-Adjusted and Disability-Adjusted Life-Years

Once an illness, condition, or disability has been described, its desirability (or lack of such) must be valued in such a manner that it can be combined with a unit of life expectancy. By convention, each measure is anchored on a scale of health of 0 to 1. QALYs are a measure of life expectancy (a benefit to be maximized), and DALYs are a measure of a health gap (a handicap to be minimized). Consequently, the scale for each measure is the reverse of the other; a valuation of 1 represents full health on the QALY scale and full disability (death) on the DALY scale, whereas 0 represents the lowest possible health state (death) on the QALY scale and no disability or full health on the DALY scale.

Preferences or values for use in QALYs are generated by a number of techniques. The most commonly used methods include standard gamble, time trade-off, and rating or visual analog scales (24). Standard gamble and time trade-off methods ask respondents to value health states by making explicit what they would be willing to sacrifice (in terms of time to death or risk for death) to return from the health state being experienced to perfect health. In rating scales or visual analog scales, respondents must designate a point on a scale that corresponds to the strength of their preference for a given health state.

In DALYs, values for diseases and other nonfatal health outcomes are obtained through an iterative, deliberative process that attempts to reconcile differences in the preferences of health professional expert groups with respect to the desirability of different conditions and injuries. The DALY valuation exercise is built on a person trade-off (PTO) method that explicitly addresses trade-offs between life and HRQL for people with different diseases (27).

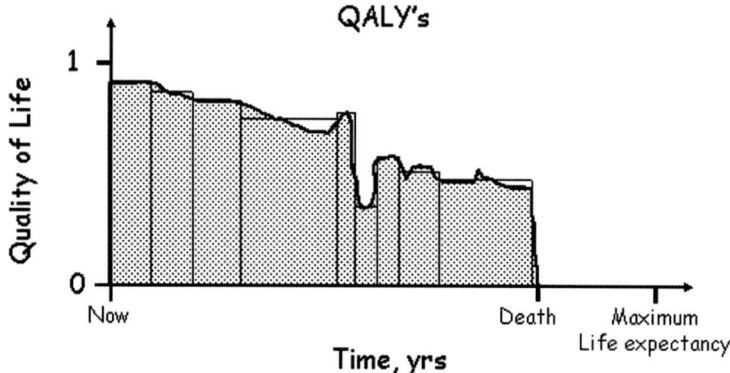

FIG. 30.4. The life path of changing health-related quality of life (HQRL) for an individual from the present until that person's death is shown by the *irregular line*. The *stippled area* indicates the quality-adjusted life-years (*QALYs*) accumulated over this portion of the person's lifetime. The area is approximated by summing the areas of the rectangles. (Reproduced from Gold MR, Stevenson D, Fryback DG. HALYs and QALYs and DALYs, oh my: similarities and differences in summary measures of population health. *Annu Rev Public Health* 2002;23:115–134, with permission.)

Combining Values for Health with Life Expectancy.

In a general sense, HALYs are created by multiplying values for health states or conditions by life expectancy.

The calculation of QALYs is explained in Figure 30.4 (13). The life path of changing HRQL for an individual from the present until death is shown by the irregular solid line. After a steady decline for some years followed by a brief improvement, the person expe-

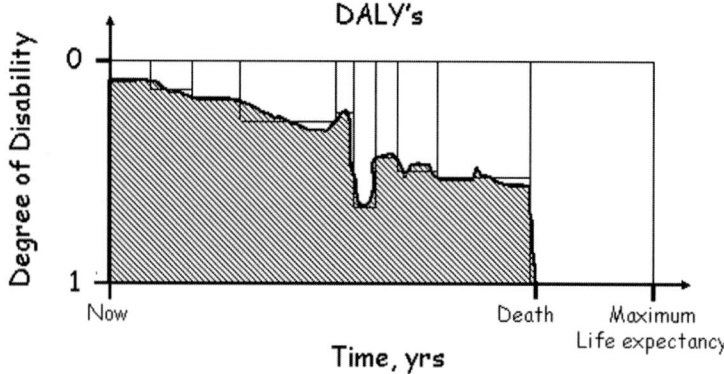

FIG. 30.5. The same life path as in Figure 30.4 is shown by the *irregular line*. Added to the graph is a point of maximal life expectancy, which is the ideal sex-specific life expectancy determined by World Health Organization researchers. To compute disability-adjusted life-years (*DALYs*), the area lost from the ideal lifetime, lived to the maximum life expectancy in full health, is computed approximately by summing the areas of the rectangles. (Reproduced from Gold MR, Stevenson D, Fryback DG. HALYs and QALYs and DALYs, oh my: similarities and differences in summary measures of population health. *Annu Rev Public Health* 2002;23: 115–134, with permission.)

riences a major event, after which some HRQL is recovered for a short time, but the recovery is followed by fluctuating HRQL until death. The area under this curve is the QALYs accumulated by the person during his or her lifetime from the present. The area is approximated by summing the areas of the rectangles.

The computation of DALYs, in principle, proceeds in the same fashion as the computation of QALYs, but as shown in Figure 30.5, the area being computed is that above the life path and extending out the ideal life expectancy, to approximate the total area lost from the ideal life path of living in perfect health for the entire ideal life expectancy.

As initially conceived, DALYs were primarily intended to document information about the comparative health of populations. At their start, QALYs focused on the evaluation of medical interventions. In a perfect measurement world, HALYs would be used at the macro level to track population health and monitor population-based interventions (e.g., health education, health-related legislative actions) and at the micro (clinical) level to assess the effectiveness of preventive, palliative, and curative therapies.

REFERENCES

1. Balaban DJ, Sagi PC, Goldfarb NI, et al. Weights for scoring the quality of well-being (QWB) instrument among rheumatoid arthritics: a comparison to general population weights. *Med Care* 1986;24:973–980.
2. Bergner M, Bobbitt RA, Carter WB, et al. The Sickness Impact Profile: development and final revision of a health status measure. *Med Care* 1981;19:787–805.
3. Bergner M, Bobbitt RA, Pollard WE, et al. The Sickness Impact Profile: validation of a health status measure. *Med Care* 1976;14:57–67.
4. Beurskens AJ, De Vet HC, Köke AJ, et al. Measuring the functional status of patients with low back pain. Assessment of the quality of four disease-specific questionnaires. *Spine* 1995;20:1017–1028.
5. Bombardier C, Hayden J, Beaton DE. Minimal clinically important difference. Low back pain: outcomes measures. *J Rheumatol* 2001;28:431–438.
6. Daltroy LH, Cats-Baril WL, Katz JN, et al. The North American Spine Society lumbar spine outcome assessment instruments: reliability and validity tests. *Spine* 1996;21:741–749.
7. De Bruin AF, Diederiks JPM, De Witte LP, et al. Assessing the responsiveness of a functional status measure: the Sickness Impact Profile versus the SIP68. *J Clin Epidemiol* 1997;50:529–540.
8. EuroQoL Group. EuroQoL: a new facility for the measurement of health-related quality of life. *Health Policy* 1990;16:199–208.
9. Fairbank JCT, Couper J, Davies JB, et al. The Oswestry Low Back Pain Disability Questionnaire. *Physiotherapy* 1980;66:271–273.
10. Fries JF, Spitz PW, Kraines RG, et al. Measurement of patient outcomes in arthritis. *Arthritis Rheum* 1980;23:137–145.
11. Fries JF, Spitz PW. The hierarchy of patient outcomes. In: Spilker B, ed. *Quality of life assessments in clinical trials*. New York: Raven Press, 1990:25–35.
12. Gold MR, Siegel JE, Russell LB, et al. *Cost-effectiveness in health and medicine*. New York: Oxford University Press, 1996:82–134.
13. Gold MR, Stevenson D, Fryback DG. HALYs and QALYs and DALYs, oh my: similarities and differences in summary measures of population health. *Annu Rev Public Health* 2002;23:115–134.
14. Greenough CG, Fraser RD. Assessment of outcome in patients with low back pain. *Spine* 1992;17:36–41.
15. Guyatt GH, Feeny DH, Patrick DL. Measuring health-related quality of life. *Ann Intern Med* 1993;118:622–629.
16. Hägg O, Fritzell P, Nordwall A. The clinical importance of changes in outcome scores after treatment for chronic low back pain. *Eur Spine J* 2003;12:12–20.
17. Hudson-Cook N, Tomes-Nicholson K, Breen A. A revised Oswestry Disability Questionnaire. In: Roland OM, Jenner JR, eds. *Back pain: new approaches to rehabilitation and education*. Manchester: University Press, 1989:187–204.
18. Hunt SM, McKenna SP, McEwen J, et al. The Nottingham Health Profile: subjective health status and medical consultations. *Soc Sci Med* 1981;15:221–229.
19. Jaeschke R, Singer J, Guyatt GH. Measurement of health status. Ascertaining the minimal clinically important difference. *Control Clin Trials* 1989;10:407–415.
20. Kopec JA, Esdaile JM, Abrahamowicz M, et al. The Quebec Back Pain Disability Scale: measurement properties. *Spine* 1995;20:341–352.
21. Kopec JA. Measuring functional outcomes in persons with back pain. A review of back-specific questionnaires. *Spine* 2000;25:3110–3114.
22. Lawlis GF, Cuencas R, Selby D, et al. The development of the Dallas Pain Questionnaire. An assessment of the impact of spinal pain on behavior. *Spine* 1989;14:511–516.

23. Lord FM. *Application of item response theory to practical testing problems*. Hillsdale, NJ: Lawrence Erlbaum Associates, 1980.
24. Mélot C. Principles of cost-benefit analysis. In: Szpalski M, Gunzburg R, Pope MH, eds. *Lumbar segmental instability*. Philadelphia: Lippincott Williams & Wilkins, 1999:259–273.
25. Manniche C, Asmussen K, Lauritsen B, et al. Low back pain rating scale: validation of a tool for assessment of low back pain. *Pain* 1994;57:317–326.
26. Million R, Nilsen KH, Jayson MIV, et al. Evaluation of low back pain and assessment of lumbar corsets with and without back supports. *Ann Rheum Dis* 1981; 40:449–454.
27. Nord E. The person trade-off approach to valuing health care programs. *Med Decis Making* 1995;15: 201–208.
28. Patrick DL, Deyo RA, Atlas SJ, et al. Assessing health-related quality of life in patients with sciatica. *Spine* 1995;20:1899–1908.
29. Patrick DL, Deyo RA. Generic and disease-specific measures in assessing health status and quality of life. *Med Care* 1989;27[Suppl]:S217–S232.
30. Rash G. *Probabilistic models for some intelligence and attainment tests*. Copenhagen: Nielsen and Lydiche, 1960.
31. Roland M, Morris R. A study of the natural history of back pain. Part I: Development of a reliable and sensitive measure of disability in low-back pain. *Spine* 1983;8:141–144.
32. Ruta DA, Garratt AM, Wardlaw D, et al. Developing a valid and reliable measure of health outcome for patients with low back pain. *Spine* 1994;19:1887–1896.
33. Waddell G, Main CJ. Assessment of severity in low-back disorders. *Spine* 1984;9:204–208.
34. Ware JE. SF-36 health survey update. *Spine* 2000;24:3130–3139.
35. Wells G, Beaton D, Shea B, et al. Minimal clinically important differences: review of methods. *J Rheumatol* 2001; 28:406–412.
36. Williams RM, Myers AM. A new approach to measuring recovery in injured workers with acute low back pain: Resumption of Activities of Daily Living Scale. *Phys Ther* 1998;78:613–623.

31

Rationale for the Surgical Treatment of Degenerative Disc Disease from the Cochrane Review

*†J. N. Alastair Gibson and ‡Gordon Waddell

*Department of Orthopedic Surgery, The University of Edinburgh;
†Spinal Unit, The Royal Infirmary of Edinburgh, Edinburgh, United Kingdom;
and ‡The Glasgow Nuffield Hospital, Glasgow, United Kingdom

Because the population of most countries in Western Europe is aging, the prevalence of back and leg pain secondary to degenerative disc disease (DDD) is likely to increase for the foreseeable future. It is therefore essential to institute rational health care programs that maximize the effectiveness of therapy and minimize its cost. It is particularly important that surgery be cost-effective when its cost will probably amount to up to one sixth of all health care costs.

During the last 5 years, we have collated data from randomized controlled trials (RCTs) as part of a Cochrane Review (14) to supply scientific evidence on different surgical interventions for DDD. Until recently, most studies were comparisons of two or more surgical treatments applied to heterogeneous groups of patients. In this chapter, we have attempted to synthesize the evidence supporting treatment for more clearly defined conditions than was previously possible. Once the benefits of surgery for a given condition are established, then separate questions relating to the type of any procedure can be addressed. In particular, it is important to know whether the use of expensive instrumentation systems, designed to facilitate fusion or perhaps retain spinal mobility, can be justified at the current time.

OBJECTIVE

The objective of our study was to determine the most appropriate treatment for specific clinical syndromes in patients with degenerative lumbar spondylosis—in essence, to test the following null hypotheses:

- There are no differences in outcome between surgical and conservative treatment.
- There are no differences in outcome between various methods of surgical treatment.
- There are no differences in the cost-effectiveness of different modes of therapy.

METHODS

Literature Search

The medical literature was searched to identify RCTs in any language. Most of the studies were found in the MEDLINE database, but EMBASE, BIOSIS, Dissertation Abstracts, and the Index to U.K. Theses were also searched. Lately, PubMed has been used to locate newly published work. In addition, *Spine* was hand-searched, and several surgeons supplied references from personal bibliographies. All references in the articles cited were checked for missed trials.

Data Analysis

Each eligible trial was subsequently entered into RevMan and sorted on the basis of inclusion and exclusion criteria. Both authors then independently extracted data from the articles and scrutinized the trials for methodologic quality, randomization method, and quality of allocation concealment.

Outcomes were tabulated from each article, as shown in Table 31.1, and any usable data were pooled with those from trials of similar type. This allowed metaanalysis and calculation of odds ratios (OR) [95% confidence internal (CI)]. Finally, it was possible to grade the evidence by applying the quality criteria recognized by the Cochrane Collaboration Back Review Group (29) as follows:

- *Level A.* Strong evidence—provided by metaanalysis of multiple high-quality RCTs.
- *Level B.* Moderate evidence—provided by one high-quality RCT and one or more low-quality RCTs, or by generally consistent findings in multiple low-quality RCTs.
- *Level C.* Limited or contradictory evidence—from only one RCT (of either high or low quality) or inconsistent findings in multiple RCTs.
- *Level D.* No evidence from RCTs.

TABLE 31.1. *Spinal fusion: instrumented fusion versus graft only (mixed disease)*

Study	Instrumented (n/N)	Noninstrumented (n/N)	Weight (%)	OR (95% CI random)
Bridwell 1993	21 / 24	3 / 10	8.7	16.33[2.66,100.26]
Fischgrund 1997	29 / 35	15 / 33	12.9	5.80[1.90,17.68]
France 1999	22 / 29	18 / 28	12.6	1.75[0.55,5.51]
Fritzell 2001	54 / 62	48 / 67	14.3	2.67[1.07,6.66]
McGuire 1993	10 / 13	10 / 14	9.1	1.33[0.24,7.56]
Moller 1999	29 / 37	24 / 37	13.4	1.96[0.70,5.52]
Thomsen 1997	42 / 62	54 / 64	14.6	0.39[0.16,0.92]
Zdeblick 1993	62 / 72	33 / 51	14.5	3.38[1.40,8.16]
Total(95%CI)	269 / 334	205 / 304	100.0	2.30[1.10,4.80]

Test for heterogeneity chi-square=24.62 df=7 p=0.0009
Test for overall effect z=2.22 p=0.03

Favours graft only   Favours instrumented

Comparison: instrumented posterolateral fusion versus graft only (mixed disease).
Outcome: fusion at 2 years.
CI, confidence interval; OR, odds ratio.

RELEVANT TRIALS

Since 2001, two theses, seven articles, and three abstracts of presented work have been published and added to the existing Cochrane Review. One abstract of work published in 1995, previously included in the Cochrane Review (14), is now excluded from the data set because no further information has been forthcoming. The clinical trials analyzed in this chapter are summarized in Table. 31.2.

Surgery for Lumbar Spinal Stenosis

Spinal stenosis affects most adults older than 65 years of age to some extent, but it is only after canal narrowing is sufficient to cause cauda equina or nerve root compression, leading to claudicant pain or neurologic symptoms, that the patient will present to a surgical clinic. Because the condition may be progressive, it is clearly important to define the timing of any surgical intervention and establish the most appropriate form of therapy.

In the original Cochrane Review published in 1999, no RCTs were identified that dealt with the efficacy of surgical decompression. However, other, non-RCT evidence in the medical literature did indicate successful results, ranging between 26% and 100% in one metaanalysis (28), and there has been little dispute among surgeons that surgery for severe stenosis is generally beneficial.

The results of a cohort study of 100 patients were published in 2000 (1). In this trial, 19 patients with severe symptoms were selected for surgical treatment and 50 patients with moderate symptoms for conservative therapy. A further 31 patients were randomized between the two treatments. At 10 years, five of 11 randomized to decompression had no or minimal pain, in comparison with four of 14 initially treated conservatively. This result, and the findings of the trial as a whole, supported the conclusion that the results of conservative therapy were better than expected, but that if treatment was deemed necessary, the results of surgery might be "good" in up to four fifths of severely affected patients. The numbers of patients who were randomized were inadequate to draw any statistically significant conclusions regarding whether surgery was actually better.

One other trial dealt specifically with patients with stenosis (16), and a further five included patients with an associated degenerative spondylolisthesis (see later discussion) (5,8,17,25,27). Postacchini et al. (25) were unable to show any difference in clinical outcome between laminectomy and multiple laminotomy, although the interpretation of the results was unfortunately limited by confounding factors. Some patients randomized to laminotomy required a laminectomy for technical reasons, and some subjects in both groups had a lateral mass fusion. The trial did not reveal any difference in progression of spondylolisthesis between the two methods. Grob et al. (16) prospectively evaluated the results of spinal decompression with or without arthrodesis. In the fusion arm of the trial, patients were allocated to decompression plus arthrodesis of only the most stenotic segment or of the whole area decompressed. The authors concluded that in the absence of instability, arthrodesis was not necessary, provided that the posterior elements were preserved at the decompression to maintain spinal stability.

At the 2002 meeting of the International Society for Surgery of the Lumbar Spine in Cleveland, OH, Zucherman et al. (31) presented the results of a randomized prospective trial that assessed the therapeutic benefits of an interspinous spacer designed to restrict lumbar spinal extension in patients with neurogenic claudication. The authors claimed a significant 82% reduction in the severity of symptoms in the patients with implants, com-

TABLE 31.2. *Characteristics of included trials*

Trial	Methods	Participants	Interventions	Outcomes
Lumbar spinal stenosis				
Amundsen et al. Norway 2000	Block randomization from table Blinding: nil Lost to follow-up: 2/31 at 4 yr 6/31 at 10 yr	31 patients: 16 male, 15 female Age 21–80 yr	Exp: Spinal decompression Ctl: Spinal orthosis	Pain rating Surgeon rating Patient rating Second procedure
Grob et al. Switzerland 1995	Quasi randomized Blinding: nil Lost to follow-up: 0/30 at 28 mo	45 patients: 21 male, 24 female Age 48–87 yr	Exp: Decompression with arthrodesis (both mono- and multisegmental) Ctl: Decompression	Patient rating Surgeon rating Second procedure —at 28 mo
Postacchini et al. Italy 1993	Alternate assignment Blinding: nil Lost to follow-up: 3/70 at 3.7 yr	70 patients: 34 male, 36 female Age 43–79 yr	Exp: Multiple laminotomy Ctl: Laminectomy	Patient rating Surgeon rating Spondylolisthesis progression Operating time Blood loss —at 3.7 yr
Zuchermann et al. U.S.A. 2002	Randomization method not stated Blinding: nil	56 patients	Exp: Interspinous spacer Ctl: Conservative therapy	Patient rating
Degenerate spondylolisthesis				
Herkowitz and Kurz U.S.A. 1991	Alternate assignment Blinding: nil Lost to follow-up: 0/50 at 3 yr	50 patients: 14 male, 36 female Age 52–84 yr	Exp: Decompression plus posterolateral fusion Ctl: Decompression	Back pain scale Leg pain scale Surgeon rating Fusion Spondylolisthesis progression —at 3 yr
Bridwell et al. U.S.A. 1993	Randomization method not stated Blinding: nil Lost to follow-up: 1/44 at 2 yr	44 patients: 10 male, 34 female Age 44–79 yr	Exp: No fusion Ctl: Posterolateral fusion with or without instrumentation	Spondylolisthesis progression Second procedure —at 2 yr

Isthmic spondylolisthesis

Study	Randomization	Patients	Groups	Outcomes
Carragee U.S.A. 1997	Randomization from sealed envelopes Blinding: nil Lost to follow-up: 2/42 at 4.5 yr	42 patients: 26 male, 16 female Age 19–51 yr	Exp: (a) Smokers with instrumented arthrodesis and decompressive laminectomy (b) Nonsmokers with graft alone and decompressive laminectomy Ctl: Same groups without decompressive laminectomy	Back pain rating Fusion Patient rating —at 3 yr
Moller and Hedlund Sweden 2000	Random choice by nurse Blinding: nil Lost to follow-up: 5/114 at 2 yr	111 patients: 57 male, 54 female Age 18–55 yr	Exp: (a) Posterolateral fusion (b) Posterolateral fusion and CD instrumentation Ctl: Physiotherapy	Patient rating Surgeon rating Disability rating index Pain index Fusion

Mechanical back pain

Study	Randomization	Patients	Groups	Outcomes
Fritzell et al. Sweden 2001	Computer-generated random number Blinding: nil Lost to follow-up: 5/294 at 2 yr	294 patients: 145 male, 149 female Age 25–64 yr	Exp: (a) Posterolateral fusion (b) Posterolateral fusion and VSP stabilization (c) As b with ALIF or PLIF Ctl: Physical therapy	Patient rating Independent observer rating Low back pain Oswestry Disability score Million score General function score Zung depression scale Fusion
Barendse et al. Holland 2001	Computer-generated randomization Blinding: double Lost to follow-up: 0/28 at 8 wk	28 patients: 10 male, 18 female Mean age 42 yrs	Exp: 90-sec 70-degree lesion Ctl: Sham procedure	Observer rating Pain VAS Oswestry Disability score
Pauza et al. U.S.A. 2002	Computer randomization in 3:2 ratio Blinding: double Lost to follow-up: 9/64 at 6 m	64 patients: 40 one level 24 two levels	Exp: IDET Ctl: Sham procedure	Pain VAS Bodily pain Oswestry Disability score Short Form 36

ALIF, anterior lumbar interbody fusion; CD, Cotrel–Dubousset; Ctl, control; Exp, experimental; IDET, intradiscal electrothermal therapy; PLIF, posterior lumbar interbody fusion; VAS, visual analog scale; VSP, variable screw placement.

pared with 10% in controls. However, it should be noted that the results were highly selected because data were analyzed from only 56 of the 236 patients who were randomized.

Nerve Root Stenosis

Currently, no RCTs have dealt specifically with surgical decompression to relieve root stenosis in the absence of a central spinal stenosis. Trials comparing natural history with intraforaminal steroid injection are not included in this surgical review.

Degenerative Spondylolisthesis

Two RCTs have specifically dealt with the management of degenerative spondylolisthesis. In 1991, Herkowitz and Kurz (17) reported the results in 50 patients studied clinically and radiographically to determine whether it was necessary to supplement decompressive laminectomy with an intertransverse spinal arthrodesis. At a minimum of 2 years of follow-up, 24 of 25 patients with an arthrodesis rated their result as "excellent" or "good," compared with only 11 of 25 without an arthrodesis ($P < 0.001$), and progressive vertebral slip was more likely to occur in the latter.

Bridwell et al. (5) subsequently reported the results of treatment in a small number of patients, but with a grossly inadequate randomization process. Patients who had an excessive "pathologic" motion on a preoperative flexion–extension radiograph (more than 10 degrees or more than 3 mm) were automatically randomized to instrumented fusion; as a result, nine patients treated conservatively were compared with 35 treated by surgery. If these data are combined with those from the trial of Herkowitz and Kurz (17) of noninstrumented fusion and those of Grob et al. (16), who included only patients with less than 5 mm of vertebral slip, then the advantage of fusion over decompression alone is no longer evident [surgeon rating: n = 138; random effects OR, 0.44; 95% CI, 0.13, 1.48]. Clearly, extreme caution is required in drawing this conclusion from such a heterogeneous set of trials. Three further RCTs including patients with degenerative spondylolisthesis also included several patients with other conditions (8,25,27).

Isthmic Spondylolisthesis

Two trials compared modes of treatment of isthmic spondylolisthesis. Moller (21,22) assessed 111 patients with isthmic spondylolisthesis. The primary objective of the RCT was to compare the outcome of posterolateral fusion with that of conservative treatment. The secondary objective was to determine whether supplementary transpedicular fixation improves the outcome of fusion. An independent assessor rated the patients, recording their return to work at 2 years and their level of pain. The findings conclusively showed that posterolateral fusion relieved pain ($P = 0.002$) and improved spinal function ($P = 0.004$) in comparison with strength training exercises, which had a limited effect, if any, on symptoms. The use of supplementary transpedicular instrumentation improved neither rate of fusion nor clinical outcome, but the mean operative time was longer and intraoperative blood loss greater ($P < 0.0001$ for both)

Carragee (7) studied patients with a grade 1 or 2 spondylolisthesis of the most caudal lumbar segment. Forty-two patients were divided according to whether or not they smoked. Posterolateral arthrodesis was performed on the spine of each patient, but decompression was randomized. Instrumentation was performed only in smokers. The results showed that the addition of decompression to an arthrodesis, whether or not the spine was instrumented, did not appear to improve the final result and might lead to a pseudarthrosis.

Mechanical Back Pain

Studies of discogenic back pain in the absence of neurologic compromise may be considered in two broad groups, depending on whether fusion and nonfusion technology was used.

Fusion

Before 2001, no RCTs of the effectiveness of fusion in patients with chronic back pain but no associated neurologic compromise had been published.

In 2001, the Swedish multicenter RCT of lumbar fusion versus nonsurgical treatment for chronic low back pain was published in *Spine* as the 2001 International Society for the Study of the Lumbar Spine Volvo Award Winner (12,13). Two hundred ninety-four patients presenting at 19 spinal centers during a 6-year period were randomized blindly to four treatment groups. Strict inclusion criteria basically limited entry to patients with back pain more pronounced than leg pain that had lasted longer than 2 years and no evidence of nerve root compression. Each patient had to have completed a course of nonsurgical treatment.

Seventy-two patients were randomized to conservative treatment and 222 to one of three different fusion techniques. Follow-up at 2 years was 98%. Twenty-five subjects did not complete treatment according to random allocation, but these "group changers" were included in the original "intention-to-treat" analysis.

At 2 years, independent assessors rated results as excellent or good in 46% of the surgical group, compared with 18% of the conservative group. More of the surgical patients rated their result as "better" or "much better" (63% vs. 29%, $P < 0.0001$). Reduction of pain (visual analog scale) and disability (Oswestry Disability Index) was greater in the surgical patients. Among the surgical patients, 47% had returned to work, compared with 33% in the group treated conservatively.

Similar numbers were treated by posterolateral fusion (n = 74), posterolateral fusion plus variable screw placement (n = 75), and posterolateral fusion plus variable screw placement plus interbody fusion (anterior lumbar interbody fusion, n = 56; posterior lumbar interbody fusion, n = 19). No difference in outcome, as rated by either the patients or an independent observer, was noted between the different surgical techniques. The instrumented fusions healed more readily than the noninstrumented fusions.

The Swedish study also provides one of the few analyses of the cost-effectiveness of spinal surgical treatment. The differences in cost between the surgical and control groups were significant, mainly because more patients went back to work in the surgical group. No significant differences were found between the individual surgical groups.

The major question about the Swedish trial concerns the nature of the conservative treatment used as the control intervention (23). We accept that the Swedish group tried to ensure that each patient understood that "no treatment method, as far as was known, was superior to any other." Nevertheless, the control group essentially received more of the same "usual nonsurgical treatment" that had already failed, and failure was one of the indications leading to consideration of surgery. In view of the likely negative patient expectations, it is hardly surprising that the results in the control group appear poorer

TABLE 31.3. *Excellent/good clinical outcome: instrumented fusion versus graft only (mixed disease)*

Study	Instrumented (n/N)	Noninstrumented (n/N)	OR (95% CI random)	Weight (%)	OR (95% CI random)
Fischgrund 1997	27 / 35	28 / 33		12.4	0.60[0.18,2.07]
France 1999	21 / 37	18 / 33		15.7	1.09[0.43,2.81]
Fritzell 2001	40 / 67	41 / 60		18.6	0.69[0.33,1.43]
McGuire 1993	10 / 13	7 / 14		8.7	3.33[0.63,17.57]
Moller 1999	31 / 37	25 / 38		13.8	2.69[0.89,8.08]
Thomsen 1997	52 / 63	49 / 66		16.9	1.64[0.70,3.85]
Zdeblick 1993	67 / 72	36 / 51		13.9	5.58[1.88,16.61]
Total(95%CI)	248 / 324	204 / 295		100.0	1.56[0.85,2.87]

Test for heterogeneity chi-square=14.42 df=6 p=0.025
Test for overall effect z=1.45 p=0.15

.1 .2 1 5 10
Favours graft only   Favours instrumented

Comparison: instrumented posterolateral fusion versus graft only (mixed disease).
Outcome: good clinical outcome.
CI, confidence interval; OR, odds ratio.

than most surgeons would expect from the natural history. This RCT did provide the first substantive evidence that fusion is more effective than continued, standard 1990s "usual care." However, as Mooney (23) pointed out, it did not answer the question of how surgery might compare with a modern exercise and rehabilitation program.

A Norwegian RCT compared fusion with what is probably the best available nonsurgical treatment in the world today—an educational intervention by Aage Indahl personally with a 3-week course of intensive exercise sessions based on cognitive behavioral principles (6). Sixty-four patients were randomized with a 97% follow-up at 1 year and intention-to-treat analysis. No differences were found in independent observer outcome ratings, pain, disability, or return to work. Radiating leg pain decreased after surgery only. Fear avoidance beliefs and forward flexion improved after conservative management only. These results suggest that fusion and a modern rehabilitation approach can produce comparable results. Clearly, questions about the scientific evidence regarding the clinical effectiveness of fusion remain unanswered. Further evidence is required, which it is hoped will be provided by RCTs being performed in England and the United States.

Several trials have addressed whether instrumentation facilitates fusion. Most of these include results from patients presenting with heterogeneous spinal pathology (10,11, 20,27,30), but if the data are combined with those extracted from the trials directed at specific pathology (5,12,21), the evidence is now strong that instrumentation facilitates fusion (evidence level A) (Table 31.3). Unfortunately, even with the inclusion of recent data (12), improvements in clinical outcome do not reach statistical significance.

Nonfusion Technology

Intradiscal Electrothermal Therapy

Radiofrequency thermocoagulation of sensory pain fibers has been used as a method of reducing facet joint pain. In the mid-1990s, surgeons speculated that this technique might also, if applied within the disc, diminish pain arising from free nerve endings in the outer annulus fibrosus. The first RCT of this technique was published in 2001.

Barendse and colleagues (2) randomized 28 patients to either radiofrequency treatment, in which a 90-second 70°C lesion was applied to the disc, or no stimulation. The trial was double-blinded, with a disinterested third party administering the stimulation. Eight weeks after treatment, only one success in the radiofrequency group (n = 13) and two in the control group (n = 15) were observed, with no difference in pain assessment or disability measured on the Oswestry Disability Index.

Concurrently with this study, others were reporting outcomes of intradiscal electrothermal therapy (IDET), which is administered for a longer time and applied over a wider area than is possible with a radiofrequency probe (9,18). Initial cohort studies were promising (26), and the results of the first double-blinded placebo-controlled randomized trial were presented to the 2002 meeting of the International Spinal Injection Society in Austin, TX (24). Sixty-four subjects (from a potential cohort of 4,253) were randomized by computer, in a ratio of 3:2, to IDET or placebo. Electrode catheters were placed in each group before the surgeon was notified of the group assignment. Postoperative protocols were identical. The results (n = 55) showed a statistically significant greater reduction in pain measured on a visual analog scale and bodily pain in the IDET group than in the placebo group. Overall disability (Oswestry Disability Index) diminished, and the Beck Depression Inventory score improved after IDET use.

It is clearly not possible to combine the results of these two RCTs, which use different treatment techniques, although they are similar in principle. The study from Texas scored higher methodologically and the results are certainly similar to those of earlier case control studies. In both trials, the patients were highly selected from a large number of eligible subjects.

Disc Arthroplasty

Intervertebral disc replacement was introduced in France in 1990. Worldwide, more than 4,000 discs have now been inserted and some excellent results reported (4,15,19). Thus far, no randomized studies comparing outcomes against natural history or conservative therapy, or outcomes between implants, have been published. The state of affairs is similar for nucleus replacement (3).

CONCLUSIONS

It is encouraging that several RCTs recently have been published, but it still remains difficult to define appropriate treatment for any specific clinical pathology. In no circumstance can we reach even a "moderate" rating of scientific evidence for any intervention.

Lumbar spinal stenosis:

- Surgical decompression may be an option in patients with severe symptoms in whom conservative treatment has failed (level C).
- The exact method of surgical decompression probably does not make much difference in regard to clinical outcome (level C).
- Fusion is probably not required provided no surgical instability is created (level C).

Degenerative spondylolisthesis:

- In patients who require surgery, clinical outcomes are better after decompressive laminectomy plus arthrodesis than after decompression alone (level C).

Isthmic spondylolisthesis:

- Posterolateral fusion may be an option in patients with severe symptoms in whom conservative treatment has failed (level C).
- Spinal decompression in addition to fusion is probably not required (level C).

"Mechanical" back pain secondary to degenerative disc disease:

- For patients with chronic pain and failed conservative treatment, fusion provides a better outcome than continued "usual care" (level C).
- Surgical fusion may not be any more effective than a modern exercise and rehabilitation program (level C).
- The evidence on IDET is conflicting, but outcome may depend on the technique used (level C).
- Disc arthroplasty is not currently supported by RCT evidence (level D).

For a metaanalysis of data that will lead to definitive guidelines and treatment protocols, further RCTs are required. The authors invite notification of any new or on-going RCTs.

REFERENCES

1. Amundsen T, Weber H, Nordal HJ, et al. Lumbar spinal stenosis: conservative or surgical management? A prospective 10-year study. *Spine* 2000;25:1424–1436.
2. Barendse GAM, Van den Berg SGM, Kessels AHF, et al. Randomized controlled trial of percutaneous intradiscal radiofrequency thermocoagulation for chronic discogenic back pain. *Spine* 2001;26:287–292.
3. Bao Q, Yuan HA. New technologies in spine. Nucleus replacement. *Spine* 2002;27:1245–1247.
4. Bertagnoli R, Kumar S. Indications for full prosthetic disc arthroplasty: a correlation of clinical outcome against a variety of indications. *Eur Spine J* 2002;11[Suppl 2]:S131–S136.
5. Bridwell KH, Sedgewick TA, O'Brien MF, et al. The role of fusion and instrumentation in the treatment of degenerative spondylolisthesis with spinal stenosis. *J Spinal Disord* 1993;6:461–472.
6. Brox JI, et al. Randomized clinical trial of lumbar instrumented fusion and cognitive intervention and exercises of patients with chronic low back pain and disc degeneration. Presented to the International Society for the Study of the Lumbar Spine, Vancouver, BC, 2003.
7. Carragee EJ. Single-level posterolateral arthrodesis, with or without posterior decompression, for the treatment of isthmic spondylolisthesis in adults. *J Bone Joint Surg Am* 1997;79:1175–1180.
8. Christensen FB, Hansen ES, Eiskjaer SP, et al. Circumferential lumbar spinal fusion with Brantigan cage versus posterolateral fusion with titanium Cotrel-Dubousset instrumentation: a prospective, randomized clinical study of 146 patients. *Spine* 2002;27:2674–2683.
9. Derby R, Eck B, Chen Y, et al. Intradiscal electrothermal annuloplasty (IDET): a novel approach for treating chronic discogenic back pain. *Neuromodulation* 2000;3:69–75.
10. Fischgrund JS, Mackay M, Herkowitz HN, et al. Degenerative lumbar spondylolisthesis with spinal stenosis. A prospective randomized study comparing decompressive laminectomy and arthrodesis with and without spinal instrumentation. *Spine* 1997;22:2807–2812.
11. France JC, Yaszemski MJ, Lauerman WC, et al. A randomized prospective study of posterolateral lumbar fusion. *Spine* 1999;24:553–560.
12. Fritzell P, Hägg O, Wessberg P, et al. Lumbar fusion versus nonsurgical treatment for chronic low back pain. A multicenter randomized controlled trial from the Swedish Lumbar Spine Study Group. *Spine* 2001;26:2521–2534.
13. Fritzell P. *Lumbar fusion for chronic low back pain. The Swedish Lumbar Spine Study* [Thesis]. Göteborg, Sweden: Göteborg University, 2002.
14. Gibson JNA, Waddell G, Grant IC. Surgery for degenerative lumbar spondylosis [Cochrane Review]. *The Cochrane Library*, Issue 1, 1999. Oxford: Update Software, 1999; *Spine* 1999;24:1820–1832.
15. Griffith SL, Shelokov AP, Buttner-Janz K, et al. A multicenter retrospective study of the clinical results of the Link® SB Charité intervertebral prosthesis. *Spine* 1994;19:1842–1849.
16. Grob D, Humke T, Dvorak J. Degenerative lumbar spinal stenosis: decompression with and without arthrodesis. *J Bone Joint Surg Am* 1995;77:1036–1041.
17. Herkowitz HN, Kurz LT. Degenerative lumbar spondylolisthesis with spinal stenosis: a prospective study comparing decompression with decompression and intertransverse process arthrodesis. *J Bone Joint Surg Am* 1991;73:802–808.

18. Karasek M, Bogduk N. Twelve-month follow-up of a controlled trial of intradiscal thermal annuloplasty for back pain due to internal disc disruption. *Spine* 2000;25:2601–2607.
19. Lemaire JP, Skalli W, Lavaste F, et al. Intervertebral disc prosthesis. *Clin Orthop* 1997;337:64–76.
20. McGuire RA, Amundson GM. The use of primary internal fixation in spondylolisthesis. *Spine* 1993;18:1662–1672.
21. Moller H. *Isthmic spondylolisthesis in adults. A randomized controlled trial* [Thesis]. Stockholm: Karolinska Institute, 1999.
22. Moller H, Hedlund R. Surgery versus conservative management in adult isthmic spondylolisthesis—a prospective randomized study: Part 1. *Spine* 2000;25:1711–1715. Instrumented and non-instrumented posterolateral fusion in adult spondylolisthesis—a prospective randomized study: Part 2. *Spine* 2000;25:1716–1721.
23. Mooney V. Point of view. *Spine* 2001; 26:2532–2534.
24. Pauza K, Howell S, Dreyfuss P, et al. *A randomized, double-blind, placebo-controlled trial evaluating the efficacy of intradiscal electrothermal anuloplasty (IDET^{TM}) for the treatment of chronic discogenic low back pain: 6-month outcomes.* Presented to the International Spinal Injection Society, Austin, TX, 2002.
25. Postacchini F, Cinotti G, Perugia D, et al. The surgical treatment of central lumbar stenosis: multiple laminotomy compared with total laminectomy. *J Bone Joint Surg [Br]* 1993;75:386–392.
26. Saal JA, Saal JS. Intradiscal electrothermal treatment for chronic discogenic low back pain. *Spine* 2002;27:966–974.
27. Thomsen K, Christensen FB, Eiskjaer SP, et al. The effect of pedicle screw instrumentation on functional outcome and fusion rates in posterolateral lumbar spinal fusion: a prospective randomized clinical study. *Spine* 1997;22:2813–2822.
28. Turner JA, Ersek M, Herron L, et al. Surgery for lumbar spinal stenosis: attempted metaanalysis of the literature 1970–1993. *Spine* 1992;17:1–8.
29. Van Tulder MW, Assendelft WJ, Koes BW, et al. Method guidelines for systematic reviews in the Cochrane Collaboration Back Review Group for Spinal Disorders. *Spine* 1997;22:2323–2330.
30. Zdeblick TA. A prospective, randomized study of lumbar fusion. *Spine* 1993;1883–1891.
31. Zuchermann J, Hsu K, Mehahe T, et al. *Multicenter randomized prospective trial for treatment of lumbar neurogenic claudication with an interspinous device: one-year results.* Presented to the International Society for Study of the Lumbar Spine, Cleveland, OH, 2002.

32

Animal Models in the Study of Degenerative Disc Disease

Robert J. Moore

Department of Pathology, The University of Adelaide; The Adelaide Centre for Spinal Research, Institute of Medical and Veterinary Science, Adelaide, Australia

Low back pain is a debilitating condition that has reached epidemic proportions in modern Western society, with substantial medical and economic consequences (40). The peak incidence of low back pain is at about 40 years of age, and although it has many likely causes, it is mostly attributed to disc degeneration and characterized by significant alterations in disc morphology (67). Paradoxically, whereas pain symptoms tend to disappear with time, disc degeneration continues unabated in the majority of cases.

The morphologic features of normal and diseased discs have been described in considerable detail through the study of surgical and cadaveric samples. Although these investigations provide insight into the range of degenerative changes encountered, they do not reveal the mechanisms that contribute to them. Only by conducting controlled experimental animal studies, in which the model mimics the changes seen in humans, is it possible to understand the pathogenesis of changes and find solutions to a major clinical problem.

Logic would suggest that the ideal animal model is one that is bipedal because the upright posture of humans is arguably one of the principal factors contributing to low back pain, yet the use of nonhuman primates in medical and scientific research is a vexed ethical issue in most countries. Accordingly, research into the pathogenesis of disc disease has for the most part been restricted to small, conventional laboratory animals, such as rabbits and dogs. This review describes how these and other animal models have been used in the study of disc degeneration.

Disc degeneration has received considerable attention since the publication of the pioneering autopsy observations of Schmorl and Junghanns (55), which showed by the age of 49 years, 60% of women and 80% of men are affected, and that 95% of all subjects are affected by the age of 70 years. These accounts of the human condition, resulting from the meticulous examination of thousands of cadaveric spines, led many workers, particularly in Europe, to use experimental animal models to investigate the pathogenesis of disc degeneration.

The embryologic and postnatal development of the discs, in addition to the basic physiologic and pathologic processes, are well documented in many animal species, and detailed descriptions compare their anatomy with that of human discs. The comprehensive review of Butler (8) described species of various sizes, ranging from mice and rats to horses and cows, but within a few years of its publication, it had become clear that larger animals, such as sheep, goats, and pigs, were needed for *in vivo* trials of the burgeoning array of implantable spinal hardware.

The earliest account of the use of animals for studies of disc degeneration originated in Germany, when Lob (39) showed that incision of the annulus fibrosus in rabbit discs resulted in gross changes similar to those seen in spondylosis deformans in humans. Two years later, Filippi (14) showed that the outer fibers of the anterior annulus in the rabbit regenerated by fibrocartilage proliferation 40 days after being incised surgically and were capable of regenerating fully within 3 months.

More than a decade passed before the first English language report of an experimental animal model of disc degeneration appeared. Key and Ford (33) created deep incisions in the posterolateral annulus fibrosus of canine discs to cause immediate prolapse of the nucleus pulposus, but in contrast to the authors of previous studies, they did not remove any nuclear material. The animals survived between 2 days and 28 weeks. Their model showed healing of the annulus only in the superficial layers, leading them to postulate that disc protrusion resulted from weakening of the thinner posterior zone of the annulus by degeneration or injury. In their opinion, degenerative changes in the nucleus were secondary to annular damage.

Using Filippi's rabbit model, but creating full-thickness annular incisions, Smith and Walmsley (61) published data from a study of 55 rabbits that survived between 1 day and 2 years. Consistent with earlier findings, they described superficial annular healing in a pattern that is typical of general histologic repair. It was postulated that the deeper part of the wound failed to heal because the inner annulus lacked a blood supply and because prolapsed nuclear material filled the defect. Based on these observations, they proposed that if early degenerative changes occurred in the human disc, the hydrostatic pressure of the nucleus combined with movement of the vertebral column would tear the inner lamellae of the annulus and allow the nucleus to escape. Such a rupture would extend to the superficial layers to produce "a tracking of the nucleus to the periphery of the disc," such as that seen in a complete disc prolapse. An incidental observation in many of the longer-term survivors was extensive ossification of the anterior annulus.

More recently, an ovine model of disc degeneration was established with only a slight but significant modification of the earlier complete annular incision techniques. Researchers already had made the critical observation that peripheral annular rim lesions were present in young human autopsy spines without any other significant pathology, leading to speculation about the role of these lesions in the pathogenesis of disc degeneration (26,68). In the sheep model, stab incisions were made in the outer one third of the annulus of lumbar discs, with care taken not to penetrate the nucleus (49). Thirty-five animals survived for periods of between 2 weeks and 2 years postoperatively. Histologic examination showed an ordered sequence of healing, with limited vascular repair in the outer annulus only and focal proliferation of blood vessels within and through the cartilage of the endplate in the early postoperative phase (45). Despite the healing response, disc degeneration was observed within 6 months, with progressive failure of the inner annular fibers and lateral displacement of the nucleus pulposus toward the site of the initial incision. The resulting radiating annular clefts, loss of disc height, loss of nuclear cells and matrix, and marginal osteophyte formation were identical to the changes seen in advanced stages of human disc degeneration (67). As in previous animal models, the inner annulus failed to heal, even after 2 years; this finding was attributed in part to the absence of a blood supply but also to possible micromotion at the interface of the cut surfaces. Fixation of a metal plate across the incised disc resulted in partial mechanical stabilization, but it failed to promote complete repair of the lesion (44). The adjacent unincised control discs from both of these studies showed no significant morphologic abnormalities.

In addition to the morphologic aspects, considerable interest has been shown in the biochemical changes associated with disc degeneration. Using the rabbit model of acute nuclear herniation, Lipson and Muir (37,38) showed that in the longer term, progressive dehydration of the incised discs was associated with a loss of aggregated proteoglycan molecules. They suggested that irreversible mechanical damage was sustained and that disc degeneration was inevitable following the loss of confined fluid mechanics. In the sheep model, biochemical changes also lagged behind the morphologic changes, with a significant loss of proteoglycans and collagen from the incised discs and a concomitant increase in noncollagenous protein levels noted after 8 months (42). Whereas the histopathology studies showed no significant differences until after 12 months, similar biochemical changes were also observed at adjacent, unincised discs within this period, indicating that disc injury may influence an area much broader than just the affected level.

It is not surprising that sheep are favored for experimental studies in Australia because they are relatively cheap and can be kept outdoors. In Europe, however, where open farmland is scarce and weather conditions are more adverse, researchers have adapted the annular incision model to the mini pig and have reported data that are almost identical to those from the sheep. Like the sheep model, porcine discs show degenerative changes similar to those seen in humans within 3 months after surgery, with elevated collagen synthesis and decreased water content, particularly in the nucleus, and marginal osteophyte formation (29,30).

The annular incision model has been used to elucidate the causes of discogenic back pain. Basic principles of wound healing would suggest that nerve fibers accompany sprouting capillaries into the granulation tissue at a site of tissue repair. Indeed, evidence suggests that several neuropeptides, including substance P, calcitonin gene–related peptide, neurofilament protein R39, protein gene product 9.5, and synaptophysin, are present in the outer two or three lamellae of the annulus in the pig (28) and the sheep (13) after outer annular incision. This finding has important implications for the treatment of back pain, including the application of intradiscal electrothermal therapy (52).

Outer annular injury in the porcine model has also been used to study the effects of nonsteroidal antiinflammatory agents on proteoglycan metabolism in the nucleus (31). The apparent cartilage-protective role of tiaprofenic acid in promoting the accumulation of proteoglycans has important implications for the treatment of injured discs because it would stimulate repair of the nuclear matrix.

Iatrogenic discitis is a condition that can develop after any procedure that violates the disc space, the most common being provocative discography and discectomy. As an experimental model, the sheep has provided compelling evidence that discitis results from the inadvertent introduction of viable bacteria, not from an aseptic process, as was once believed. In the first of these studies, the deliberate injection of suspensions of bacteria into the disc, along with chymopapain, resulted in typical radiographic and pathologic features of discitis after 6 weeks (15). In another group of sheep, radiographic contrast deliberately contaminated with bacteria was injected during discography, with similar consequences (16). This pioneering work showed the importance of prophylactic antibiotics in minimizing the incidence of iatrogenic discitis and limiting the vertebral body destruction associated with the disease process (17). Although the benefits of prophylactic antibiotics remain questionable in some quarters, inasmuch as discitis generally resolves once the infection spreads to the vertebral body marrow and activates the immune system, early detection is still important. Work in the sheep model indicates that discitis can be detected reliably by some magnetic resonance imaging sequences as early as 6 days after inoculation, and this may provide sufficient time for diagnosis and the initiation of antibiotic therapy (46).

Degenerative disc disease (DDD) can cause mechanical instability and pain in a spinal motion segment. Spinal arthrodesis (fusion) aims to eliminate abnormal movement and relieve pain symptoms by creating bony union across unstable levels. Since the pioneering study of Albee (2), published almost a century ago, animals have been used extensively to investigate spinal fusion. There is no question that dogs have been the animal model most commonly used, although many studies have also used rabbits, guinea pigs, and rats (54). These smaller animals are relatively cheap and convenient to handle in the laboratory, and they generally achieve fusion readily within a short period of time. This may be an advantage because larger groups can provide more data sooner. On the other hand, many of these species continue to grow through adult life, never reaching skeletal maturity, and therefore they do not mimic the human situation exactly. Studies with dogs in particular have been criticized because dogs show a tendency to fuse in almost every case, even after simple decortication (9). Nevertheless, although larger animals better simulate the relatively large human spine and therefore are able to accommodate fixation devices, they offer no significant advantage over the dog from a biologic perspective. In fact, if nothing else, they can be considerably more costly to maintain.

Goats have been used for *in vivo* studies to examine the radiologic, biomechanical, and histologic effects of a range of grafting and fixation methods of cervical spine fusion (4,51,72). Although none of these studies specifically validated the suitability of the goat spine as a model of the human spine, they nonetheless provided valuable information about the biology of fusion and the merits of various surgical approaches.

It is uncommon for nonhuman primates to be used for spinal research, even though these animals are genetically similar to humans. The baboon has been viewed as a potential model of the human upper cervical spine, and apart from some minor differences, it was shown to have identical anatomic components in similar proportions and with a similar geometric configuration (12). The anatomy and biomechanical behavior of the baboon were sufficiently similar for it to be deemed a valid model for the study of human atlantoaxial biomechanics and pathology.

In the last decade, monkeys have been used to develop new lumbar spinal fusion techniques, mainly with a view to examining the role of an osteoinductive growth factor, recombinant human bone morphogenetic protein-2 (rhBMP-2), in promoting fusion (5,6,25,62). In these animals, as in humans, it takes many months to achieve fusion, but despite the high maintenance costs, the similarities in anatomy, biology, and biomechanical characteristics make them valid models for preclinical testing (53).

It is not unusual to encounter criticism of biomechanical studies that use quadrupedal animals as models of the human spine, on the grounds that the physiologic loading pattern is not comparable. Although it is true that quadrupedal animals have longer, thinner, and denser vertebral bodies than humans, the orientation of the trabeculae in several species indicates that they experience mainly axial compressive forces in the same way as humans (10,60,70). Furthermore, the range of motion and stiffness of the calf (71) and the sheep (69) spine are sufficiently similar to those of the human to make them valid models.

One problem with larger animals is that surgical intervention is required to induce experimental disc degeneration. In most cases, even the earliest signs of degeneration are not seen for at least 3 months, and the animals often must be maintained for years before significant changes develop. Therefore, the maintenance costs of such studies are high. However, some animals appear to undergo spontaneous disc degeneration. At about the same time that annular incision was being used to study the pathogenesis of disc prolapse, it was shown that beagles, dachshunds, and basset hounds are susceptible to spontaneous prolapse early in life without any surgical intervention (23). These "chondrodystrophoid" breeds, as they are known, are interesting because they show abnormal development of the epiphyseal cartilage during endochondral ossification, and a chondroid metamorphosis reliably appears in the nucleus within the first few years of life (24). During this process, chondrocyte-like cells replace the normal population of notochord cells in the nucleus, and the collagen content in the matrix increases to levels higher than usual. These features are morphologically and biochemically similar to those of the adult human disc (20).

DDD also has been reported to occur naturally in macaque monkeys (36). In a cohort of 192 female monkeys between 5 and 30 years of age, radiologic disc narrowing and osteophytosis were observed along the length of the thoracolumbar spine from an early age, consistent with changes seen in humans. In addition, degeneration increased with advancing age in the quadrupedal animal model, although relative to humans, the prevalence was greater in the oldest age group. The authors concluded that the similarity between these two species indicates that a bipedal habit is not the only, and probably not the most important, biomechanical contributor to the onset and progression of DDD.

A model of spontaneous disc degeneration in an even smaller laboratory animal may have economic advantages. The sand rat (*Psammomys obesus*) is one such animal. Age-related changes in the discs of this small animal were first described by Silberberg et al. (58), and their report was followed by a series of studies characterizing histologic and morphometric (1,47,56,57) and biochemical (59,73) changes from the age of 3 months. By 12 months of age, the majority of these animals show radiologic disc space narrowing and wedging, subchondral endplate sclerosis that increases with age, and marked osteophytic spur formation similar to that seen in diffuse idiopathic skeletal hyperostosis syndrome (22). Microscopic analysis also shows changes similar to those seen in the aging human, with chondrone formation and generalized tissue necrosis and ossification. Although the sand rat must be fed a special low-caloric diet to prevent the development of diabetes, it is otherwise a useful animal that can be kept for long periods at relatively low cost.

A mutant strain (SAMP-1) of the senescence-accelerated mouse, which displays normal growth but rapidly progressive senescence and death within about 12 months after birth, has been used to investigate the role of BMP-2/4 and its receptors in disc degeneration (64). Following normal maturation, expression of BMP-2/4 and its receptors moved from the hyaline cartilage of the endplate to fibrous cells within the annulus and also to the calcified cartilage at the site of enthesis, where in the latter case they presumably play a role in osteophyte formation. Furthermore, in an experimental murine spondylosis model, disc degeneration, including complete loss of the endplate, was accompanied by increased apoptosis in endplate chondrocytes in comparison with naturally aged mice, suggesting that apoptosis plays a role in age-related change of the disc (3).

Segmental spinal defects resulting from degenerative conditions, tumor, trauma, and developmental abnormalities can cause pain, instability, deformity, or neurologic deficit. The traditional treatment for these conditions is fusion, but this is associated with problems of morbidity at the donor site, altered biomechanical function, accelerated degeneration at the adjacent levels, and the risk for hardware failure. Vertebral column allografting was tried as an alternative to fusion in a study of 11 dogs (48). In the immediate postoperative radiographs, the allografts lost 5% of their length. This was followed by a further 10% loss after 3 months and an additional 5% loss during the next 15 months. No significant difference in stiffness of the allograft levels during compression, flexion, and extension testing was noted in comparisons with intact controls. Histologic examination showed incorporation of the cranial and caudal margins of the three-level thoracic allografts in almost all cases, but in only about half of the intervening portions. The disc allografts showed substantial deterioration with loss of disc height during 18 months. Similar results were recorded in subsequent disc allografting studies in which dogs were maintained for 4 months (18) and 1 year (32), and sheep were maintained for 3 months (50). These studies suggest that allografting procedures are associated with many technical problems, including adequate preparation of the graft site and appropriate treatment of the graft between harvest and transplant; as a result, the morphology and metabolism of the disc and facet joints are compromised, even in the short term. It would appear that this procedure is some way from clinical application.

Total disc arthroplasty appears to be a promising alternative to interbody arthrodesis for the surgical treatment of DDD. The main goals of disc arthroplasty are to replace a painful degenerate disc with a device that restores biomechanical function while protecting important neurovascular structures. Although it would seem prudent to use animal models for functionality and biocompatibility testing before clinical trials are undertaken, this has actually been done with very few of the dozens of devices that have been proposed (63).

One of the earliest prototypes was tested in chimpanzees (66). This device consisted of a central silicone core sandwiched between two layers of woven Dacron mesh. Eight discs were inserted into four adult chimpanzees, which survived for up to 1 year. Despite being confounded by several factors, including disc space infections and improperly fitting devices, this study reported generally favorable outcomes on radiology, biomechanical testing, and histological examination.

A scaled-down version of a prototype Kostuik disc prosthesis, consisting of a titanium alloy spring approximating normal stiffness, screws for immediate fixation to the vertebral bodies, and cobalt–chromium alloy bearing surfaces with a porous coat, was tested in six ewes (34). All six devices were well fixed in position, but substantially better bony ingrowth was noted after 6 months. No evidence of any adverse tissue reaction was found, either around the prosthesis or in the lymph nodes.

In vivo trials of a scaled-down version of an artificial disc (3-DF), consisting of a triaxial three-dimensional fabric woven with an ultra–high-molecular-weight polyethylene fiber bundle, have been reported in a series of 23 sheep (35). The 3-DF discs were coated with either sintered hydroxyapatite or apatite-wollastonite glass ceramic granules and implanted in the sheep with or without fixation. Bony integration was reported in approximately one third of the implanted levels after 4 months and in two thirds after 6 months, although it is not clear whether this was influenced by either fixation or the type of surface coating. Importantly, however, no histologic evidence of material debris or foreign body reaction was found, and the device was seen as having "potential for future clinical application." The authors conceded that comparisons of biomechanical behavior between the quadrupedal model and the human may have some limitations. In a parallel study, they reported increasing segmental stiffness with time, attributed to scar and osteophyte formation, and an accompanying commentary warned that this device could behave more as a fusion device rather than as a functional disc unit (65).

The AcroFlex lumbar disc (DePuy AcroMed, Raynham, MA, U.S.A.) was tested in particulate form for up to 6 months in 90 rats and 18 sheep (43) and *in vivo* as a functional device in 20 baboons for up to 12 months (11). In the baboon study, excellent trabecular lamellar bone integration was observed at the implant–bone interface, with no radiographic lucency or other evidence of loosening. After 6 months, the peak range of motion in axial compression in the implanted levels was not significantly different from that in autografted or unoperated control levels, although the autografted levels were significantly stiffer in axial rotation. Range of motion was greater in the intact level than in the AcroFlex level, where, in turn, the range of motion was greater than in the autograft level during flexion–extension and lateral bending tests at 6 months. After 12 months, neither the AcroFlex nor autograft levels were significantly different from the intact levels during axial compression testing, but both were significantly stiffer than the intact level in all other testing modalities. The decreased range of motion in the second half of the study was attributed to periannular calcification caused by the smaller footprint of the custom-made device on the endplate. Despite this decreased flexibility, no radiographic or macroscopic evidence of component failure was found. Minor foreign body reactions to polyolefin particles were reported in both studies, in addition to other insignificant pathology that was attributed to factors such as the housing environment or iatrogenic infection rather than to the implant. Testing of the AcroFlex device produced a satisfactory outcome in both animal models.

These investigators also reported favorable results after *in vivo* tests of the SB Charité III (Link Spine Group, Branford, CT, U.S.A.) hydroxyapatite-coated total disc prosthesis in a series of seven baboons (41). No radiographic evidence of lucency or loosening of the vertebral endplate was noted after 6 months, and extensive biomechanical testing showed no significant difference in range of motion between the prosthesis and unoperated levels. Histomorphometric analysis also showed bony ingrowth across almost half of the endplate, which is much better than what has been reported for cementless femoral components and is attributed to more sustained compression across the metal–bone interface.

One further development that is emerging as a potential treatment of DDD is intervertebral disc cell transplantation. This treatment has already proved successful in treating deep cartilage defects in knees (7). One of the earliest indications of disc degeneration is decreased disc height associated with loss of matrix within the nucleus. The notion that chondrocytes can be harvested from an individual, expanded *in vitro*, and subsequently transplanted into the nucleus of an affected disc in the same individual therefore presents exciting possibilities for a safe and effective treatment of this condition. As for artificial disc prostheses, clinical trials are in progress in several centers; experimental studies in animals have also been reported.

In one study, ear cartilage was harvested from five New Zealand white rabbits, cultured *in vitro*, and transplanted into the nuclear cavities of discs that had been "emptied" during previous surgery (27). After 6 months, most of the discs contained viable chondrocytes surrounded by newly synthesized hyaline matrix. In another study, lumbar disc tissue was removed from 15 sand rats, and autologous chondrocytes were transplanted in cubes of Gelfoam carrier into the same discs after *in vitro* culture and cell labeling (21). Successful engraftment was observed up to 33 weeks later with normal matrix surrounding the transplanted cells that showed appropriate cell morphology. In a canine model (19), cells were harvested from the inner annulus and nucleus of two lumbar discs during microdiscectomy to induce degeneration, cultured *in vitro*, and transplanted into one of the discs either 5 or 12 weeks later. Measurements from radiographs taken at 3-month intervals showed a trend that disc height was maintained in the transplanted levels. The magnetic resonance imaging signal was reduced in both operated levels after 1 year in comparison with the unoperated control, but it was reduced more in the nontransplant control disc. Microscopically, the transplanted cells appeared to survive, populate, produce matrix, and suppress an inflammatory reaction in the adjacent bone marrow.

Despite some technical difficulties associated with the harvest procedure (which is described as aggressive and a likely cause of disc damage and osteophyte formation), these studies suggest that the transplantation of cultured cells into the degenerate nucleus results in the survival and proliferation of cells with a phenotype similar to that of the resident cell population. In light of the unwanted secondary effects associated with harvesting cells from the disc, it might be worth considering a source of chondrocytes other than the disc. In theory, this is an attractive procedure for the treatment of disc degeneration because unlike interbody fusion, it should not affect normal motion at either the operated or adjacent spinal levels.

We have benefited enormously from the early animal models that demonstrated the mechanisms of DDD, but the emphasis has now changed from understanding the pathogenesis of degeneration to developing living systems in which to test the biocompatibility, function, and longevity of new surgical devices. As a result, larger animal models are more appropriate. If animal models are to be used at all, however, certain fundamental considerations are still as applicable to any testing system as they are to the study of spinal fusion (54). The model must be relevant to human biology, anatomy, and pathology. Its breeding characteristics should be uniform, so that study conditions can be reproduced. The model should be available at reasonable cost and easily handled under all experimental conditions. Finally, the choice of any animal model must be supported by a large database of biologic information, so that results and interactions can be understood and explained.

Humans are privileged to be able to use animals to undertake scientific studies in pursuit of their own well-being, and that privilege should be respected by making careful and appropriate choices.

REFERENCES

1. Adler JH, Schoenbaum M, Silberberg R. Early onset of disk degeneration and spondylosis in sand rats (*Psammomys obesus*). *Vet Pathol* 1983;20:13–22.
2. Albee FH. An experimental study of bone growth and the spinal bone transplant. *JAMA* 1913;60:1044–1049.
3. Ariga K, Miyamoto S, Nakase T, et al. The relationship between apoptosis of endplate chondrocytes and aging and degeneration of the intervertebral disc. *Spine* 2001;26:2412–2420.
4. Baisden J, Voo LM, Cusick JF, et al. Evaluation of cervical laminectomy and laminoplasty. A longitudinal study in the goat model. *Spine* 1999;24:1283–1289.
5. Boden SD, Martin GJ Jr, Horton WC, et al. Laparoscopic anterior spinal arthrodesis with rhBMP-2 in a titanium interbody threaded cage. *J Spinal Disord* 1998;11:95–101.
6. Boden SD, Moskovitz PA, Morone MA, et al. Video-assisted lateral intertransverse process arthrodesis. Validation of a new minimally invasive lumbar spinal fusion technique in the rabbit and nonhuman primate (rhesus) models. *Spine* 1996;21:2689–2697.
7. Brittberg M, Lindahl A, Nillson A. Treatment of deep cartilage defects in the knee with autologous chondrocyte transplantation. *N Engl J Med* 1994;331:889–895.
8. Butler WF. Comparative anatomy and development of the intervertebral disc. In: Ghosh P, ed. *The biology of the intervertebral disc*. Boca Raton, FL: CRC Press, 1988:83–108.
9. Callewart CC, Kanim LEA, Dawson EG. *Evaluation of the canine spinal fusion method*. Presented to the annual meeting of the North American Spine Society, San Diego, CA, 1993.
10. Cotterill PC, Kostuik JP, D'Angelo G, et al. An anatomical comparison of the human and bovine thoracolumbar spine. *J Orthop Res* 1986;4:298–303.
11. Cunningham BW, Lowery GL, Serhan HA, et al. Total disc replacement arthroplasty using the AcroFlex lumbar disc: a non-human primate model. *Eur Spine J* 2002;11[Suppl 2]:S115–S123.
12. Dickman CA, Crawford NR, Tominaga T, et al. Morphology and kinematics of the baboon upper cervical spine. A model of the atlantoaxial complex. *Spine* 1994;19:2518–2523.

13. Fagan AB, Fraser RD, Moore RJ. *The three-dimensional structure of annular innervation.* Presented to the annual meeting of the International Society for the Study of the Lumbar Spine, Adelaide, Australia, 2000.
14. Filippi A. La guarigione del disco intervertebrale dopo asportazione del nucleus pulposus negli animali da esperimento. *Chir Organi Mov* 1935;20:1–9.
15. Fraser RD, Osti OL, Vernon-Roberts B. Discitis following chemo-nucleolysis. *Spine* 1986;11:34–43.
16. Fraser RD, Osti OL, Vernon-Roberts B. Discitis after discography II: an experimental study. *J Bone Joint Surg Br* 1987;69:31–35.
17. Fraser RD, Osti OL, Vernon-Roberts B. Iatrogenic discitis. The role of intravenous antibiotics in prevention and treatment: an experimental study. *Spine* 1989;14:1025–1032.
18. Frick SL, Edward NH Jr. Lumbar intervertebral disc transfer: a canine study. *Spine* 1994;19:1826–1835.
19. Ganey TM, Meisel HJ. A potential role for cell-based therapeutics in the treatment of intervertebral disc herniation. *Eur Spine J* 2002;11[Suppl 2]:S206–S214.
20. Ghosh P, Taylor TKF, Braund KG. The variation of the glycosaminoglycans of the canine intervertebral disc with ageing. 1. Chondrodystrophoid breed. *Gerontology* 1977;23:87–98.
21. Gruber HE, Johnson TL, Leslie K, et al. Autologous intervertebral disc cell implantation. *Spine* 2002;27:1626–1633.
22. Gruber HE, Johnson T, Norton HJ, et al. The sand rat model for disc degeneration: radiologic characterization of age-related changes. Cross-sectional and prospective analyses. *Spine* 2002;27:230–234.
23. Hansen H-J. A pathologic-anatomical study on disc degeneration in dogs. *Acta Orthop Scand* 1952;11[Suppl]:1–117.
24. Hansen H-J. Comparative views on the pathology of disk degeneration in animals. *Lab Invest* 1959;8:1242–1265.
25. Hecht BP, Fischgrund JS, Herkowitz HN, et al. The use of recombinant human bone morphogenetic protein 2 (rhBMP-2) to promote spinal fusion in a nonhuman primate anterior interbody fusion model. *Spine* 1999;24:629–636.
26. Hilton RC, Ball J. Vertebral rim lesions in the dorsolumbar spine. *Ann Rheum Dis* 1984;43:302–307.
27. Joksimovic C, Cör A, Jeras M et al. *Histological analysis of intervertebral disc regeneration using cultured autologous and allogenic elastic cartilage derived from chondrocytes as implants.* Presented to the annual meeting of the International Cartilage Repair Society, Toronto, Quebec, Canada, 2002.
28. Kaapa E, Gronblad M, Holm S, et al. Neural elements in the normal and experimentally injured porcine intervertebral disk. *Eur Spine J* 1994;3:137–142.
29. Kaapa E, Han X, Holm S, et al. Collagen synthesis and types I, III, IV, and VI collagens in an animal model of disc degeneration. *Spine* 1995;20:59–66.
30. Kaapa E, Holm S, Han X, et al. Collagens in the injured porcine intervertebral disc. *J Orthop Res* 1994;12:93–102.
31. Karppinen J, Inkinen RI, Kaapa E, et al. Effects of tiaprofenic acid and indomethacin on proteoglycans in the degenerating porcine intervertebral disc. *Spine* 1995;15:1170–1177.
32. Katsuura A, Hukuda S. Experimental study of intervertebral disc allografting in the dog. *Spine* 1994;19:2426–2432.
33. Key JA, Ford LT. Experimental intervertebral-disc lesions. *J Bone Joint Surg Am* 1948;30:621–629.
34. Kostuik JP. Intervertebral disc replacement. Experimental study. *Clin Orthop* 1997;337:27–41.
35. Kotani Y, Abumi K, Shikinami Y, et al. Artificial intervertebral disc replacement using bioactive three-dimensional fabric. Design, development, and preliminary animal study. *Spine* 2002;27:929–936.
36. Kramer PA, Newell-Morris LL, Simkin PA. Spinal degenerative disk disease (DDD) in female macaque monkeys: epidemiology and comparison with women. *J Orthop Res* 2002;20:399–408.
37. Lipson S, Muir H. Proteoglycans in experimental disc degeneration. *Spine* 1981;6:194–210.
38. Lipson S, Muir H. Experimental intervertebral disc degeneration: morphologic and proteoglycan changes over time. *Arthritis Rheum* 1981;24:12–21.
39. Lob A. Die zusammenhange zwischen den verletzungen der bandscheiben und der spondylosis deformans in tierversuch. *Dtsch Z Chir* 1933;240:421–440.
40. Maetzel A, Li L. The economic burden of low back pain: a review of studies published between 1996 and 2001. *Best Prac Res Clin Rheumatol* 2002;16:23–30.
41. McAfee PC, Cunningham BW, Sefter JC, et al. *General principles of porous ingrowth total disc replacement arthroplasty: a nonhuman primate model.* Presented at the annual meeting of the International Society for the Study of the Lumbar Spine, Cleveland, OH, 2002.
42. Melrose J, Ghosh P, Taylor TKF, et al. A longitudinal study of the matrix changes induced in the intervertebral disc by surgical damage to the annulus fibrosus. *J Orthop Res* 1992;10:665–676.
43. Moore RJ, Fraser RD, Vernon-Roberts B, et al. The biologic response to particles from a lumbar disc prosthesis. *Spine* 2002;27:2088–2094.
44. Moore RJ, Latham JM, Vernon-Roberts B, et al. Does plate fixation prevent disc degeneration after a lateral annulus tear? *Spine* 1994;19:2787–2790.
45. Moore RJ, Osti OL, Vernon-Roberts B, et al. Changes in endplate vascularity following an outer annular tear. *Spine* 1992;17:874–878.
46. Moore RJ, Taylor DJ, Hutchinson JM, et al. *How can early discitis be detected using MRI?* Presented to the annual meeting of the International Society for the Study of the Lumbar Spine, Adelaide, Australia, 2000.

47. Moskowitz RW, Ziv I, Denko CW, et al. Spondylosis in sand rats: a model of intervertebral disc degeneration and hyperostosis. *J Orthop Res* 1990;8:401–411.
48. Olson EJ, Hanley EN, Rudert MJ et al. Vertebral column allografts for the treatment of segmental spinal defects. An experimental investigation in dogs. *Spine* 1991;16:1081–1088.
49. Osti OL, Vernon-Roberts B, Fraser RD. Annulus tears and intervertebral disc degeneration. An experimental study using an animal model. *Spine* 1990;15:762–767.
50. Penta M. *Allograft intervertebral disc transplantation in the sheep* [Thesis]. Adelaide, Australia: University of Adelaide, 1995.
51. Pintar FA, Maiman DJ, Hollowell JP, et al. Fusion rate and biomechanical stiffness of hydroxylapatite versus autogenous bone grafts for anterior discectomy. An in vivo animal study. *Spine* 1994;19:2524–2528.
52. Saal JA, Saal JS. Intradiscal electrothermal therapy for the treatment of chronic discogenic low back pain. *Operative Techniques Orthop* 2000;10:271–281.
53. Sandhu HS, Khan SN. Animal models for preclinical assessment of bone morphogenetic proteins in the spine. *Spine* 2002;27:532–538.
54. Schimandle JH, Boden SD. The use of animal models to study spinal fusion. *Spine* 1994;19:1998–2006.
55. Schmorl G, Junghanns H. *The human spine in health and disease*, 2nd American ed. Besemann EF, trans. New York: Grune & Stratton, 1971.
56. Silberberg R. Histologic and morphometric observations on vertebral bone of aging sand rats. *Spine* 1988;13:202–208.
57. Silberberg R, Adler JH. Comparison of truncal and caudal lesions in the vertebral column of the sand rat (*Psammomys obesus*). *Isr J Med Sci* 1983;19:1064–1071.
58. Silberberg R, Aufdermaur M, Adler JH. Degeneration of the intervertebral disks and spondylosis in aging sand rats. *Arch Pathol Lab Med* 1979;103:231–235.
59. Silberberg R, Meier-Ruge W, Odermatt B. Age-related changes in fibronectin in annulus fibrosus of the sand rat (*Psammomys obesus*). *Exp Cell Biol* 1989;57:233–237.
60. Smit TH. The use of a quadruped as an in vivo model for the study of the spine—biomechanical considerations. *Eur Spine J* 2002;11:137–144.
61. Smith JW, Walmsley R. Experimental incision of the intervertebral disc. *J Bone Joint Surg Br* 1951;33:512–525.
62. Suh DY, Boden SD, Louis Ugbo J, et al. Delivery of recombinant human bone morphogenetic protein-2 using a compression-resistant matrix in posterolateral spine fusion in the rabbit and in the non-human primate. *Spine* 2002;27:353–360.
63. Szpalski M, Gunzburg R, Mayer M. Spine arthroplasty: a historical review. *Eur Spine J* 2002;11[Suppl.2]:S65–S84.
64. Takae R, Matsunaga S, Origuchi N, et al. Immunolocalization of bone morphogenetic protein and its receptors in degeneration of intervertebral disc. *Spine* 1999;24:1397–1401.
65. Toth JM. Point of view. *Spine* 2002;27:935–936.
66. Urbaniak JR, Bright DS, Hopkins JE. Replacement of intervertebral discs in chimpanzees by silicon-Dacron implants: a preliminary report. *J Biomed Mater Res* 1973;7:165–186.
67. Vernon-Roberts B. Age-related and degenerative pathology of intervertebral discs and apophyseal joints. In: Jayson MIV, ed. *The lumbar spine and back pain*, 4th ed. Edinburgh: Churchill Livingstone, 1992:17–41.
68. Vernon-Roberts B, Pirie CJ. Degenerative changes in the intervertebral discs of the lumbar spine and their sequelae. *Rheum Rehabil* 1977;16:13–21.
69. Wilke HJ, Kettler A, Claes L. Are sheep spines a valid model for human spines? *Spine* 1997;22:2365–2374.
70. Wilke HJ, Kettler A, Wenger KH, et al. Anatomy of the sheep spine and its comparison to the human spine. *Anat Rec* 1997;247:542–555.
71. Wilke HJ, Krischak S, Claes L. Biomechanical comparison of calf and human spines. *J Orthop Res* 1996;14:500–503.
72. Zdeblick TA, Cooke ME, Wilson D, et al. Anterior cervical discectomy, fusion, and plating. A comparative animal study. *Spine* 1993;18:1974–1983.
73. Ziv I, Moskowitz RW, Kraise I, et al. Physicochemical properties of the aging and diabetic sand rat intervertebral disc. *J Orthop Res* 1992;10:205–210.

33

Epidemiology, Outcome, and Costs of Surgery for Lumbar Disc Herniation

Marc G. Du Bois and Peter Donceel

Department of Occupational and Insurance Medicine, School of Public Health, Catholic University of Leuven, Leuven, Belgium

The epidemiologic and economic impact of low back pain (LBP) and herniated discs in industrialized countries is enormous. LBP affects up to 80% of adults at some point during their lifetime. Of these, about 1% become totally disabled, the LBP becomes chronic in 10%, and the rest recover uneventfully, with 80% returning to work in 8 to 10 weeks. In the Netherlands, approximately 7.5% of the population have either chronic spinal disorders lasting longer than 3 months or a herniated disc at some point. In the United States in 1989, the rate of disability exceeded the rate of population growth by a factor of 14, and the estimated total workers' compensation cost for LBP was $11.4 billion (1,8,10).

In approximately 2% of cases, LBP results from the acute herniation of an intervertebral disc. Herniated nucleus pulposus is one of the indications most frequently leading to temporary absence from work. Furthermore, herniated discs are one of the most frequent causes of entitlement to disability benefits.

In some patients with a herniated disc, symptoms persist despite conservative treatment. They may become candidates for surgery. Outcome studies of lumbar disc surgery have documented success rates between 23% and 95%. Rates of return to work vary between 50% and 90% (5). It is generally assumed that reported outcomes in patients undergoing surgical procedures for lumbar disc herniation are poorer those receiving workers' compensation. The present study has been performed to investigate the situation in the Belgian population.

In Belgium, as in other Western countries, awareness of the social and economic burden that common and chronic diseases impose on society is increasing. Providers, payers, and regulatory authorities are focusing on advancing the quality of care within restricted budgets by emphasizing patient outcomes and evaluating physicians' practices. In this sense, lumbar disc herniation is a case in point in an increasingly restricted health care environment.

The present study was carried out to determine the rates of surgery for lumbar disc herniation in Belgium. A second objective was to describe the surgical results and predictors of outcomes in terms of hospital stay, return to work, and use of medication. A third objective was to analyze the social security costs related to surgery for lumbar disc herniation.

MATERIALS AND METHODS

The study was a retrospective cohort design. Records from the National Sickness and Invalidity Authority were used to calculate trends in the rates of surgery for lumbar disc herniation from 1989 to 2001. Surgical rates were calculated by dividing the number of treated patients by the year-specific total Belgian population. Rates were not adjusted for demographic parameters.

All medical and compensation payments in addition to patients' medical files from the Christian Sickness Fund were reviewed to delineate the outcome of surgery. The Christian Sickness Fund is the largest sickness fund in Belgium, covering approximately 45% of the mandatory insured population. Between January 1999 and January 2000, 1,431 enrollees in the Christian Sickness Fund underwent surgery for lumbar disc herniation. Of these, 8% underwent combined discectomy and fusion.

We recorded the following variables for each patient: age, gender, type of surgery, occupation, period of work incapacity before surgery, length of hospital stay, use of medication, and period of work incapacity after surgery. Patients were evaluated by medical advisers of the Christian Sickness Fund. Their judgment of fitness for work is based on the patient's last job during the first 6 months of work incapacity. After 6 months of incapacity, the evaluation considers all occupations in which the patient may have engaged according to professional career and education.

To assess the outcome of treatment, patients were classified into two outcome categories. A bad outcome was defined as the inability resume work 1 year after surgery. Outcome was also measured in terms of the use of opioids 3 months before and 3 months after surgery. Hospital stay was used as a parameter to measure the process of surgery for disc herniation.

The cost assessment phase of the study determined the social security cost in the first year after surgery. Costs were calculated based on the official fees applicable in 1999. Costs attributable to lost productivity were not taken into account. The study more specifically compared the social security expenses of standard surgery with those of combined discectomy and fusion. During a review of the Christian Sickness Fund financial data, the medical costs of patients undergoing surgical treatment were broken down into hospital costs, surgeon's fees, and costs of anesthesia, radiology, office visits, and follow-up rehabilitation. The expenses were converted into 2001 euros.

STATISTICAL ANALYSIS

Microsoft Excel 97-SR2 and SPSS 10.0 for Windows were used to perform statistical analysis. Multiple factors were evaluated in a single variable model for their relationship to fitness for work after surgery. Potentially significant factors were then entered into a multivariate logistic regression model. The odds ratio was calculated for significant outcome predictors. The level used to determine statistical significance was a P value of less than 0.05.

RESULTS

Trends in Surgery Rates

Figure 33.1 shows the trend in surgery rates from 1989 to 2001. The rate of combined discectomy and fusion more than doubled during the 13-year period. The last 3 years saw a substantial decline in standard surgery in favor of combined discectomy and fusion. The

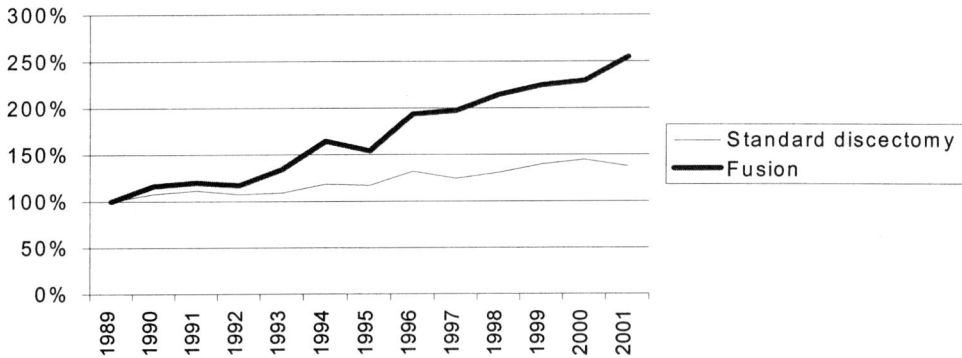

FIG. 33.1. Evolution of rates of surgery for lumbar disc herniation in Belgium (1989 = 100%).

annual rate for standard discectomy was 94 interventions per 100,000 enrollees. For combined discectomy and fusion, we found an annual rate of 12 operations per 100,000 enrollees.

Hospital Stay

The median duration of the hospital stay after standard surgery was 8 days. For combined discectomy and fusion, we found a median hospital stay of 13 days. The hospital stay varied greatly within the major Belgian hospitals. The duration of hospitalization ranged from 4 to 12 days for standard surgery and from 8 to 18 days for combined discectomy and fusion.

Fitness for Work

A total of 1,431 patients were treated for lumbar disc herniation. Of these, 65% were men and 35% were women (Table 33.1). The average age of the entire population was 41 years. The median duration of work incapacity before surgery for lumbar disc herniation was 6 months.

Combined discectomy and fusion were performed in 8% of the patients. Combined discectomy and fusion resulted in a worse outcome than standard discectomy. Of the patients who underwent combined discectomy and fusion, 20.2% were classified as hav-

TABLE 33.1. *Patient data*

Gender	
Male	65%
Female	35%
Occupation	
Self-employed	6%
Blue collar worker	60%
White collar worker	34%
Surgery	
Standard surgery	91%
Discectomy and fusion	8%
Age, mean	41 y
Duration of work incapacity before surgery, mean	6 mo

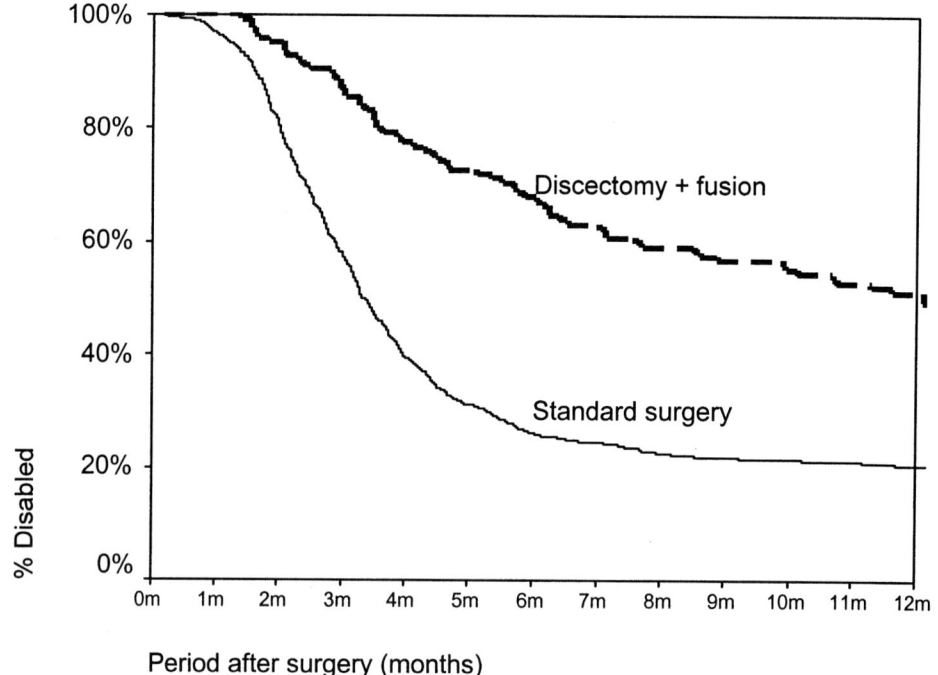

FIG. 33.2. Incapacity for work after surgery for lumbar disc herniation (n = 1,431).

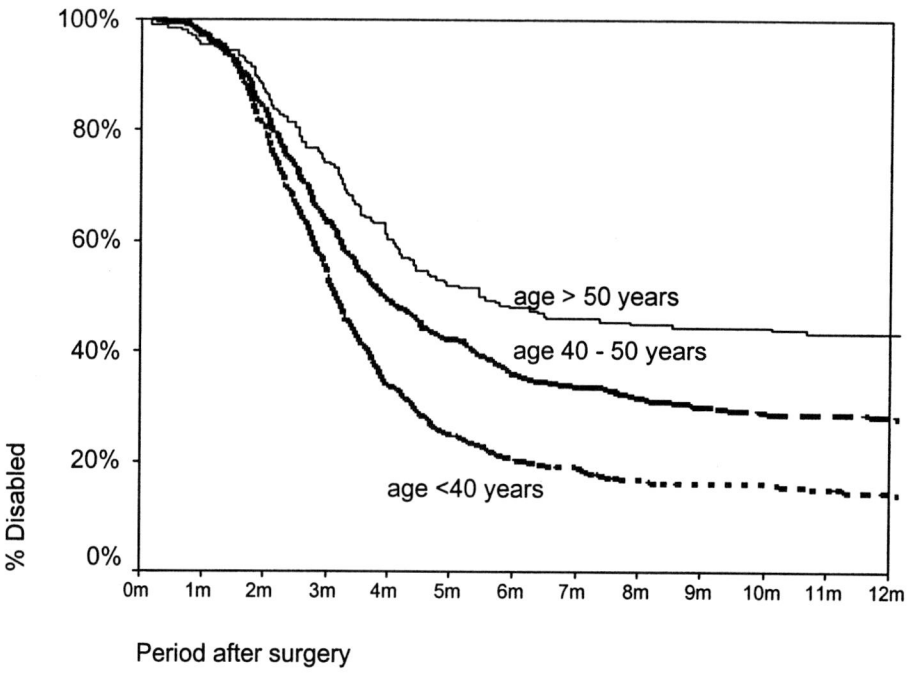

FIG. 33.3. Incapacity for work after surgery for lumbar disc herniation. Outflow curves for subgroups in different age categories (older than 50 years, 40 to 50 years, and younger than 40 years of age).

TABLE 33.2. *Summary results of the studied variables in a logistic regression model*

	Variables in the equation					
	B	SE	Wald	df	Sig	Exp(B)
[a]Work incapacity			290.076	2	0.000	
Work incapacity 0–1 mo	0.522	0.212	6.049	1	0.014	1.686
Work incapacity >3 mo	−2.572	0.212	147.629	1	0.000	0.076
Age			51.035	2	0.000	
Age 40–50 y	−1.595	0.230	48.086	1	0.000	0.203
Age >50 y	−0.790	0.179	19.494	1	0.000	0.454
Woman	0.792	0.178	19.757	1	0.000	2.208
Occupation			12.515	2	0.002	
Blue collar	0.761	0.318	5.741	1	0.017	2.141
White collar	1.178	0.343	11.797	1	0.001	3.248
Standard surgery	1.380	0.245	31.711	1	0.000	3.974
Constant	−0.152	0.423	0.129	1	0.720	0.859

[a]B, parameter estimate; SE, standard error of the parameter estimate; Wald, Wald statistic; df, degree of freedom; Sig, significance level for the Wald statistic; Exp(B), factor by which the odds change when the independent variable increases by one unit.

ing a poor result because they were not able to resume work 1 year after surgery. For combined discectomy and fusion, we found a poor outcome in 55.4% of the cases (Fig. 33.2).

The duration of work incapacity before surgery was significantly associated with return to work. Of the patients whose work incapacity had lasted longer than 3 months before surgery, 70% were unable to resume work 1 year after surgery.

The relationship between age and the disability rate is shown in Figure 33.3. The rates of disability were highest in the oldest patients. Conversely, the rates of disability after surgery were lowest in the patients younger than 40 years. Significantly more of the patients who were not able to resume work within 1 year after surgery were blue collar workers.

The final regression model showed that a short period of work incapacity before surgery, younger age, male gender, white collar work status, and standard surgery were significant predictors of the likelihood of fitness for work 1 year after surgery (Table 33.2).

Use of Narcotics

A reduction in the use of narcotic pain medication after surgery was considered an indirect parameter of postoperative pain relief. Before standard surgery, 236 (59%) of the patients were using opioids. Three months after standard surgery, 104 (26%) were still using narcotic pain medication. This finding demonstrates that standard surgery significantly affected the preoperative pain level.

Social Security Costs

Table 33.3 shows the direct social security costs associated with surgery for lumbar disc herniation. The cost of standard lumbar disc surgery, including hospitalization and the cost of the procedure itself, was found to be approximately 3,487 euros. However, significant differences in cost were found between standard lumbar discectomy and combined discectomy and fusion. The direct postoperative cost of combined discectomy and fusion, including the cost of follow-up physician visits and physiotherapy, was 7,762 euros.

TABLE 33.3. *Mean social security expenditures during a one-year period after surgery for lumbar disc herniation*

	Office visits (euros)	Orthopedics (euros)	Radiology (euros)	In-hospital nursing (euros)
Standard	166	399	207	1,497
Fusion	212	734	334	2,454

DISCUSSION

This study was retrospective and based on the administrative files of patients' records from the largest sickness fund in Belgium. Important limitations of the present study include a lack of information on individual patients regarding preoperative and postoperative clinical manifestations, imaging study findings, and specific complaints. The advantages of analyzing the record files of an active population in Belgium include a uniform method for determining disability compensation, 100% postoperative follow-up, independent third-party evaluation, and a uniform reimbursement schedule based on the National Sickness and Invalidity Authority.

We noted an increasing rate of surgery for lumbar disc hernia. In particular, procedures combining discectomy and fusion are on the rise. In Belgium, the annual rate was 12 operations per 100,000 enrollees. Traditionally, spinal fusion surgery has been the treatment of choice for persons who have not obtained relief of chronic back pain through conservative treatment. Lumbar discectomy is one of the surgical procedures most commonly performed in the United States, where in 1992, the rate of lumbar spinal fusion operations for degenerative spine conditions was estimated to be 30.9 per 100,000. The rate is substantially higher today. The growing trend in spinal surgery mirrors the excellent results already obtained in addition to further developments in spinal technology (4,8).

An objective analysis of the outcome in patients undergoing lumbar disc surgery is difficult because most of the criteria used in the evaluation are based on problems of LBP, persistent radicular symptoms, limitations in physical activity, and lack of a feeling of well-being. The objective of lumbar disc surgery is to relieve pain and restore the patient to normal life. We attempted to measure the experience of pain according to the use of opioids before and after surgery and concluded that standard surgery relieves pain.

However, pain is subjective and difficult to assess quantitatively. In our study, outcome was therefore mainly measured in terms of fitness for work. Outcome was assessed by a medical adviser. This may be an advantage because patients tend to report better results to the surgeon or the surgeon's representatives than to a third party. Additionally, the evaluation of disability was uniform because it was based on the same compensation law. Medical advisers are physicians employed by sickness funds. Their main task is to evaluate work incapacity. Objectively, the criterion for fitness for work is that patients must be able to perform the duties of their previous job or employment according to their level of education. When patients are judged unable to resume work, they are entitled to a monthly income. Additionally, if they cannot work for 1 year or longer, they are entitled to less expensive medical care.

Our results showed that 20% of all patients were still unable to resume work 1 year after standard surgery. For combined discectomy and fusion, this percentage increased to 55%. In a retrospective study, Saal (12) found that 90% of patients who underwent surgery for herniated disc associated with sciatica reported a satisfactory outcome; their rate of return to work was 92% at an average follow-up of 31 months. In the international literature, rates of return to work vary from 50% to 90%. Variations in surgical results relate more to selection factors than to either the quality of surgery or specific measures of outcome.

Our current finding is in agreement with the assumption that reported outcomes in patients undergoing surgical procedures for lumbar disc herniation are poorer in those receiving compensation or involved in litigation. A thorough assessment of the role of the social security system is difficult because of differences in disability benefits and legislation (7,21).

Whether to perform fusion in association with disc excision remains controversial. Several investigators have compared the results of disc excision alone with those of disc excision plus fusion. Some authors, such as Vaughan et al. (18), have reported that performing lumbar fusion at the time of disc excision yields better results. In contrast, White et al. (20) and others (15,17) have reported that fusion is rarely indicated because equally satisfactory results can be obtained by disc excision alone.

We found female gender and older age to be associated with a poor outcome. Both female gender and lower income have been associated with a poor outcome in other studies. In the studies of Junge et al. (6) and Rasmussen (11), a poor outcome of lumbar disc surgery was associated with lower levels of education and income, among other factors.

Blue collar employment was significantly associated with a smaller chance of return to work. This finding may be a function of the more strenuous physical tasks required of blue collar workers. The difference may also be related to differences in job satisfaction and career commitment. Davis (5) and Schade et al. (13) found that manual laborers reported persistent or recurrent pain more often than persons performing more sedentary tasks (5,13).

When the data were subjected to multivariable analysis, the duration of work incapacity before surgery was the most important significant factor associated with fitness for work. This variable can be viewed as a feasible approach for predicting patients' fitness for work after lumbar discectomy or combined discectomy and fusion.

Our study indicates that patients who are being considered for lumbar disc surgery should be screened for long periods of work incapacity before surgery. Surgeons must consider preoperatively any psychologic factors that may be affected by a period of work incapacity before surgery. It is becoming increasingly evident that a poor outcome of lumbar disc surgery is most often a consequence of poor selection for surgery. Physicians agree that almost all patients with LBP and sciatica caused by a herniated disc require less than 10 to 12 weeks of conservative therapy for recovery. The only absolute indication for surgery for lumbar disc disease is cauda equina syndrome. Lumbar discectomy is justified if a patient has persistent sciatica, neurologic signs or signs of nerve root tension, and imaging study findings that correlate exactly with the clinical findings (2,3,19).

The median duration of the hospital stay after standard surgery was 8 days, and after combined discectomy and fusion, it was 13 days. In the United States, a standard procedure for lumbar disc hernia is followed by a very short inpatient hospital stay of 1 to 3 days. Some authors have questioned whether an inpatient stay is necessary after elective uncomplicated discectomy. Advances in anesthesia and surgical techniques have contributed to an increase in the number of discectomy procedures performed on an outpatient basis.

The average social security cost of combined discectomy and fusion was approximately double that of standard surgery. The difference was largely explained by the cost of implants and in-hospital nursing. In the present study, the greater economic burden of combined discectomy and fusion was evident. Given the substantial economic impact of herniated lumbar discs, the clinical and economic consequences should be taken into consideration by health care policy makers and physicians. Patients with a poor outcome of a first surgical intervention pose a medical challenge to physicians and are an economic concern because they rarely experience complete pain relief and are at high risk for long-term disability

In view of these economic concerns, increasing the success rate of lumbar disc surgery by placing a major emphasis on "careful" patient selection to avoid costly failures should be a primary objective in a responsible health care environment (9,14,16).

REFERENCES

1. Andersson GB, Weinstein JN. Disc herniation. *Spine* 1996;21[24 Suppl]:1S.
2. Andersson GB, Brown MD, Dvorak J, et al. Consensus summary of the diagnosis and treatment of lumbar disc herniation. *Spine* 1996;21[24 Suppl]:75S–78S.
3. Chen TY. The clinical presentation of uppermost cervical disc protrusion. *Spine* 2000;25:439–442.
4. Cherkin DC, Deyo RA, Loeser JD, et al. An international comparison of back surgery rates. *Spine* 1994;19:1201–1206.
5. Davis RA. A long-term outcome analysis of 984 surgically treated herniated lumbar discs. *J Neurosurg* 1994;80:415–421.
6. Junge A, Dvorak J, Ahrens S. Predictors of bad and good outcomes of lumbar disc surgery. A prospective clinical study with recommendations for screening to avoid bad outcomes. *Spine* 1995;20:460–468.
7. Kaptan GJ, Shaffrey CI, Alden TD, et al. Secondary gain influences the outcome of lumbar but not cervical disc surgery. *Spine* 1999;52:217–225.
8. Katz JN. Lumbar spinal fusion. Surgical rates, costs and complications. *Spine* 1995;20[24 Suppl]:78S–83S.
9. Maniadakis N, Gray A. Heath economics and orthopaedics. *J Bone Joint Surg Br* 2000;82:2–7.
10. McCulloch JA. Focus issue on lumbar disc herniation: macro- and microdiscectomy. *Spine* 1996;21[24 Suppl]:45S–56S.
11. Rasmussen C. Lumbar disc herniation: social and demographic factors determining duration of disease. *Eur Spine J* 1996;5:225–228.
12. Saal AJ. Natural history and nonoperative treatment of lumbar disc herniation. *Spine* 1996;21[24 Suppl]:2S–9S.
13. Schade V, Semmer N, Main CJ, et al. The impact of clinical, morphological, psychosocial and work-related factors on the outcome of lumbar discectomy. *Pain* 1999;80:239–249.
14. Schwicker D. Cost effectiveness of lumbar disc surgery and of a preventive treatment for peridural fibrosis. *Eur Spine J* 1996;5[Suppl 1]:S21–S25.
15. Sonntag VKH, Klara P. Controversy in spine care. Is fusion necessary after anterior cervical discectomy? *Spine* 1996;21:1111–1113.
16. Stevenson RC, McCabe CJ, Findlay AM. An economic evaluation of a clinical trial to compare automated percutaneous lumbar discectomy with microdiscectomy in the treatment of contained lumbar disc herniation. *Spine* 1995;20:739–742.
17. Takeshima T, Kambara K, Miyata S et al. Clinical and radiographic evaluation of disc excision for lumbar disc herniation with and without posterolateral fusion. *Spine* 2000;25:450–456.
18. Vaughan PA, Malcolm BW, Maistrelli GL. Results of L4-L5 disc excision alone versus disc excision and fusion. *Spine* 1988;13:690–695.
19. Vucetic N, Astrand P, Güntner P. Diagnosis and prognosis in lumbar disc herniation. *Clin Orthop* 1999;361:116–122.
20. White AH, Von Rogov P, Zucherman J, et al. Lumbar laminectomy for herniated disc: a prospective controlled comparison with internal fixation fusion. *Spine* 1987;12:305–307.
21. Young JN, Shaffrey CI, Laws ER. Lumbar disc surgery in a fixed compensation population: a model for influence of secondary gain on surgical outcome. *Surg Neurol* 1997;48:552–559.

34

Clinical Outcome, Measurements, and Languages: Some Cultural Aspects

Margareta Nordin

Departments of Orthopedic and Environmental Medicine, School of Medicine, New York University; and Occupational and Industrial Orthopedic Center, Hospital for Joint Diseases, New York, New York

Society is changing as the multicultural population increases. In the United States, estimates based on the 2000 census reveal continuous changes in the composition of the U.S. population (15). The Hispanic population between 1990 and 2000 grew 58% according to census data for these 10 years. Hispanics and African-American are now the largest minority groups in the United States. In California, for example, non-Hispanic whites are now a minority. In California and Florida, according to the 2000 census, Hispanics outnumber African-Americans.

The census also revealed a problem of identifying individuals as belonging to a certain group. Given the option to identify their ethnic background, 2.4% of the U.S. population, or nearly 7 million persons, categorized themselves as multiethnic.

Because of differences in beliefs about health and acceptance of care, changes in the composition of a population make it more challenging for a health care system to manage care effectively. The design and effective delivery of interventions for alleviating pain and other treatments to culturally diverse patients can be a complicated task for the health care system (10). In the United States, the newest immigrants come from increasingly untraditional regions, such as Southeast Asia and Latin America. Lasch (10) describes the current group as more heterogeneous than their predecessors at the time of World War I and World War II and in 1980, the most recent periods of peak immigration. Our new immigrants often do not speak English and frequently face numerous social, economic, and health problems. Substantial proportions of persons are former refugees with experiences of resettlement camps and war (6). Similar situations are found in Europe and elsewhere in the world. It is beyond the intent of this chapter to describe the problems of other nations; however, population changes are a common contemporary phenomenon and do not belong only to the past. The change in the composition of the U.S. population is presented as an example to increase awareness of this problem. The delivery of care to culturally specific populations places specific demands on health care providers. This chapter focuses on some of the cultural aspects and outcome.

DEFINITION OF THE CONCEPT OF CULTURE IN THIS TEXT

The term *culture* is derived from a Latin word meaning development, improvement, or refinement of the mind, emotions, interests, manners, and taste, or of the ideas, customs, skills, and arts of a given people in a given period. Culture also represents a civilization (17). Culture has been defined in many different ways and by many authors, and its meaning has enlarged with time. Culture refers to the behavioral norms, attitudes, and meaning systems of a group of people (10). Communities, neighborhoods, patient advocacy groups, immigrants, religious groups, and others can all represent a specific culture. In this chapter, culture relates to health beliefs, which usually comprise an individual's beliefs about sickness, the behavior related to sickness, the perception of disability, and expectation of treatment. Culture in this context also refers to the delivery of health care and includes the responses of the individual's family, health care providers, and work environment.

Several authors have studied the influence of culture on illness, health beliefs and behaviors, care-seeking activities, care delivery and practice, and receptivity to medical interventions (5,7,9,13). Lasch (10) states, "Western trained clinicians will view the medical care system as technologically sophisticated and helpful in the curing process; patients may fear hospitals as a place to die and may distrust a simple routine blood test because of their beliefs about blood and the wholeness of the body." Western medicine has been concerned mostly with the biomedical aspects of illness and injury. However, patients acquire their own idiosyncratic lay theories of illness and causation. This is a complex process that the caregiver cannot always understand, and it may result in poor adherence to treatment or just a change of health care provider until the patient finds a provider who shares similar theories. It may very well also be that in a given culture, a specific disease carries a totally different weight, even a stigma.

Schweder (11) emphasizes the importance of extending the distinction between illness—what the patient experiences—and disease—what the health care provider diagnoses.

Cultural aspects have influenced the experience of back pain throughout history. In a brief section on history, Waddell (16) cites Paracelsus (1493–1541) as one of the first leaders of modern medicine. Paracelsus promoted "clinical freedom by treating each patient on the basis of his own observation and diagnosis." These observations today on the part of a health care provider can include a clinical evaluation, diagnostics, and usually a psychosocial evaluation for persistent low back pain. For patients with pain in the spine, the psychosocial intervention has been shown to be particularly important because cultural aspects and expectations are included. Gaps, even major gaps, are still found in the explanatory models of spine pain that health care providers offer to patients. For example, nonspecific low back pain is often explained as strain or sprain of a structure in the spine, which may be an unacceptable explanation for a patient who cannot recall a strenuous event.

The view of Helman (7) of the divergence of the explanatory model between patients and health care providers is compelling. He argues that the way that lay and medical explanatory models interact in clinical situations is influenced not only by the physical context in which they occur, such as hospitals, clinics, or centers, but also by the social class and gender of the two parties involved. The power invested in clinicians by virtue of their background, training, and experience may allow them to mold the patient's explanatory model to make the patient "fit" into the medical model of disease, rather than allow the patient's own perspective of the illness to emerge and be discussed.

Remolding or reshaping the patient's model does not facilitate communication; in brief, the patient does not recognize or accept the explanation given by the clinician. Should patient and clinician belong to two wholly different cultural groups, then conflict between them may be unavoidable if the cultural differences are not acknowledged. Remolding a health belief takes time and may or may not be successful (4). The reason for accepting a treatment from a patient's point of view is still little explored in nonfatal diseases.

TABLE 34.1. *Questions suggested by Helman to elicit patient's health beliefs and explanatory model*

1. What has happened?
2. Why has it happened?
3. Why has it happened to me?
4. Why now?
5. What will happen to me if nothing is done about it?
6. What are the likely effects on other people (family, friends, employers, workmates) if nothing is done about it?
7. What should I do about it—or to whom should I turn for further help?

From Helman CG. *Culture, health and illness.* London: Butterworth-Heinemann, 1993:95–105, with permission.

CROSS-CULTURAL ASSESSMENT

Diversity is found both within and between cultures. The importance here is not to make stereotyped judgments in a world that is continually becoming more multicultural and ethnically diverse. Two tools are described to ascertain a patient's health belief, one generic and one for chronic pain. Helman (7) suggests seven questions that the clinician can ask about an illness to elicit the patient's health belief and own explanatory model (Table 34.1). Lasch (10) has proposed a tool to elicit a patient's health belief about chronic pain (Table 34.2). Tables 34.1 and 34.2 can be used as guides to understand the explanatory model of a patient from a population with a different culture. These guides may also be helpful to the clinician in selecting an acceptable treatment for such a patient.

Standardized measures of patient outcomes are being used increasingly in clinical daily practice. If we assume that language is one expression of culture, then cross-cultural issues must be addressed in health outcome measures (3,8). Health outcome measures can be helpful in clinical practice to identify the perception of well-being or disability in a patient. They are essential to evaluate the outcome of a proposed treatment, in addition to adherence to and acceptance of a treatment. Outcome measures are also highly relevant as health care and research issues become globalized. The exclusion of certain population groups because of cultural or language differences may lead to a systematic bias (8).

TABLE 34.2. *A tool to elicit health beliefs about chronic pain*

1. What words would you use to describe your pain?
2. Where do you think this pain comes from?
3a. Why do you think it happened when it did?
   3b. Why do you think it lasted this long?
4a Do you think this pain will go away?
   4b. If it goes away, what will make it happen?
5. What are the main problems your pain causes for you?
6a. Have you gone to a healer for this pain?
   6b. With what remedies did they try to help you?
   6c. Are you still using what they recommended?
   6d. Do you still see them?
7a. Who, if anyone, in your family or circle of friends knows about your pain and its treatment?
   7b. What do they know?
   7c. What do you want them to know?
8a. How do your family and friends react to your pain?
   8b. What do they think about it?

Adapted from Lasch KE. Sociocultural considerations in pain and its management. In: Wittink H, Hosbins Michel T, eds. *Chronic pain management for physical therapists,* 2nd ed. Boston: Butterworth-Heinemann, Elsevier Science, 2002:23–36, with permission.

DEVELOPMENT OF A PATIENT SELF-ADMINISTERED OUTCOME MEASURE

Different approaches are used to develop outcome measures in cross-cultural settings. It is beyond the aim of this chapter to describe these approaches. However, a short description of some methodologic difficulties will be described.

Methodologic Problems

Methodologic problems affecting cross-cultural outcome measures can be divided into *technical*, *conceptual*, and *linguistic* problems (8).

Technical Problems

An example of a technical problem is illiteracy. Asking a patient to use a self-administered instrument assumes a satisfactory level of literacy and familiarity with the method of data collection. Many populations still retain a high level of illiteracy, particularly among the elderly and certain ethnic minorities. In this case, the use of a trained interviewer is necessary and may introduce a new set of problems.

Conceptual Problems

An example of a conceptual problem is the description of health. West Indians of African descent consider health to mean being strong and fit, whereas Asians see it as one's ability to perform everyday activities. Health beliefs differ extensively between populations and groups. The experience of an illness is a cultural phenomenon reflecting beliefs about etiology, illness behavior, and assigned role in addition to type of treatment and social system. Showing emotional distress, anxiety, or depression is discouraged in certain cultures, whereas in others, it is normal to meet with a psychologist to solve weekly problems.

Cultural differences must be taken into account before an existing instrument is adapted or a new one is developed. If these have not been satisfactorily considered, an instrument should be used with great caution.

Linguistic Problems

A linguistic problem can be illustrated by a question about depression (8). An English health care provider may ask a patient, "Last week, were you depressed?" The same question in an African language may be phrased as, "Recently, have you felt like a branch hanging from a tree?" An item in an instrument can be translated from one language to another semantically; however, the translation may still have a different meaning in the target language. The item in one culture will not represent the same thing in another culture.

CROSS-CULTURAL EQUIVALENCE

Five areas have been cited for judging the criteria for cross-cultural equivalence in the development of an instrument (3,8): *content* equivalence (e.g., regarding different social or leisure activities in different cultures); *semantic* equivalence (e.g., more important to translate the meaning than to provide a direct literal translation); *conceptual* equivalence (e.g., the concepts of social support and family may have very different meanings in different languages); *technical* equivalence (e.g., self-administered data collection versus structured interview); and *criterion* equivalence (e.g., reliability and validity in cross-cultural settings).

Examples of Cross-Cultural Studies and Back Pain

Skovron et al. (12) studied the prevalence of back pain among speakers (n = 2,660) of Flemish and French in Belgium, a bicultural and economically diverse society with a national security system and single payer health care reimbursement. In multivariate analyses controlling for social class, rural or urban location, and occupation and work status, they found that increasing age, female gender, and speaking the French language were associated with reporting a history of back pain (i.e., ever having had back pain). Speaking the French language and female gender predicted a first episode of back pain, language being the strongest predictor. When daily back pain was explored, the factors that emerged as predictors, other than age and gender, were social class, living in a large city, and being an unskilled worker. These predictors are largely social but could also be cultural if immigrant groups did most of the unskilled work. The study does not discuss this point of view. Thus, in this study, it appears that cultural factors may influence rates of reporting a first episode of back pain; however, persistent pain appears to be unrelated to culture.

Szpalski et al. (14), in the same sample, studied health care use among speakers of Flemish and French. All forms of health care use examined were associated with health beliefs in both language groups. Reference categories for the multivariate analysis were gender, age, language, habitat, social class, working status, good health, and lifelong problems. Language was not associated with any current health care behavior, such as bed rest, use of medication, surgery, or a history of radiographic studies. These results indicate that the cultural differences here expressed as language may not be carried over into health care behaviors in a system where universal access to health services is available, as in Belgium. Health beliefs in both language groups were important determinants of health care behavior. The belief that low back pain would be a lifelong problem was associated with an increased likelihood of seeing a health care provider, resting in bed, taking medication, undergoing surgery, or having a history of radiographic studies. When these results were controlled for frequency of low back pain and other covariant factors, the adjusted odds ratios remained increased from OR 2.86 to OR 1.96.

A well-controlled study by Bates et al. (2) from a single multidisciplinary center for pain management reported variability in pain reporting among "old Americans, at least third-generation U.S.–born non-Hispanic whites," and Hispanic, Irish, Italian, French Canadian, and Polish subjects. Most of the subjects experienced chronic low back pain, and no significant differences in diagnosis or mean number and types of medication were found between the ethnic groups. Hispanics reported the highest levels of pain, measured by the Total Pain Rating Index from the McGill Pain Questionnaire. In multiple regression analysis, both ethnic identity and perceived "locus of control" were significantly associated with perception of pain after the data were controlled for age. Variation within ethnic groups was also found to be related in a complex way to the degree to which individuals identified with their ethnic group. This study showed that differences attributed to ethnicity should be interpreted cautiously because variations exist within the "cultural group"; furthermore, the Hispanic group in this study had a significantly lower level of education.

A few well-designed cross-cultural studies related to diseases and disorders of the spine have been performed. Culture and expression of pain or specific diseases have been studied extensively, but not nearly enough studies are related to the spine and its ailments.

WORKING CROSS-CULTURALLY AND CULTURAL SENSITIVITY

Working cross-culturally and being culturally sensitive may require a change of health care practice and a willingness to change. Communication and access to care issues may prevent patients from diverse cultures and especially from minority cultures from receiving appropriate preventive and curative care. It is helpful to develop standardized clinical approaches and outcome measures in different languages, and training clinical staff members in cultural sensitivity and cultural competence is becoming more important as contact among cultures increases. Interest in cross-cultural health care is emerging. For example, the American Medical Association has provided a *Cultural Competence Compendium*, which focuses on the ability to provide culturally competent care to patients (1).

In 2000–2001, the World Health Organization (18) stated in its budget plan that "cultural insensitivity and the proliferation of myths on certain health-related matters have hampered the flow of health information" and further that "in disseminating information, cultural sensitivity is important to ensure that health messages sent to countries are acceptable and effective."

CONCLUSIONS

Working cross-culturally is enormously rewarding; however, it is also difficult and energy-consuming because it requires engaging in mutuality and seeking unconventional solutions and acceptance by the patient. Unsuccessful adherence to a treatment may stem from a different or opposite culture and beliefs regarding health and illness and the practice of care. Such differences remaining between the health care seeker and health care provider may determine the success or failure of a suggested treatment.

REFERENCES

1. American Medical Association. *Cultural competence compendium*. Chicago: American Medical Association, 1999. www.ama-assn.org.
2. Bates MS, Edwards WT, Anderson KO. Ethnocultural influences on variation in chronic pain perception. *Pain* 1993;52:101–112.
3. Beaton DE, Bombardier C, Guillemin F, et al. Guidelines for the process of cross-cultural adaptation of self-report measures. *Spine* 2000;25:3186–3191.
4. Cedraschi C, Robert J, Perrin E. The role of congruence between patient and therapist in chronic low back pain patients. *J Manipulative Physiol Ther* 1996;19:244–249.
5. Dimou N. Illness and culture: learning differences. In: Assal J-P, Visser AP, eds. *New trends in patient education*. Amsterdam: Elsevier Science, 1995:153–157.
6. Espenshade TJ, Fu H. An analysis of English-language proficiency among United States immigrants. *Am Sociol Rev* 1987;68:288–305.
7. Helman CG. *Culture, health and illness*. London: Butterworth-Heinemann, 1993:95–105.
8. Hutchinson A, Bentzen N, Konig-Zahn C. *Cross-cultural health outcome assessment: a user's guide*. European Research Group on Health Outcomes, 1996.
9. Kleineman A. *Patients and healers in the context of culture*. Berkeley, CA: University of California Press, 1980.
10. Lasch KE. Sociocultural considerations in chronic pain and its management. In: Wittink H, Hoskins Michel T, eds. *Chronic pain management for physical therapists*, 2nd ed. Boston: Butterworth-Heinemann, Elsevier Science, 2002:23–36.
11. Schweder R. *Thinking through cultures*. Boston: Harvard University Press, 1986.
12. Skovron ML, Szpalski M, Nordin M, et al. Sociocultural factors and back pain: a population study in Belgian adults. *Spine* 1994;19:129–137.
13. Spector RE. *Cultural diversity in health and illness*. Stamford, CT: Appleton & Lange, 1991.
14. Szpalski M, Nordin M, Skovron ML, et al. Health care utilization for low back pain in Belgium. *Spine* 1995;20:431–442.
15. U.S. Census Bureau, U.S. Department of Commerce. www.census.gov.
16. Waddell G. *The back pain revolution*. Edinburgh: Churchill Livingstone, 1999:45–66.
17. *Webster new world dictionary of the American language*, 2nd college ed. Cleveland, OH: Simon & Schuster, 1982.
18. World Health Organization, budget 2000–2001. www.who.org.

Subject Index

Note: page numbers followed by *f* indicate figures. Page numbers followed by *t* indicate tables.

A

Aberdeen Low Back Pain Scale, 284
AcroFlex lumbar disc, 308
Acupuncture, 264, 265, 269, 270
Adenovirus, 137
Adolescents
 disc degeneration in, 121–124
 disc herniation in, 125
 scoliosis in, 125–126
Advanced glycation end-product (AGE), 16
Aggrecan, 16, 17, 134
Aggrecanases, 20–21
Aging
 changes to endplates with, 9
 disc degeneration and, 3
ALIF procedure, 157 158, 175–178, 235–236
Allograft bone
 bone grafting and, 141–142
 DBM and, 142
 implant materials and, 208
 implant of, 210*f*
American Academy of Orthopedic Surgeons, 285
American Society for Testing and Materials (ASTM), 216, 217, 219*f*
Animal models
 allograft studies of, 307–308
 baboon, 306, 309
 background, 303
 chimpanzees, 308
 conclusion about, 310
 cost issues, 306, 307
 disc degeneration and, 303–304
 goats, 306
 monkeys, 306–307
 ovine, 304
 rabbit, 304, 309
 sand rat, 307
 sheep, 304–305
 spinal devices used for, 308–309
 in vivo and *in vitro* testing of, 309–310
Annular incision model, 304–305
Annular injection, 102*f*
Anterior lumbar interbody fusion (ALIF)
 advantages and disadvantages of, 178
 for DDD, 175–178
 DYNESYS system and, 235–236
 rhBMPs and, 157–158
Anterior–posterior procedure, 215
Anterior spinal fixation. *See* K-Centrum anterior spinal fixation system
Antibiotics, 305
Antidepressants, 268
Antiinflammatory drugs, 265
Apoptosis, 28
Arthrodesis, 184, 293, 296, 306, 308
Arthroplasty, 299, 308
Autogenous iliac crest bone, 176
Autologous bone graft, 140–141
Autologous Growth Factors (AGF), 151
Autopsy studies, disc degeneration, 121–123
Avascular disc, 9
Awkward postures, 39–40

B

BAK cages, 177, 178
Batson plexus, 66*f*
Beck Depression Inventory, 299
Bed rest, 270
Behavioral therapy
 for LBP, 266, 269
 for neck pain, 270, 271
Belgium disc herniation studies
 background, 313
 cost issues, 314
 discussion about, 318–320
 materials and methods, 314
 results of, 314–315, 316*f*, 317
 statistical analysis, 314

SUBJECT INDEX

Bioactivity
  defined, 211
  of spinal implant materials, 211–213
Biofeedback, LBP and, 269
Blood oxygen level–dependent (BOLD) effect, 3
Blue collar employment, 319
Body weight, IDD and, 68
Bone formation
  BMPs and, 156–159
  gene therapy and, 160
  SB Charité III disc replacement and, 246
Bone grafting
  ALIF procedure and, 176
  allograft bone and, 141–142
  autologous, 140–141
  biodegradable polymers and, 151
  BMPs and, 147–151
  ceramics for, 142–146
  composite grafts and, 146–147
  DBM and, 142
  gene therapy and, 151–152
  growth factor enhancements and, 151
  K-Centrum and, 219
  OptiMesh devices and, 190
  principles of, 139–140
Bone marrow
  aspirate, 141, 145
  disc degeneration and, 82, 85
Bone morphogenetic proteins (BMPs)
  animal models and, 307
  applications of, 147–149
  biodegradable polymers and, 151
  bone grafting and, 140
  chemistry of, 155–156
  clinical studies with, 158–160
  disc degeneration and, 134
  gene therapy and, 135, 136
  preclinical studies with, 156–158
  properties of, 147
  rhBMP-7 safety and, 150–151
  rhOP-1 use and, 150

C

Calcium phosphate crystals, 211, 212f, 213
Carbon fiber–reinforced polyetheretherketone (CF/PEEK), 207, 208
Cartilage endplates. *See* Endplates
Cell(s)
  death, 28–29, 45
  disc, 26
  energy metabolism, 27–28
  mechanical stress and, 30

Ceramics
  for bone grafting, 142–143
  cements, 146
  commercially available, 143–145
  disadvantages of, 143–144
  types of, 143
Cervical spine, MRI of, 2t
Children. *See also* Spinal disorders
  disc calcifications in, 128
  disc degeneration in, 121–124
  scoliosis in, 125–126
Chondrocyte death, 9
"Chondrodystrophoid" breeds, 307
Christian Sickness Fund, 314
Circumferential reciprocating reamer, 191
Clinical Back Pain Questionnaire, 284
Cochrane Collaboration Back Review Group, 263, 292
Colchicine, 268
Collagen
  alternations in, 20
  bone grafting and, 146–147
  function of, 15–16
  IDET therapy and, 164–165
  loss of, 305
  network, 24–25
  role of, 23–24
  types of, 15, 134
Collagraft, 146–147
Complementary DNA (cDNA), 160
Computed tomography (CT)
  back pain and, 264
  for DDD, 171
  for disc degeneration, 77–78, 79f–80f
  discography, 102f–103f
  for IDD, 68
  SB Charité III disc replacement and, 246, 247
  of spinal lesions, 88
Continued activity, LBP and, 270
Cooling spray, 270
Coralline hydroxyapatite, 143
Corpectomy, 219, 220
Cultural issues
  concept of culture and, 321–323
  cross-cultural assessment and, 323
  cross-cultural equivalence and, 324–325
  multicultural population and, 321
  patient self-administered outcome measure, 324
  working cross-culturally and, 326
Cytokines
  DDD and, 18

disc cells and, 30–31, 135
disc herniation and, 113, 114f

D

Dallas Pain Questionnaire, 285
"Da Vinci" position, 251
Degenerative disc disease (DDD). *See also*
 Randomized controlled trials (RCTs)
 animal models of, 306–310
 awkward postures and, 39–40
 biologic evidence of, 45–46
 BMPs for, 147
 changes in, 170
 diagnosis of, 170–173
 disc replacement and, 247
 DYNESYS system for, 228–231
 features of, 257
 heavy physical work and, 36
 IDET therapy for, 163–167
 L4-5 fusion for, 224f
 lifting and forceful movements and, 37–38
 mechanical evidence of, 46–47
 MRI for, 42
 new concepts for, 186
 OptiMesh system and, 194f
 pathophysiology of, 99–100
 plain films for, 75, 76f
 Rhakoss-C device for, 239–243
 stages of, 46
 treatment of, 173, 174f, 175–178
 whole-body vibration and, 40–43
Degenerative spondylolisthesis, 293, 294t, 296, 299
Demineralized bone matrix (DBM)
 allograft bone and, 141–142
 preclinical studies with, 156
Depression, 67
Devices. *See* Spinal devices
Diabetes, 139
Diastrophic dysplasia, 128
Disability-adjusted life-years (DALYs), 286, 287, 288f
Disability rate, 313, 317
Disc(s)
 allografting, 308
 arthroplasty, 299, 308
 cells, 26, 28–29
 components of, 7, 18, 133–134
 erect and supine images of, 93, 94f–95f
 fetal and infantile, 122
 homeostasis and, 18
 implanted, 258f
 innervated, 115
 under load, 24–25
 nutrition, 8, 27–28
 porcine, 305
 structural molecules of, 15–18
 surgery, 47
Disc calcifications
 in children, 128
 differential diagnosis of, 78, 79f
Disc degeneration. *See also* Animal models
 alternations in collagen in, 20
 autopsy studies, 121–123
 biochemical changes related to, 305
 biologic approaches to treat, 134–135
 diastrophic dysplasia and, 128
 different grades of, 82f
 Down syndrome and, 127
 enzymes in, 20–21
 experimental, 54–58
 gene therapy for, 135–137
 Klippel–Feil syndrome and, 128
 LBP and, 114–116, 133, 181–182
 loading on, 55
 loss of PG in, 18–19, 25–26
 MRI for, 42, 63, 80–87, 116–117, 123–124
 nociception and, 111
 nutrient supply and, 28
 radicular pain and, 111–114
 radiographs showing, 1, 3
 Scheuermann disease and, 126–127
 in scoliosis, 125–126
 spina bifida occulta and, 128
 spondylolisthesis and, 126
 thalidomide-induced embryopathy and, 128–129
 therapeutic developments for, 21
 transitional vertebra and, 127
 vertebral fractures and, 127
Discectomy
 lumbar, 177, 318
 social security cost of, 319
 spinal fusion and, 314, 315
 surgical, 182f
Disc herniation
 in adolescents, 125
 Belgium studies, 313–319
 IDET therapy and, 165
 MRI for, 87, 88
 nerve root compression and, 112
 surgery for, 265–266, 271, 314–315, 318
 T2-weighted images, 94f–95f
 work incapacity and, 314

Disc injection
  images of, 103
  pain as a result of, 99, 104
  pressure recording at time of, 104
Discitis
  differential diagnosis with, 81f
  following discography, 101, 104–105
  iatrogenic, 305
  osteomyelitis and, 69
Discogenic pain syndrome. See Degenerative disc disease (DDD); Internal disc disruption (IDD)
Discography
  background, 99
  complications of, 104–105
  for DDD, 173
  findings in, 102–104
  for IDD, 68–69
  indications for, 100
  LBP and, 3, 106–107, 182
  relevance of, 107
  technique, 100–101
  validity of, 105–106
Disc replacement
  background, 245
  discussion about, 247
  patient selection for, 245–246
  results of, 246–247
  SB Charité III, 245–248
Disc space
  ProDisc implant and, 251, 254f
  Rhakoss-C device and, 240, 241
Distress and Risk Assessment Method (DRAM), 245, 246
Down syndrome, 127
DRAM score, 245, 246
Driving, low back pain and, 41–42
Dynagraft, 142
Dynamic neutralization system (DYNESYS)
  case presentation, 231, 232f–234f
  discussion about, 235–236
  features of, 228
  implants, 230
  results of, 230–231
  selecting patients for, 228–229
  technique, 229
  testing of, 230
Dysstability. See Segmental instability

E

Ehlers–Danlos syndrome type IV, 129
Elastin, composition of, 17
Electromagnetic therapy, 270
Electromyographic activity, 60–61
Endplates. See also Disc(s)
  background, 7
  changes to, 9–10
  deflection, 100
  disc degeneration and, 88
  features of, 7–8
  implantation of, 251
  mechanical failure of, 10
  Schmorl nodes in, 10
  sclerosis, 171
  spinal devices and, 11
  vertebral, 116, 309
Energy dispersive spectroscopy (EDS), 211
Energy metabolism, 27–28
Enzymes, 18, 20–21
European Federation of National Associations of Orthopaedics (EFORT), 274
European Spine Registry, 275–277
EuroQoL EQ-5D, 283
Expanding reamer, 190
Ex vivo gene therapy, 136

F

Facet joints
  arthrosis, 247
  LBP and, 181
  pain, 298
Flexion–extension movement, 60
Flexion–relaxation phenomenon, 54
Fluoroscopy, 251
Fourier transform infrared spectroscopy (FTIR), 211
"Fusion disease", 176
Fusion procedure. See Spinal fusion/operation

G

Gadolinium, 104
Gelfoam, 309
Gene therapy
  bone formation and, 160
  delivery mechanism, 136–137
  for disc degeneration, 135–136
  osteoinductive molecules and, 160
  for spinal fusion, 151–152
Glycosaminoglycan (GAG) chains, 17, 18f
Graf ligamentoplasty
  clinical results of, 198–199
  conclusion about, 199
  Graf band and, 198
  indications for, 197–198
  intervertebral stability and, 204–205
  lumbar instability and, 197

vs. other surgical procedures, 199
sample case, 199, 200f
Grafton Allogenic Bone Matrix, 142
Growth factors, 18, 30–31

H

Health-adjusted life expectancy (HALE), 279
Health-adjusted life-years (HALYs), 279, 286–289
Health beliefs
  eliciting patient's, 323t, 324
  influence of culture on, 322
Health-related quality of life (HQRL)
  life path of changing, 288f
  measurement of, 279
Health resorts, 269
Health status, measurement instruments for, 280, 282–283
Heavy physical work, 35–37, 47
Hemicorpectomy, 223
Hemilaminotomy, 259
Herniated nucleus pulposus (HNP)
  awkward postures and, 39
    lifting and forceful movements and, 37, 38
    whole-body vibration and, 41
Heterodimers, 156
High-intensity zone (HIZ), 116
Homeostasis, 18
Homodimers, 156
Hospital stay, disc herniation and, 314, 315, 319
Hydrostatic properties, loss of, 26
Hydroxyapatite, 211
Hysteresis, 57

I

Illiteracy, cross-cultural assessment and, 324
Illness, influence of culture on, 322
Imaging studies. *See* Computed tomography (CT); Magnetic resonance imaging (MRI)
Immobilization, 228
Immunocytochemistry, 114
Implants/implantation. *See also* ProDisc implant
  of allograft bone, 210f
  documentation, 277–278
  of endplates, 11, 251
  spinal, 208, 211–213, 278
Infections, bone grafting and, 141

Information technology innovations, 274–275
Infrared light, 270
Injection(s)
  for LBP, 268
  tube, 191
Injuries
  disc degeneration and, 30
  in intervertebral joint, 57–58
Institute for Evaluative Research in Orthopaedic Surgery, 274
Interbody fusion device (IBFD)
  bioactivity of, 211, 212f, 213
  features of, 207
  implant materials, 207–210
  purpose of, 177, 207
  Rhakoss-C, 239–243
Interbody grafting, 220
Internal disc disruption (IDD)
  background, 63–65
  body weight changes in, 68
  diagnosis of, 68–70
  evolution of, 65
  loss of energy in, 68
  neurologic signs in, 67
  psychologic factors related to, 67–68
  rehabilitation for, 71–72
  symptom production in, 65–67
  treatment of, 70–71, 173, 174f, 175–178
  upper lumbar lesions in, 70
International Documentation and Evaluation System (IDES), 274
International Society for Surgery of the Lumbar Spine, 293
International Society for the Study of the Lumbar Spine (ISSLS), 297
International Spinal Injection Society, 299
International Standardization Organization (ISO), 250, 275
Intervertebral disc. *See also* Disc(s)
  cell transplantation, 309
  nociceptive nerve fibers in, 114
Intervertebral joint
  kinematics of, 55
  pattern of motion in, 57–58
Intervertebral motion device/patterns
  development of, 55, 56f
  in humans, 60
Intervertebral osteochondrosis, 75
Intervertebral stability
  ligamentoplasty and, 204–205
  posterolateral fusion and, 201, 202f–203f
  purpose and principles of, 201

Intradiscal electrothermal therapy (IDET)
  background, 163
  mechanism of action, 164–165
  postoperative care in, 167
  procedure, 163–164
  results of, 166
  selecting patients for, 165–166
  trials for, 298–299
Intradiscal pressure (IDP), 38, 44
Intradiscal thermal annuloplasty, 106
Isolated disc resorption (IDR), 64, 170
Isthmic spondylolisthesis, 295t, 296–297, 300

K

K-Centrum anterior spinal fixation system
  background, 215–216
  bench testing of, 216–217
  case examples, 221–221, 222f, 223–224
  clinical results of, 221
  components of, 218f
  features of, 216
  technique, 220
  in vitro testing of, 219–220
Klippel–Feil syndrome, 128
Kostuik disc prosthesis, 308

L

Laparoscopic procedure, 177–178
Laparotomy, 251
Laser treatment, 270
Life expectancy, 279, 288–289
Lifting
  low back pain and, 37–39
  postures and, 40
Lifting strength rating (LSR), 37
Limb pain, 65
LIM mineralization protein-1 (LMP-1), 136, 160–161
Linguistic problems, cross-cultural assessment and, 324
Loading
  disc degeneration and, 46, 96
  on lumbar spine, 44
Low Back Outcome Score, 284
Low back pain (LBP). *See also* Degenerative disc disease (DDD); Endplates
  assessment of, 264
  behavior therapy for, 266
  cross-cultural studies and, 322, 325
  diagnosis of, 116–118
  discogenic, 114–116, 165
  discography and, 3, 106–107
  disc replacement for, 245–248

DYNESYS system and, 233f
etiology of, 181–183
evidence base for, 263
heavy physical work and, 35–37, 47
influence of social factors on, 266–268
lifting and forceful movements and, 37–39
MCID for, 285, 286t
measurement instruments for, 283–285
mechanical, 295t, 297, 300
OptiMesh system and, 194f
PDN device for, 257–262
postures and, 39–40, 43–45
primary care for, 267
spinal arthrodesis for, 245
total disc replacement for, 249–252, 254–255
treatment of, 184–186, 264–266, 268–270
whole-body vibration and, 40–43
Low Back Pain Rating Scale, 285
Lumbar disc disease, 87
Lumbar discectomy, 177
Lumbar fusion
  complications of, 184–186
  indications for, 181, 184
  MRI findings and, 183
  sagittal alignment in patients undergoing, 185
  trials for, 297–298
Lumbar instability syndrome, 197
Lumbar pain, 227
Lumbar spinal stenosis
  conclusion about, 299
  surgery for, 293, 296
  trials for, 294t
Lumbar spine
  degenerative changes in, 57–58
  electromyographic recording of, 60
  loading on, 44, 96
  MRI of, 2t, 92–93, 123–124
Lumbar Spine Questionnaire, 285

M

Magnetic resonance imaging (MRI)
  back pain and, 183, 264
  of cervical and lumbar spine, 2t
  for disc degeneration, 42, 63, 80–87, 116–117, 123–124, 172–173
  in flexed and extended positions, 91–93, 96
  for IDD, 69–70
  of spinal disorders, 125–128
Manipulation for LBP, 269
Manual materials handling (MMH), 37
Manual therapy
  for LBP, 269

for neck pain, 270
Marker gene experiments, 137
Matrix
　effect of degenerative changes in, 25–26
　synthesis and turnover, 29–31, 134
Matrix metalloproteinases (MMPs)
　development of, 122
　disc herniation and, 112
　role of, 23–26, 113
　types of, 20
Maurice E. Müller Center for Education and Documentation (MEM-CED), 274, 275, 276, 278
Medical Outcome Study, 283
Metabolism, disc composition and, 133–134
Metal mesh cages, 221
Minimal clinically important difference (MCID), 285–286
Mobilization, LBP and, 269
Modic lesions, 186
Modified Somatic Perception Questionnaire (MSPQ), 245
Morphogens, disc cells and, 135
Muscle relaxant drugs
　for LBP, 265, 268
　for neck pain, 270
Myelography, 171
Myelopathy, 240

N

Narcotics, 317
National Sickness and Invalidity Authority, 314, 318
Neck Disability Index (NDI), 240, 242
Neck pain
　assessment of, 264
　influence of social factors on, 266–268
　treatment of, 265, 266, 270–271
Nerve roots
　pain and, 101, 112
　stenosis, 296
　TNF-α application to, 113
Neurogenic inflammation, 115–116
Neuropathy, inflammatory, 113
Nociceptive nerve fibers, 114
Nonfusion technology, 298–299
Nonsteroidal antiinflammatory drugs (NSAIDs), 268
Norian cement, 146
North American Spine Society, 273, 285
Nottingham Health Profile, 283
Nucleus pulposus
　degenerative lesions and, 122

detecting changes within, 172
　glycosaminoglycan content in, 123
　herniated, 313
　pain and, 112
　PDN device and, 259f
Nutrition
　cell energy metabolism and, 27–29
　matrix turnover and, 30

O

Occupational factors
　awkward postures, 39–40
　heavy physical work, 35–37
　lifting and forceful movements, 37–39
　static work postures, 43–45
　whole-body vibration, 40–43
Odds ratio (OR)
　awkward postures and, 39
　disc degeneration and, 35
　heavy physical work and, 36
　lifting and forceful movements and, 37
　whole-body vibration and, 40–41
Opioids, 314
Opteform, 142
OptiMesh system
　biologic testing with, 192
　clinical studies with, 192, 193f, 194–195
　defined, 189–190
　for fractures, 192
　preclinical studies with, 190
　tools, 191
　vs. traditional spinal devices, 190
Orthoglobe, 274, 275
Orthovita, 208
Osteoconduction, defined, 139
Osteofil, 142
Osteogenesis, defined, 139
Osteogenic cells, 140
Osteoinduction, defined, 139
Osteoinductive molecules
　background, 155
　BMPs and, 155–160
　gene therapy and, 160
　LMP-1 and, 160–161
Osteophytes, 36, 76f, 78f
Oswestry Disability Index (ODI)
　BMPs and, 147, 150, 159
　DYNESYS system and, 229, 231, 235, 236
　Graf ligamentoplasty and, 198–199
　IDET therapy and, 166, 299
　LBP and, 265, 283–284
　lumbar fusion and, 184
　PDN device and, 261, 262

Oswestry Disability Index (ODI) (*contd.*)
  ProDisc implant and, 255
  SB Charité III disc replacement and, 245, 246, 247
Ovine model, disc degeneration and, 304

P

Pain. *See also* Low back pain (LBP)
  behavioral therapy for, 270, 271
  disc herniation and, 318
  discography and, 100, 104, 106
  eliciting patient's health beliefs about, 323*t*
  facet joints, 298
  in IDD, 67
  radicular, 111–114
  as a result of disc injection, 99, 104
Pantaloon cast, 184
Patient education, neck pain and, 270
Patient outcomes. *See also* Quality of life
  cross-cultural assessment and, 323
  dimensions of, 280, 281*f*
  HALYs and, 286–289
  hierarchy of, 279–280, 281*f*
Patient selection
  for disc replacement, 245–246
  for Rhakoss-C device, 239–240
Pattern of motion
  in intervertebral joint, 57–58
  segmental instability and, 58–59
PDN device
  design of, 257–259
  discussion about, 261–262
  implantation of, 260
  modifications in, 261
  purpose of, 257
  results of, 260
Pedicle fixation, 184
Pentosidine, 16
Permeability barrier, loss of, 26
Person trade-off (PTO) method, 287
Physical training, 271
Physiotherapy, 270
PLIF procedure, 173, 174*f*, 175–176
Polyglycolic acid (PGA), 151
Polylactic acid (PLA), 151
Polymethyl-methacrylate (PMMA), 220, 221
Porcine model, disc degeneration and, 305
Posterior lumbar interbody fusion (PLIF)
  advantages and disadvantages of, 178
  for DDD, 173, 174*f*, 175–176
Posterolateral fusion
  Graf ligamentoplasty and, 199
  intervertebral stability and, 201, 202*f*–203*f*
  results of, 184, 186
Postures
  awkward, 39–40
  flexed, 40
  spinal, 201, 203*f*
  standing and supine, 92
  static work, 43–45
ProDisc implant
  background, 249
  design of, 249–250
  discussion about, 255
  patients for, 254–255
  results of, 255
  technique, 251–252, 253*f*–254*f*
Prolo scores, 261, 262
Pro Osteon, 143, 144
Proteoglycan molecules
  common type of, 16–17
  loss of, 18–19, 25–26, 305
  role of, 8, 9, 23–24

Q

Quality-adjusted life-years (QALYs), 286, 287, 288*f*, 289
Quality of life
  background, 279–280
  MCID and, 285–286
  measurement instruments for, 280, 282–283, 286
Quality of Well-Being, 283
Quebec Back Pain Disability Scale, 285

R

Rabbit model, disc degeneration and, 304
Radial annular tears, 170
Radicular pain, 111–114
Radiculopathy, 240
Radiofrequency thermocoagulation, 298–299
Radiographs
  of allograft bone, 210*f*
  showing disc degeneration, 1, 3
  showing disc space, 241*f*
  showing titanium cages, 177*f*
Randomized controlled trials (RCTs)
  analysis of, 294*t*–295*t*
  background, 291
  conclusion about, 299–300
  methods, 292
  objective, 291
  relevant, 293, 296–299
Range of motion, 201, 203*f*–204*f*, 309
Rehabilitation, 71–72

Resumption of Activities of Daily Living Scale, 285
Retrovirus vectors, 137
Rhakoss-C device
  discussion about, 242–243
  patient selection for, 239–240
  results of, 240–242
Rhakoss Synthetic Bone Spinal Implant
  bioactive nature of, 213
  calcium phosphate on surface of, 212f
  features of, 208
  FTIR showing close match of, 211f
  histologic section of, 213f
  radiopacity of, 209f
RhBMP-2, 147, 149
RhBMP-7, 147, 149
rhOP-1, 147, 149f–150f
Roentgenography, 182, 221, 224, 252, 253f
Roland–Morris Disability Questionnaire (RMDQ), 284

S
SB Charité III, 246, 247, 248
Scanning electron microscopy (SEM), 211, 212f
Scheuermann disease, 10, 126–127
Schmorl nodes, 10, 75, 85
Sciatica
  disc herniation and, 318
  treatment of, 265–266
Scoliosis
  ceramics for, 143, 144
  disc degeneration in, 125–126
Secure data integration concept (SEDICO), 278
Sedentary work, 43–45
Segmental instability
  background, 53–54
  Graf ligamentoplasty and, 199
  LBP and, 182
  pattern of motion and, 58–59
Sheep model, disc degeneration and, 304–305
Sickness Impact Profile (SIP), 282–283
Smoking, fusion rates and, 139
Social security costs, 314, 317–319
Spina bifida occulta, 128
Spinal arthrodesis, 245
Spinal devices, 190, 308–309
Spinal disorders. See also OptiMesh system
  calcification, 128
  diastrophic dysplasia, 128
  disc herniation, 125
  Down syndrome, 127
  fractures, 127
  Klippel–Feil syndrome, 128
  Scheuermann disease, 126–127
  scoliosis, 125–126
  spina bifida occulta, 128
  spondylolisthesis, 126
  thalidomide-induced embryopathy, 128–129
  transitional vertebra, 127
Spinal fusion/operation. See also Interbody fusion device (IBFD); Total disc replacement
  animal models of, 306
  Belgium studies, 314–317, 319
  BMP-induced, 149
  bone grafting and, 139–142
  ceramics for, 143–145
  DBM and, 156
  for DDD, 175
  disadvantages of, 257
  gene therapy for, 151–152
  for IDD, 70–71
  instrumented fusion vs. graft, 292t
  LMP-1 and, 161
  rehabilitation after, 71–72
  rhBMPs for, 156–160
  trials for, 297–298
Spinal implant materials
  bioactivity of, 211, 212f, 213
  properties of, 209–210
  radiopacity of, 208
  types of, 207–208
Spinal lesions, 88
Spinal stenosis
  conclusion about, 299
  surgery for, 293, 296
  trials for, 294t
Spine registry
  background, 273–274
  European, 275–277
  implant documentation and, 277–278
  information technology innovations and, 274–275
  Spine Tango and, 274, 277f
Spine Society of Europe, 274
SpineView software, 199, 201
Spondylolisthesis, 93
  ceramics for, 143
  disc degeneration and, 126
  isthmic, 295t, 300
  lumbar fusion and, 186
  spinal fusion and, 175
  trials for, 293, 294–295t, 296, 299
Spondylosis deformans, 75, 77
St. Thomas Questionnaire, 284

Standing, low back pain and, 44
Stenosis
 IDET therapy and, 166
 spinal fusion and, 175
Steroid injections, 268, 270
Stretching for neck pain, 270
Structural autograft, 208
Sulfated glycosaminoglycan (sGAG), 134, 136
Supportive devices, 269
Swedish Hip Registry, 273
Synthetic ceramics. *See* Ceramics

T

T1/T2 weighted images
 axial, 80
 bone marrow changes and, 82, 85
 hypointensity on, 84*f*–87*f*
 posterior high-intensity zone on, 83*f*
 sagittal, 105*f*
 signal intensity on, 172–173
 in supine and erect positions, 92–93, 94*f*–95*f*
TENS. *See* Transcutaneous electric nerve stimulation (TENS)
Thalidomide-induced embryopathy, 128–129
Thermography, 264
Thoracic lumbar sacral orthosis (TLSO), 223
Titanium, 208
Total disc arthroplasty, 308
Total disc replacement
 background, 249
 discussion about, 255
 patients for, 254–255
 ProDisc implant for, 249–251
 results of, 255
 technique, 251–252, 253*f*–254*f*
Total Pain Rating Index, 325
Traction
 for LBP, 269
 for neck pain, 270
Transcutaneous electric nerve stimulation (TENS), 264, 265, 269, 270
Transitional vertebra, 127
Trunk motion, testing, 59*f*
Tumor necrosis factor-α (TNF-α), 113

U

Ultra-high-molecular weight polyethylene (UHMWPE)
 animal models and, 308
 K-Centrum and, 216
 PDN device and, 258
 ProDisc implant and, 249, 250*f*, 252, 255
Ultrasonography, 264
Upper lumbar lesions, 70

V

Vehicle driving. *See* Driving
Versican, 17
Vertebral bodies, 65, 66*f*
Vertebral column allografting, 307–308
Vertebral fractures
 disc degeneration and, 127
 OptiMesh system for, 192, 194
Visual analog scale (VAS)
 DYNESYS system and, 235
 IDET therapy and, 166
 LBP and, 265, 284
 PDN device and, 261, 262
 ProDisc implant and, 255
 Rhakoss-C device and, 240, 241, 242
Vitoss, 144–145, 146*f*

W

Waddell Disability Index, 284
Waddell signs, 170
Whole-body vibration, 40–43
Worker compensation claims/costs
 LBP and, 313
 manual materials handling and, 38
Work incapacity, 314, 315, 316*f*, 317, 319
World Health Organization, 326

Z

Z-Plate Thoraco-Lumbar device, 216